Laparoscopic Colectomy

Sharon L. Stein • Regan R. Lawson
Editors

Laparoscopic Colectomy

A Step by Step Guide

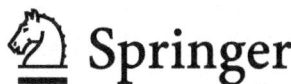

Editors
Sharon L. Stein
University Hospital Cleveland
Medical Center
Cleveland, OH
USA

Regan R. Lawson
Exponent
Philadelphia, PA
USA

ISBN 978-3-030-39557-5   ISBN 978-3-030-39559-9   (eBook)
https://doi.org/10.1007/978-3-030-39559-9

This Springer imprint is published by the registered company Springer Nature Switzerland AG
The registered company address is: Gewerbestrasse 11, 6330 Cham, Switzerland

Preface

Minimally invasive surgery has become a standard approach to surgical problems including colon and rectal surgery. While minimally invasive surgery provides significant benefits to the patient, appreciating the challenges of anatomy from a laparoscopic perspective has created new challenges for both educators and trainees. This book was designed specifically to help equip new surgeons with the anatomical and technical knowledge to supplement hands-on experience in minimally invasive colon and rectal surgery.

There are multiple colorectal surgeries which distinctly lend themselves to the use of the laparoscopic approach. To assist the junior surgeon who is embarking on a career in surgery, we enlisted the help of expert surgeons and educators in the field of colon and rectal surgery from around the country to author the chapters included in this book. Our goal was to impart the mastery of these experts to help the junior surgeon optimize minimally invasive surgery.

We asked our authors to describe key elements of each surgery, including the order of surgery and when and how they created tension, rotated the patient, and optimized flow of the surgery. We turned to the adage "Skill comes from experience, but not all that experience needs to be yours." In addition to the key elements of each surgery, the authors have provided the reader with tips and pitfalls to guide and warn the junior surgeon. These tips and pitfalls are the "trade secrets" that are not always explicitly presented when describing a surgical approach as they tend to be situational, not occurring in every surgery. It is our hope that the addition of such information, presented in separate text boxes, will arm junior surgeons with a diverse tool-kit in which to draw upon. Each chapter is also full of new illustrations to show the direction of traction, the line of dissection, and the anatomy of the colon and presents tools in a color-coded format to clearly distinguish between the surgeon and the assistant's tools.

We hope that this book will be one that residents and junior attendings turn to often when mastering laparoscopic colon and rectal surgery – a book that conveys the experience of our talented authors and surgeons, as if they were in the room with you, guiding you through the surgery.

Cleveland, OH, USA   Sharon L. Stein
Philadelphia, PA, USA   Regan R. Lawson

Acknowledgments

This book was an enormous effort and we would like to thank our authors for their time, experience, and expertise. It is not an easy task to translate the actions they engage in during their surgeries into text descriptions, and they have done tremendous and thoughtful work in presenting their approaches in a very accessible manner. We would also like to thank the illustrators who worked with us through multiple revisions in our attempt to provide you with the most informative representation of each surgery. We would like to thank our families and friends who supported us through this project, the challenges and triumphs. And we would like to thank each other for adding perspective and richness to this text and for the synergy that always seems to happen when we get together.

Contents

Contributors

Joshua I. S. Bleier Department of Surgery, Division of Colon & Rectal Surgery, Perelman School of Medicine, Pennsylvania Hospital, Philadelphia, PA, USA

Raul M. Bosio Division of Surgery, ProMedica Health & Wellness Center, Sylvania, OH, USA

Bradley J. Champagne Department of Surgery, Cleveland Clinic Fairview Hospital, Cleveland, OH, USA

Meagan M. Costedio Division of Colorectal Surgery, University Hospitals, Cleveland, OH, USA

Lisa Coviello Center for Colorectal Surgery, Tidewater Physicians Multi-specialty Group, Newport News, VA, USA

Kurt G. Davis Section of Colon and Rectal Surgery, LSUHSC, LA, USA

Anthony L. DeRoss Pediatric Surgery, Cleveland Clinic, Cleveland, OH, USA

Todd D. Francone Division of Colon & Rectal Surgery at Newton-Wellesley Hospital, Newton, MA, USA

Kevin R. Kniery Department of Surgery, Madigan Army Medical Center, Tacoma, WA, USA

Ron G. Landmann MD Anderson Cancer Center - Baptist Medical Center, Jacksonville, FL, USA

Colon and Rectal Surgery, Mayo Clinic, Jacksonville, FL, USA

Mark L. Manwaring Saint Thomas Medical Partners in Murfreesboro, Greenville, TN, USA

Justin A. Maykel Department of Colon and Rectal Surgery, University of Massachusetts Medical School, Worcester, MA, USA

Jason S. Mizell University of Arkansas for Medical Sciences, Division of Colon and Rectal Surgery, Little Rock, AR, USA

Michael J. Mulcahy Tripler Army Medical Center, Honolulu, HI, USA

Govind Nandakumar Department of Surgery, Weill Cornell Medical College New York, New York, NY, USA

Tushar Samdani Department of Surgery, Medstar Saint Mary's Hospital, Leonardtown, MD, USA

Andrew T. Schlussel Division of Surgery, Madigan Army Medical Center, Tacoma, WA, USA

Skandan Shanmugan Department of Surgery, Division of Colon & Rectal Surgery, Penn Presbyterian Medical Center, Philadelphia, PA, USA

Scott R. Steele Department of Colorectal Surgery, Digestive Disease and Surgery Institute, Cleveland Clinic, Cleveland, OH, USA

Sharon L. Stein Division of Colon and Rectal Surgery, Department of Surgery, University Hospital Cleveland Medical Center, Cleveland, OH, USA

David B. Stewart Colorectal Surgery, University of Arizona – Banner University Medical Center, Tucson, AZ, USA

About the Editors

Content Editor and Contributing Author

Sharon L. Stein, M.D., is a board certified colon and rectal and general surgeon. She is Associate Professor of Surgery and the Murdough Master Clinician of Colon and Rectal Surgery at the University Hospital Cleveland Medical Center, Cleveland, Ohio. She serves as the Director of UH Research in Surgical Outcomes and Effectiveness (UH-RISES) and the Program Director of the Colon and Rectal Surgery Residency at university hospitals in Cleveland, OH. Dr. Stein has published over 100 articles, abstracts, and book chapters and is frequently invited to speak nationally and internationally about minimally invasive surgery. She is an active leader in multiple surgical societies including the American Society of Colon and Rectal Surgeons (ASCRS), American College of Surgeons, and Society of American Gastrointestinal and Endoscopic Surgeons and is the current President of the Association of Women Surgeons.

Educational Editor

Regan R. Lawson, Ph.D., has a doctorate in Applied Physiology with a focus on cognitive motor control and motor learning and Master of Arts in Secondary Science Education. She has spent over 25 years in the educational field working with students of all ranges including undergraduate and graduate neuroscience students. Her publications have focused on the motor learning during prosthetic use. She has been invited to provide multiple lectures and presentations for neuroscience, science education, curriculum development, and teacher training. Regardless of the learner, her focus is on presenting information in formats which capitalize on educational pedagogy and neuroscientific learning principles. She is an active member of the Society for Neuroscience and the Human Factors and Ergonomics Society. Dr. Lawson currently works at Exponent as a Human Factors Scientist providing consulting services in a variety of areas including those associated with improving how users learn to effectively and safely use a product.

Tools

Kurt G. Davis and Lisa Coviello

Introduction

Goals for setup in the operating room should focus on:

- Preparation
- Visibility
- Operative strategy
- Easy access to instrumentation

The importance of ergonomics cannot be overimpressed as repetitive use injury and musculoskeletal strain certainly are underreported and underappreciated in the surgical community. Setup considerations begin far before the day of operation.

- *General approach*: General approach should be decided (total laparoscopic, hand-assisted, intercorporeal vs. extracorporeal anastomosis, extraction point).
- *Communication*: Communication with the team and evaluations of any comorbidities which may affect the course of the operation must be established (steroid use, radiation,

prior surgeries, obesity, cardiac limitations, pulmonary disease sensitive to increased intra-abdominal pressures, etc.).

- *Secondary plan*: As patient factors increase the complexity of the operation, it is extremely important to have a secondary (or even tertiary) plan already thought out well in advance if the primary approach is no longer feasible.

Choices in the OR for laparoscopic colectomy should be developed for maximal efficiency while minimizing excessive cost; however, safety or operative objectives should never be sacrificed.

Preoperative Preparation

Patients should undergo an appropriate disease-specific evaluation prior to undergoing laparoscopic colon and rectal surgery. Although the details of staging and surgical decision-making prior to surgery will not be covered in this book, some general principles particularly applicable to laparoscopic surgery will be reviewed.

Bowel Prep

There has been extensive discussion of bowel preparation, its necessity, and its benefits in the literature. Although there is debate regarding the utility of mechanical bowel preparation in

K. G. Davis (✉)
Section of Colon and Rectal Surgery,
LSUHSC, LA, USA
e-mail: kdav26@lsuhsc.edu

L. Coviello
Center for Colorectal Surgery, Tidewater Physicians
Multi-specialty Group, Newport News, VA, USA

© Springer Nature Switzerland AG 2020
S. L. Stein, R. R. Lawson (eds.), *Laparoscopic Colectomy*,
https://doi.org/10.1007/978-3-030-39559-9_1

open surgery, the improved ability to manipulate stool-filled intestine laparoscopically as well as reported dangers associated with using diathermy on unprepared bowel makes mechanical bowel prep prudent. The option of intraoperative endoscopy for localization of pathology is possible after mechanical bowel preparation. Generally, a mechanical preparation is coupled with oral antibiotics to reduce the risk of infection.

Patient Setup

There are several considerations for positioning during laparoscopic colon and rectal surgery. While patient safety is always paramount, the patient must also be positioned to optimize the surgeon's ability to perform the surgery. The patient will often be placed in extremes of positioning, particularly when operating in the pelvis. To help facilitate the case, prior to starting the operation, it is wise to ensure that the bed is electrically manipulated and is functioning properly.

Details of patient setup are included in each chapter; however, the surgeon is responsible to ensure that the patient is safely secured to the bed and will not move during the operation. Surgeons may choose between gel pads, bean bags, and commercial devices, such as the Pink Pad® (Xodus Medical Inc., New Kensington, PA). The goal of each of these devices is to prevent the patient from sliding on the operative table during the extremes of positioning during laparoscopic surgery. Surgeons may have personal preference, but there is no data recommending one technique over the other. To ensure the patient is adequately stable, it is suggested to move the patient into steep Trendelenburg position and airplane from side to side prior to starting the case (see Fig. 1.1). Some surgeons also place tape across the chest to prevent the patient from moving.

During the case, lithotomy position is used for many patients. This provides access to the perineum, for possible endoscopy, or stapled anastomosis, allowing the surgeon to operate from between the legs, which may be particularly helpful when mobilizing the transverse colon and splenic flexure. It also provides an additional location of fixation of the patient to the table. Padded stirrups, such as the yellow fin stirrups, provide stable secure placement of the legs. The surgeon must be cognizant of the alignment of the hips, knees, and ankles, to ensure there is no torque on the patient's joints during the operation. The stirrups should also be set up to prevent hyperextension at the hips.

Arms are often tucked at the patient's sides. If an arm is left out on an arm board, it limits surgeon mobility around the table and can prevent full access to all quadrants. When tucked, care should be taken to ensure that the ulnar nerve, located under the elbow (see Fig. 1.2), is well padded. The hands should also be protected, particularly when lithotomy position is used as they may be close to the stirrups. Prior to prepping, it is crucial to ensure that the IVs are working well, the blood pressure cuff is functioning, and the anesthesia team has appropriate access.

Lines and Tubes

Prior to starting the surgery, it is important to ensure placement of all tubes which will be used during the surgery. Most commonly, these include (1) a nasogastric or orogastric tube, (2) a urinary catheter, and (3) sequential compression devices. Placement of a nasogastric or orogastric tube ensures the stomach is decompressed and limits injury. Similarly, placement of a urinary catheter prior to starting the surgery provides important information and prevents a bladder injury. Generally, sequential compression devices are placed on bilateral legs to prevent thromboembolic events.

During many operations, both the surgeon and the assistant will change locations, moving from one side to another. This is particularly true if performing lysis of adhesions or for a multiquadrant surgery such as subtotal colectomy. Having the arms tucked helps to facilitate this transfer of position. Running all lines and tubes off the shoulder of the patient is also useful, to allow for full mobility. Laparoscopic drapes with pockets are ideal to allow for storage of instru-

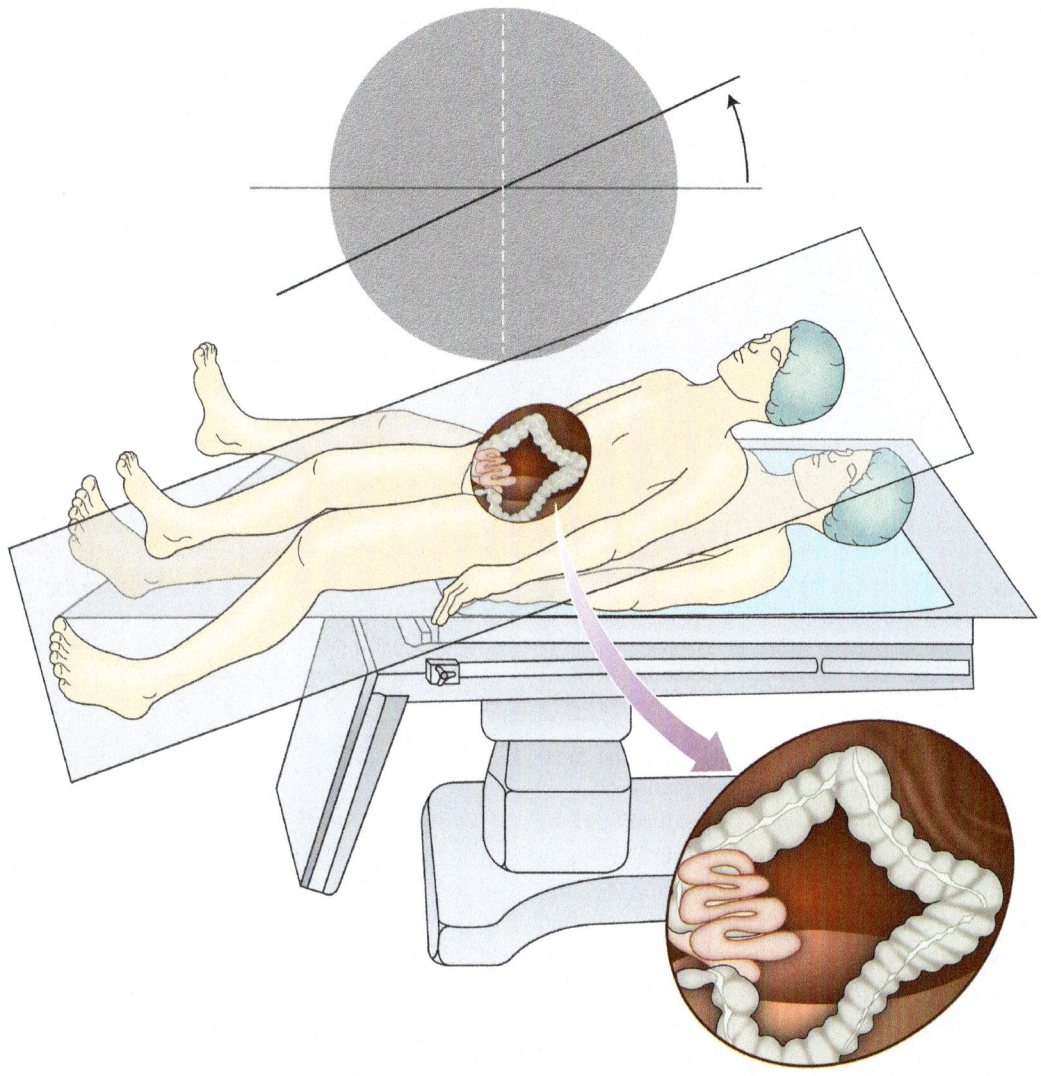

Fig. 1.1 Securing the patient to the table adequately is vital to optimizing visualization during the case. Using extremes of positioning facilitates the use of gravity as a retractor, helping to move the bowel out of the operating field

ments when they are not used. All heat source cords, light cords, and insufflation tubing should be handed off the field and secured to the drapes at the beginning of the case prior to making the first incision.

Accessing the Abdomen

Entry into the abdomen can be performed via open Hassan technique, Veress needle, or alternatively with an optical trocar. All entry techniques are associated with defined morbidity and potential complications. Debate over the safest entry technique continues, and there is no consensus regarding the superiority of any one technique. Most data points to the fact that laparoscopic surgeons are best served by finding and adhering to the technique with which they are most comfortable and can safely perform. Challenges to entry are particularly great in patients who are obese, have a history of prior abdominal surgery, or prior mesh placement. In these cases, significant experience with a variety of laparoscopic

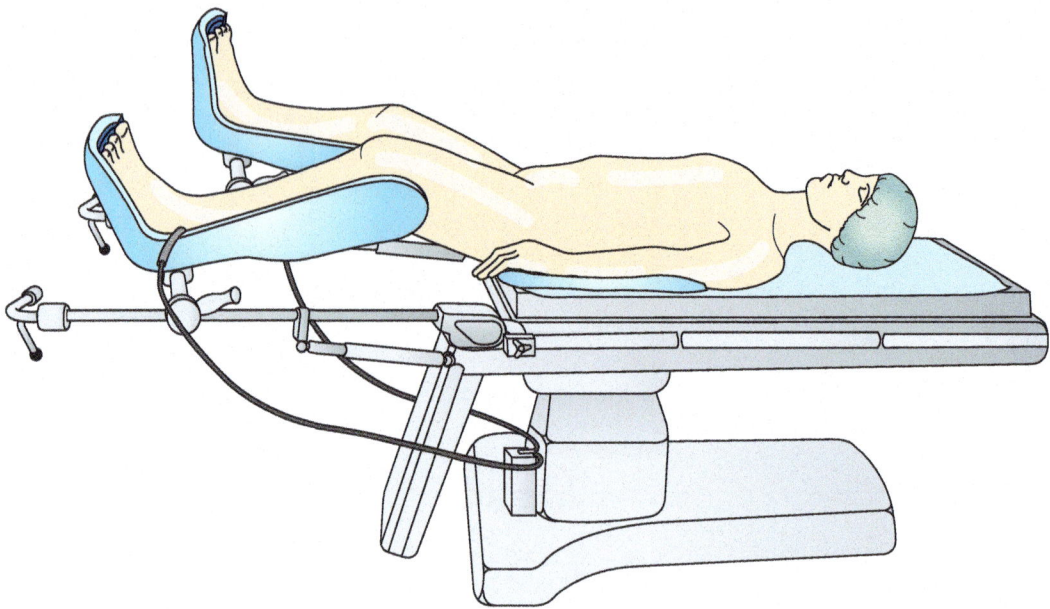

Fig. 1.2 Arms needed to be tucked and pressure points padded to ensure that the ulnar nerve is protected adequately. Legs should be placed into stirrups and checked to ensure they will not be hyperextended during the case

techniques can be helpful in selecting the most appropriate technique.

For all techniques, the surgeon should be cognizant of initial opening pressure. Prior to insufflation, a pressure of 8 mmHg or less signals appropriate intra-abdominal placement. If the pressure is higher than this, the surgeon should recheck placement and ensure that the abdominal compartment has been appropriately entered.

Open Hassan Technique

The umbilicus provides a reliable and central location that facilitates most procedures, and it is the authors' preference (see Tip 1.1). Generally, an incision of approximately 1–1.5 cm in length is made superior to the umbilicus. The umbilical stalk is then grasped with a Kocher clamp and raised superiorly and anteriorly putting the fascia on stretch. Small retractors, such as the S-shaped retractors, are used to retract the skin and subcutaneous tissue, while the fascia is scored. Once the anterior fascia has been scored, the peritoneum must be identified and sharply opened. This provides access to the abdomen.

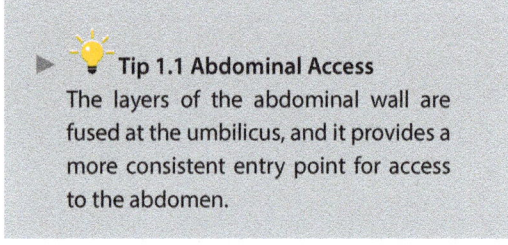

▶ **Tip 1.1 Abdominal Access**
The layers of the abdominal wall are fused at the umbilicus, and it provides a more consistent entry point for access to the abdomen.

Choices of trocar type are varied and include traditional beveled Hassan trocars, balloon ports, or traditional straight ports. Hassan trocars and balloon ports provide greater diameter to "plug" the hole created during entry. The ports can be anchored to the fascia with placement of fascial sutures prior to insertion (see Fig. 1.3). These sutures can then be used to close the incision at the end of the case.

Veress Entry

Veress entry is a blind entry using a spring-loaded retractable needle. Needles come in two lengths, allowing for entry into obese patients.

Selecting the location of entry is critical. The needle should be inserted away from prior incisions as well as away from prior surgical sites.

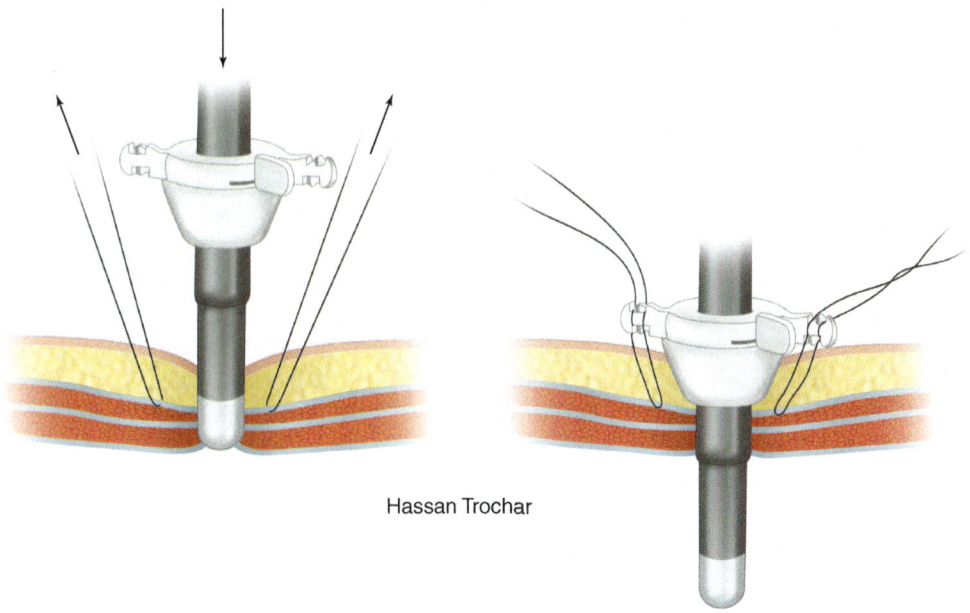

Fig. 1.3 Hassan trocar is introduced to the abdomen and secured with bilateral sutures

The two most common locations are the left upper quadrant, at Palmer's point (see Tip 1.2) and infraumbilical. In morbidly obese patients, towel clamps can be placed on either side of the insertion site to elevate the abdominal wall during insertion.

> 💡 **Tip 1.2 Palmer's Point**
> Palmer's point in the left upper quadrant is an ideal alternate for optical trocar entry due to the avoidance of unprotected liver and anterior elevation of the abdominal wall by the ribs. One must ensure optical entry is inserted mid-rectus muscle so that identification of each layer of fascia and muscle is extremely clear.

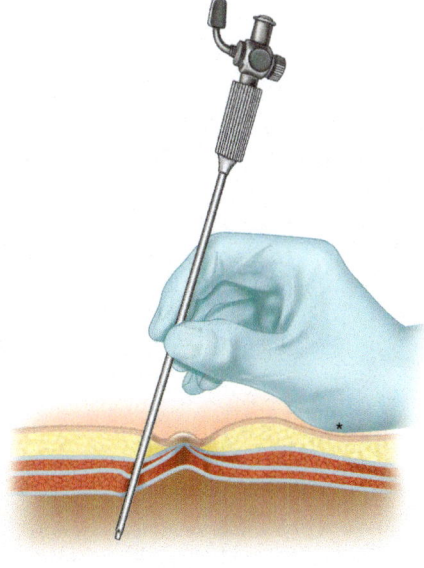

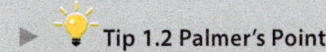

Veress entry

Fig. 1.4 The Veress needle is carefully inserted through the fascia and into the abdomen. The needle should be angled away from vital structures to prevent injury

A 1 mm incision is generally made with a #11 scalpel. During insertion, the needle is slowly advanced. A thorough understanding of anatomy is crucial, to avoid injury to underlying structures. The needle should be inserted through two distinct planes, which represent the anterior and posterior fascia. The surgeon should have a sense of free space when the needle is advanced appropriately (see Fig. 1.4).

Prior to insufflation, a 10 cc syringe filled with saline is placed on the needle. The saline should be injected freely without resistance. The needle should then be refilled with saline and should drop into the abdomen freely, if the placement is correct. Aspiration of blood or succus is a sign of incorrect placement and should be dealt with immediately.

Insufflation tubing is then attached to the Veress needle. The intra-abdominal pressure should be 8 mmHg or less on initial testing. Higher pressure signals incorrect placement, and the needle should be repositioned prior to insufflation. Under low flow, insufflation should begin. After obtaining insufflation, an additional port for camera placement can be placed either at the location of Veress entry or in an alternative location.

Visual Entry System

The visual entry cannula system uses a zero-degree scope through a clear optical trocar during initial entry. Similar to the Veress needle, entry should be away from prior incisions and surgical procedures. A 1 cm skin incision is made, and the laparoscope is inserted into the trocar. The path of entry is then visualized, passing through the subcutaneous, anterior fascia, muscle, posterior fascia, and finally into the peritoneum. The abdominal wall must be elevated during insertion to prevent direct entry into the abdominal organs.

Trocars

After safe entry into the abdomen has occurred, the surgeon has a choice of trocar types and placements. Specific recommendations for each procedure are given within the chapters. Typically, these ports come in either 5 or 10–12 mm sizes. Most instruments are manufactured in the 5 mm size, allowing the freedom to change port sites if necessary. One notable exception is the laparoscopic stapling devices that require larger ports, generally a 12 mm port or larger. The surgeon should give special consideration to where the stapler will be best utilized and plan port placement accordingly. Advancements in technology have provided a superior 5 mm camera and allow minimizing of port sizes. Consideration for increasing the number of larger ports must be made if the institution maintains only 10 mm cameras (see Fig. 1.5).

The number of ports can be varied with experience or need/type of assistance. A rule of thumb is to keep ports a hand's breadth apart and avoid placement in line with the camera port which would make it difficult to use. The periumbilical port should be placed in a vertical orientation in case conversion to open should occur. The lateral port placement should be outside the rectus

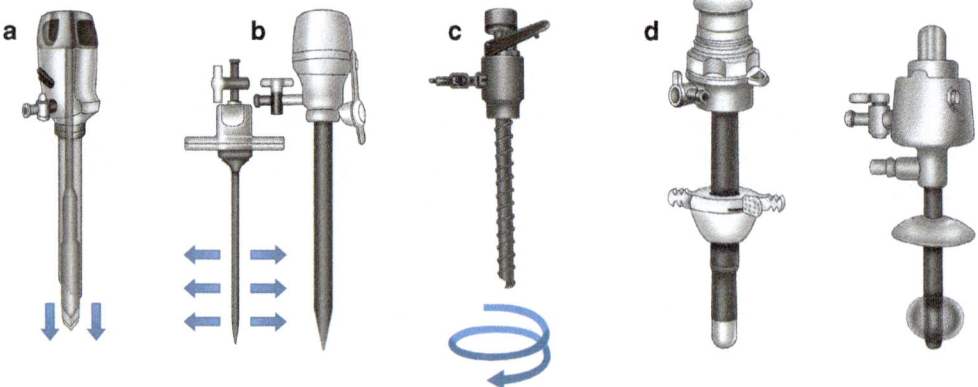

Fig. 1.5 These are examples of trocars, each with their own unique method of remaining in the abdominal wall to prevent sliding in and out when instruments are exchanged. (**a**) Bladed or Cutting Trocar (**b**) Expandable Sheath Type Trocar (**c**) Threaded or Ribbed Type Trocar (**d**) Hasson Type or Suture Secured Trocar

sheath to avoid epigastric vessel injury. While general principles are addressed here, ideal specific port placement for each approach will be described in detail in each chapter.

It is important to consider the position of an ostomy prior to operation. Marking of a possible ostomy site in the typical standing/sitting fashion is recommended. In the operating room, the port placement may be altered to allow for utilization of a port site as the ostomy site, minimizing the number of incisions/scars.

Changing Ports in the Obese/Large Patient/Tall Patient/Redundant Pannus

While it may be tempting to address the concern of variation in abdominal size, and not having access to all areas, with additional ports, preoperative adjustments in port placements can be made in anticipation of body habitus challenges.

- In taller patients (with a longer abdomen), all ports need to be adjusted from the arrangements described in later chapters in either a cephalad or caudal direction depending on the area of focus. The distance between the umbilicus and the xiphoid process or pubic symphysis can be significantly varied, and the umbilicus is not always located midway between the two.
- In obese or large patients, the umbilicus is frequently in a much lower position. In that case, the "umbilical" port may have to be placed several centimeters cephalad to the umbilicus for effective camera placement.

Positioning of the subsequent ports may be decided after insufflation is completed. In protuberant abdomens, the volume of gas required for insufflation may be larger and increase the surface area of the abdominal wall. Assessing the internal surface area after insufflation and area of pathology may cause a change in port placement to a more appropriate location.

Techniques for Surgery

Types of Bowel Graspers

Blunt instruments are generally preferred to prevent inadvertent injury to the bowel. Kittners are also useful especially in shifting the small bowel out of the field of view. Graspers come in a variety of types: with teeth, wavy, babcock, "duckbill," fenestrated, Alice, atraumatic, etc. (see Fig. 1.6). Respect for tissues is prudent at all times, and

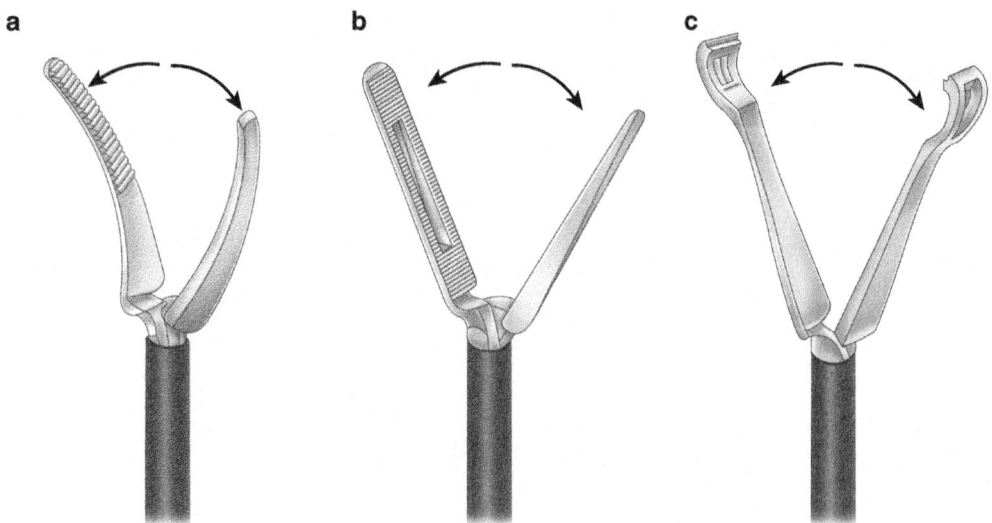

Fig. 1.6 Various types of graspers can be used, depending on surgeon preference. Each grasper has different characteristics which enable fine dissection, gross control, or decreased trauma depending on the situation. (**a**) Maryland Grasper (**b**) Glassman Forceps (**c**) Babcock Forceps

grasping bowel should be avoided unless it will be part of the specimen removed. If running of the bowel is required, atraumatic graspers with very gentle pressure and no tension should be utilized. Careful attention to the amount of pressure and what is grasped must be maintained in order to avoid serious damage to tissues. Longer instruments tend to disperse the pressure over a larger length of the bowel and decrease the risk of injury to the bowel.

Running of the Bowel

One important technique utilized to examine the bowel is running the bowel. Running the bowel is done in a "hand over hand" technique

(see Fig. 1.7). The operator needs to be facile and fluid with both hands utilizing instruments. One must keep in mind how hands function in the normal environment. Frequently, hands will cross one another to accomplish certain tasks of day-to-day activities. This movement must be reproduced inside the abdomen. Effective use of hand over hand technique is critical to efficient and successful laparoscopic colectomy. Sometimes, hand over hand involves blunt pushing, and other times the action involves grasping tissue. The surgeon needs to know the length of an open instrument to measure the length of the bowel laparoscopically. This can be important in cases of Crohn's disease where quantifying the amount of normal and disease bowel can be crucial in determining treatment.

Fig. 1.7 Running the small bowel allows for measuring the remaining bowel, identification of pathology, and unlooping of volvulus or internal hernia. Particular care should be taken when handling distended bowel as it can be easily damaged. Two methodologies of running the bowel exist: (**a**) an accordion-like running of the bowel, where the distal bowel is brought more proximally segment by segment without crossing of the hands, and (**b**) hand over hand, where the right hand repeatedly crosses the left to move distally on the bowel

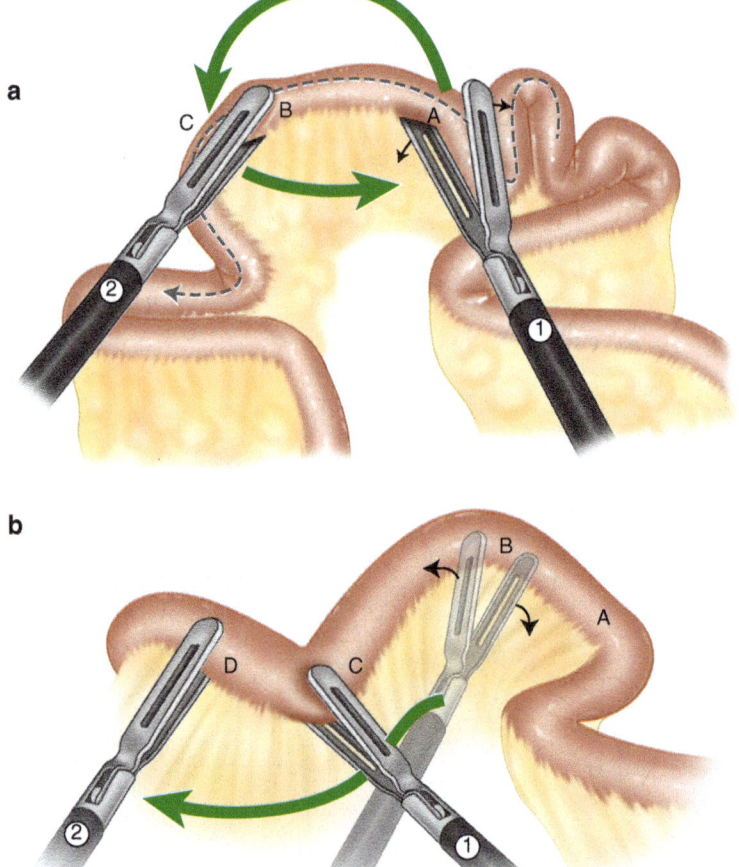

Energy Instrumentation

The most commonly employed electrical device is monopolar currency. Using monopolar technology, a current travels from the device to the tissue and returns to the generator via a pad placed on the patient, away from the operative field. Monopolar current can be used with a device specifically for this purpose such as a cautery device. In addition, cautery can be attached to several laparoscopic instruments via an external cord connection knob that is located at the proximal end of the instrument, above the handles. The surgeon then controls the activation of the energy with a foot pedal. The surgeon should always maintain control of the cautery and not abdicate this task when moving from one position to another. The surgeon using the instrument should always be the person in control of delivering the energy. The volume of these devices, signaling activation, should be increased so that it is easily audible to all members of the team, and any distracting conversations and music should be minimized so that inadvertent energy delivery can be averted (see Pitfall 1.1).

 Pitfall 1.1
Commonly a suction-irrigation-cautery device is used. The sheath to cover the cautery on these devices can be problematic. When the device is advanced through the trocar to its maximum, usually in an attempt to suction blood or irrigation fluid in a difficult location, the sheath can be inadvertently retracted, exposing the cautery hook. This error not only exposes risk of thermal spread but also can cause serious bleeding or unseen viscous violation.

There are two broad categorical settings on monopolar devices: cut and coagulation. The cut setting delivers an unmodulated, continuous current, whereas the coagulation setting delivers a modulated, interrupted current. The cut setting is more appropriate for dissection, while the coagulation setting performs better for vessel sealing. In addition, the cut setting can also be placed in a blended setting that gives more coagulation than in the pure cut mode but less than with coagulation. The coagulation setting can also be placed in fulguration or spray mode. This is ideal for noncontact coagulation when the current jumps from the active electrode to tissue that is not in direct contact with the device, causing fulguration. Monopolar instruments are varied and include hook, standard tip, and hot shears. While each provides fast dissection of planes, they carry more risk of thermal spread and injury if one is not attentive.

Bipolar devices are also commonly employed in laparoscopic colon and rectal surgery (see Fig. 1.8). In bipolar electrocautery, electric current passes from one jaw of a grasper, the active electrode equivalent, and passes to the other jaw, the return electrode equivalent. The active and passive jaws alternate, giving a more even, and localized, distribution of the thermal effect. In addition, bipolar devices obviate the need for a return pad on the patient. These bipolar devices can also seal larger blood vessels, up to 7 mm in diameter, making them ideally suited for laparoscopic colon surgery.

Ultrasonic shears are another commonly employed device in laparoscopic colon sur-

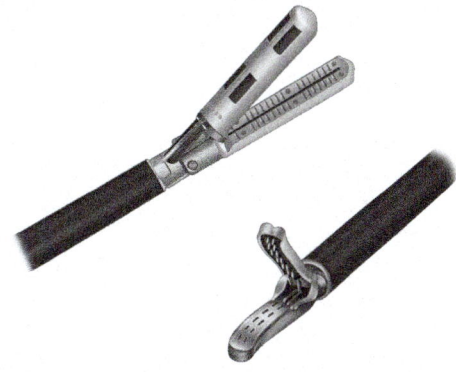

Fig. 1.8 Bipolar devices apply heat to a wider segment of tissue and generally have a blade for cutting tissue after desiccation

gery. The tissue effects obtained with ultrasonic energy are similar to those achieved with contact monopolar or bipolar electrocautery. Ultrasonic devices produce tissue effects using vibrations. These vibrations produce shearing effects on the tissues, allowing dissection and hemostasis.

Choice of energy instrument is quite personal to each surgeon and may have been developed at the institution of training. Despite the fact that there are numerous electrical devices to aid in surgery, they are only tools in the surgeon's armamentarium and are not substitutes for sound surgical technique and judgment. It is critical for the surgeon to become familiar with the particular devices available at their institution and to not be swayed or tempted to employ new technology in a haphazard fashion.

Laparoscopic electrosurgical injuries are also not an uncommon occurrence. In addition to surgeon error, injuries can occur when there are problems with the laparoscopic equipment. There can be inadvertent current leakage from the active electrode instrument when there is an insulation failure of the instrument or when direct coupling occurs. When these injuries do occur, they are often not recognized intraoperatively. As a result, there is no accurate estimation of these injuries (see Pitfall 1.2). Ensuring that the whole length of electrocautery instruments is monitored while in use can help prevent and injury and spot one, should it occur.

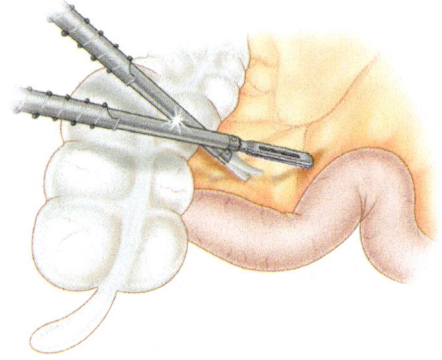

Fig. 1.9 Electrical injuries may occur if instruments are not appropriately insulated. All instruments should be checked prior to insertion into the abdomen and replaced if damage is found

Stray current injury can occur if there is a defect in the insulation material covering the active electrode, allowing current to flow to tissues or other instruments in close proximity to the break in insulation (see Fig. 1.9). There is evidence that as many as 15% of laparoscopic instruments demonstrate an insulation failure. An even higher incidence of insulation failure has been detected in dedicated monopolar instruments such as hooks and scissors. Direct coupling can occur when current from the active electrode passes to another instrument that is in contact with tissues away from this electrode. For example, if the active electrode inadvertently touches another metal instrument or metal trocar, the current will be conducted to any tissues contacting this instrument or trocar. The entire operative team should be familiar with and regularly inspect the equipment prior to the operative procedure and maintain vigilant throughout the operative procedure.

Intraoperative Endoscopy

Endoscopy

Almost every elective colon surgery is preceded by an endoscopic evaluation. Prior to taking

 **Pitfall 1.2**
Wrapping electrical cords around clamps can cause abnormal function of electrical current. Also be aware while placing clamps onto drapes so as to not catch the wire in the jaws of the clamp or violate the protective sheath over the wire. This exposes significant electrical risk and is usually out of the surgeon's direct view. By the time the violation is identified, the patient can have suffered a tremendous burn.

the patient to the operating room for laparoscopic surgery, the surgeon should review the endoscopic report and images. It is critical to determine the location of pathology, the extent of pathology, and the presence of synchronous lesions. If there is any question, the examination should be repeated to create a comprehensive operative plan.

Preoperative marking of any lesion to be removed is critical in patients with lesions not well visualized on imaging, such as computed tomography. Endoscopic localization is inaccurate for lesions located anywhere but the cecum or rectum. Laparoscopic surgery precludes the ability to palpate a lesion, and, as a result, there needs to be a definitive way for the surgeon to visually identify these lesions intraoperatively. The most common method of marking a lesion is tattooing with India ink. Tattooing the colon in three areas around the circumference is wise in order to ensure that the tattoo is visible laparoscopically. When only one location is tattooed, the tattoo may fall within the mesentery, obstructing visualization during surgery. By convention, lesions should always be marked on the distal end (closer to the anus). This assists the surgeon in identifying the distal extent of the tumor (see Fig. 1.10).

Other methods available include placing clips or the use of intraoperative colonoscopy. Clips will not be visualized intraoperatively but can help the surgeon locate the tumor by using X-rays. X-rays must be obtained prior to surgery but can identify the general region of the colon where the tumor is located. Intraoperative colonoscopy can be employed if the tattoo is not visualized. This requires that the patient has a bowel prep during surgery.

If intraoperative endoscopy is required, insufflation with carbon dioxide needs to be utilized for faster reabsorption of intraluminal gas. As insufflation is continued, intra-abdominal visibility will become completely obscured making completion of the operation laparoscopically virtually impossible. This problem can be minimized by:

- Employing the shortest duration of endoscopy possible
- Using an atraumatic grasper or other blunt instrument to carefully compress the colon or terminal ileum obstructing flow to areas proximal to the lesion.

Insufflation of the small bowel, if flow is not obstructed and an incompetent ileocecal valve is present (reported in approximately 30% of cases), can be especially problematic and probably force conversion to open surgery. Loop formation can be minimized by desufflation of the abdomen which permits external compression for advancement of the endoscope. Once the area of concern has been identified, it should be marked intra-abdominally with a clip or a suture for future reference.

Wound Protectors

Incisions/Wound Protectors

With laparoscopic colectomy, there is the requirement to make an incision large enough to extract the specimen and also ample enough to make an anastomosis if this is to be performed in an extracorporeal fashion. There are numerous options for making this incision. The options are typically impacted by factors such as (1) the colon to be resected, (2) the type of anastomosis to be performed, and (3) the body habitus of the patient. Using an existing hand port

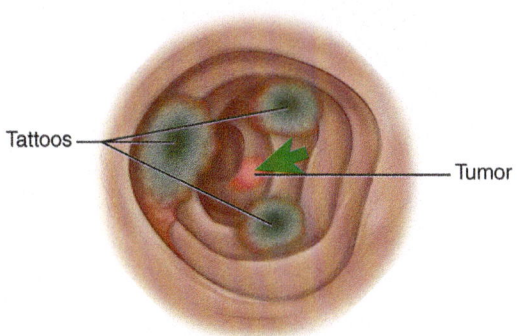

Fig. 1.10 Endoscopic tattooing of the colon in three locations, distal to the tumor

is one obvious option, as is extending any existing port incision to allow adequate operative exposure. When using a hand-assisted incision, care should be taken to ensure it is a good distance away from the quadrant of interest. Dissection becomes technically challenging if the hand port incision is located just over the area of focus. The arm and hand will tend to obscure visibility as well.

One incision that is well suited for pelvic operations is the Pfannenstiel incision. This versatile incision allows operative exposure of the pelvis if additional dissection is necessary and allows direct visualization when transecting bowel in the pelvis as well as completing the low pelvic anastomosis. It is believed that this incision has less pain and is more cosmetic for patients. In addition, non-midline incisions are associated with decreased postoperative incisional hernia rates than the more traditional midline incisions. However, if there is any thought that conversion may be a possibility, a vertically oriented incision is preferred.

Regardless of the incision that is chosen, it is important to protect the skin edges while removing bowel or performing an anastomosis (see Fig. 1.11). Several commercially available

wound protectors work well for this purpose and have been demonstrated to reduce the incidence of surgical site infections in colorectal surgical procedures. Wound protectors can be used in conjunction with a hand assist device at the beginning of the case or at the end for extraction. Several wound protector products (usually in conjunction with hand assist devices) have the ability to offer re-insufflation after extraction to complete the case. Other techniques employed with basic wound protectors involve using a large peon clamp under the external ring in order to reestablish a pneumoperitoneum. This is useful to ensure your anastomosis or ostomy did not become twisted in the process of creation or to ensure hemostasis at the end of the case.

Wound Closure

Any incision, 10 mm in size or greater, should be closed at the end of the operation. The fascia should be closed to prevent hernia and incarceration. There are multiple commercially available devices to assist with closure, which allow for visualization of the closure prior to removal of the laparoscope (see Fig. 1.12). Key to this technique is ensuring that a solid bite of

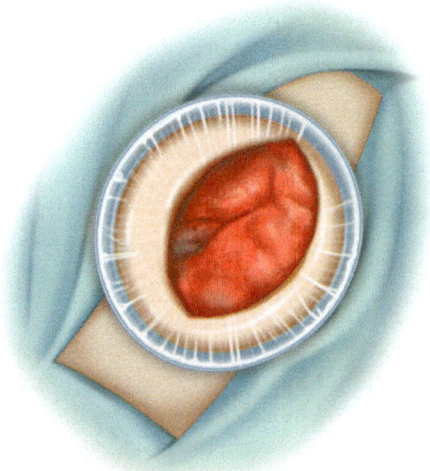

Fig. 1.11 Wound protectors help by optimizing retraction of the wound, enabling removal of specimen, or creating extracorporeal anastomoses in appropriate cases. The also prevent soilage into the subcutaneous tissue, with the intent of decreasing wound infection rates

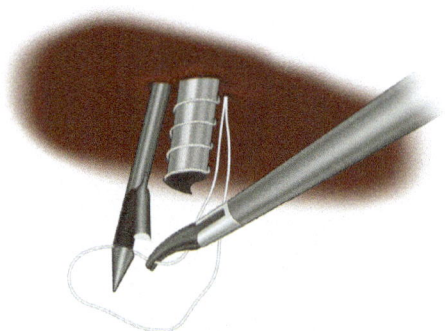

Carter Thomason

Fig. 1.12 Carter-Thomason endoscopic suture passer is used to pass the suture from one side of the wound to the other while guided laparoscopically. A 5 mm camera is generally used through a lateral port to facilitate visualization

fascia is obtained on both sides of the incision, and the fascia is completely closed. The Carter-Thomason close suture system (Inlet Medical, Inc. Eden Prarie, MN, USA) is one such device. Generally, a 0 or 2–0 polyglactin suture is used for closure. A snap is placed on one end of the suture. The Carter-Thomason device is then loaded with the other end of the suture. It is passed through the skin incision, into the fascia lateral to the fascial incision. The assistant uses a second port site to grasp the suture and pull it into the abdomen. The empty Carter-Thomason is then passed through the contralateral side of the fascia. The suture is passed to the empty device and then pulled out of the incision. Generally, a figure of eight suture is used, covering left superior to right superior, and then left inferior to right inferior.

Laparoscopic colectomy, as in all surgery, involves a great deal of forethought and familiarity with equipment. Approach varies widely from surgeon to surgeon, and the goals here are to provide one with guidance, tips, and pitfalls to ensure success.

Laparoscopic Right Colectomy

Raul M. Bosio and Sharon L. Stein

Introduction

Laparoscopic right colectomy involves resection of the terminal ileum and right colon with creation of an ileocolic anastomosis. It is performed for pathology of the terminal ileum or right colon such as neoplasia, volvulus, arterial venous malformations, or Crohn's disease.

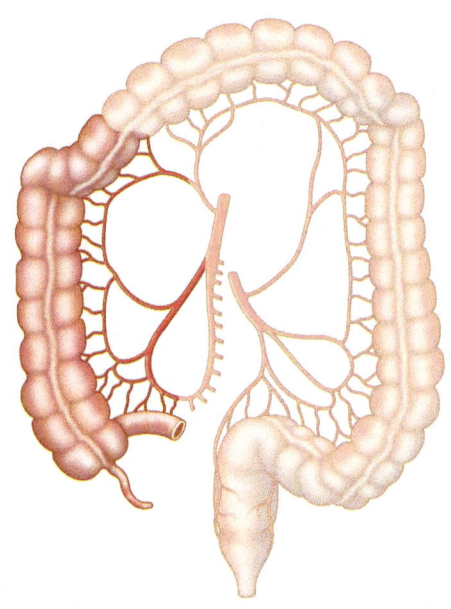

Indications
- Neoplasia (benign or malignant) of the right colon
- Crohn's disease of the terminal ileum or right colon
- Cecal volvulus
- Ischemia
- Right-sided diverticula
- Perforated appendicitis requiring cecectomy

Preoperative Planning
- Colonoscopy to confirm diagnosis, relevant anatomy, synchronous lesions, and tattooing if appropriate
- Preoperative staging for malignancy:
  - CT scan of chest abdomen and pelvis
  - Carcinoembryonic antigen serum level
- Deep venous thrombosis prophylaxis
- Preoperative antibiotics
- Mechanical bowel prep, if indicated

R. M. Bosio
Division of Surgery, ProMedica Health & Wellness Center, Sylvania, OH, USA

S. L. Stein (✉)
Division of Colon and Rectal Surgery, Department of Surgery, University Hospital Cleveland Medical Center, Cleveland, OH, USA
e-mail: Sharon.stein@uhhospitals.org

© Springer Nature Switzerland AG 2020
S. L. Stein, R. R. Lawson (eds.), *Laparoscopic Colectomy*,
https://doi.org/10.1007/978-3-030-39559-9_2

Steps of the Operation

Patient positioning

1. Step 1: Port placement
2. Step 2: Staging laparoscopy and restoration of anatomy (if necessary)
3. Step 3: Identification of pathology
4. Step 4: Identification and transection of the ileocolic pedicle
5. Step 5: Dissection of the retroperitoneal plane
6. Step 6: Identification and transection of the middle colic arteries
7. Step 7: Transverse mesenteric transection
8. Step 8: Entry into the lesser sac
9. Step 9: Hepatic flexure mobilization
10. Step 10: Lateral mobilization
11. Step 11: Attachments to the terminal ileum
12. Step 12: Externalization of specimen
13. Step 13: Anastomosis
14. Step 14: Closure

Tools of the Operation

- 5 mm ports (3)
- 12 mm Hassan (entry) port (1)
- 10 mm 30-degree camera (1)
- Laparoscopic bowel graspers (3)
- Scissors with electrocautery (1)
- Energy instrument for vessel ligation (1)
- Stapler for vessel ligation (optional)
- Endoloop® (Ethicon, optional)
- Wound protector
- Two firings of the linear intestinal stapler for extracorporeal anastomosis

Patient Positioning for Laparoscopic Laparoscopic Right Colectomy

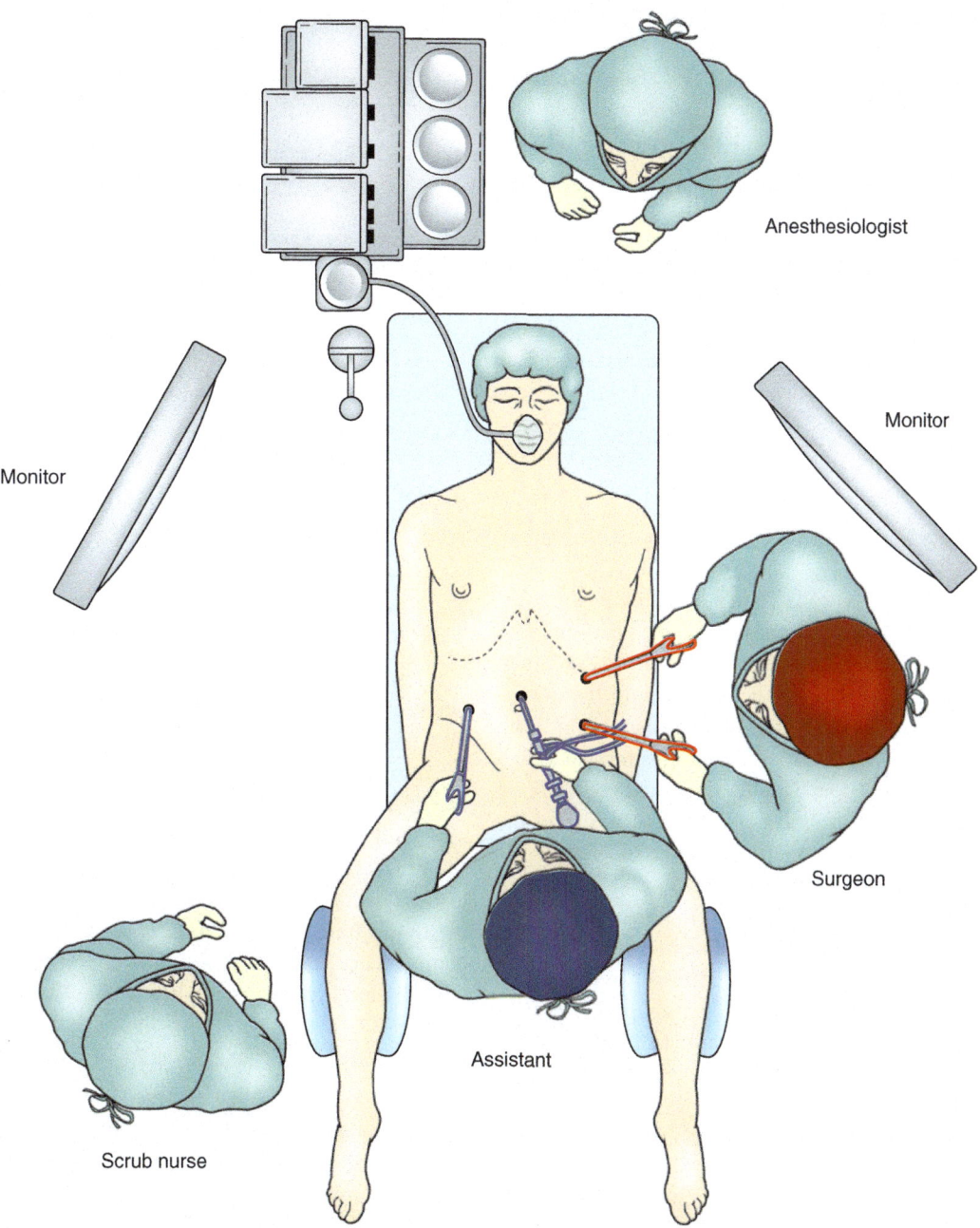

Patient position: The patient is placed in modified lithotomy position with both arms tucked. All lines/tubes are run off the top of the table to allow the surgeon to move easily around the table if needed. Video monitors are placed on the left and right side of the patient, toward the patient's head and anesthesia

The patient is positioned in modified lithotomy position as detailed in Chap. 1. Both arms are tucked to allow for surgeon position and manipulation of instruments. If necessary, the right arm may be placed on an arm board. However, leaving the right arm out may limit the ability to dissect adhesions if encountered upon entry into the abdomen.

The surgeon will stand primarily on the patient's left side. The primary video monitor is positioned off the patient's right shoulder to allow for triangulation between camera, instrument ports, and pathology. The assistant will generally stand between the patient's legs.

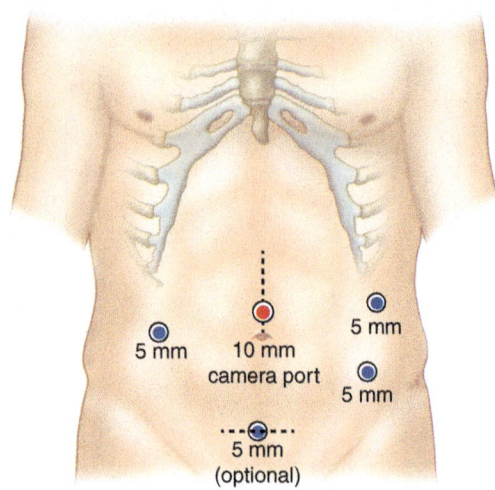

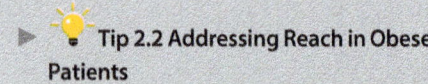

Fig. 2.1 Port placement: The camera port is a supraumbilical 10 mm port, as this will often be the extraction site for the specimen. Additional 5 mm ports are placed in the right upper, right lower, and left lower quadrants. Choice of extraction sites includes the upper midline or Pfannenstiel and depends on surgeon preference

Operative Strategy

Step 1: Port Placement

Abdominal entry is via a supraumbilical/umbilical incision in the midline via open Hassan technique. Because multiple layers of the abdomen are fixed at the umbilicus, access to the peritoneum is relatively straightforward at this location even in obese patients. The skin is incised with a vertical incision. This incision will generally be enlarged for specimen extraction at the end of the case. A Kocher clamp is used to elevate the umbilical stump, and the fascia is scored. S-shaped retractors are used to retract tissue. The posterior sheath and peritoneum are lifted and incised. Entry into the abdominal cavity is confirmed by visualization of the free space or bowel. A suture is placed in a purse string fashion around the anterior fascia to secure the trocar. A Hassan trocar is placed through the umbilical incision, and pneumoperitoneum is obtained (see Tip 2.1).

The camera is used to evaluate the area directly below the access point immediately upon entry into the abdomen. Vascular and bowel injuries are most likely to be seen prior to adjustment of the table or manipulation of bowel and can be identified and treated at this point.

Additional ports (5 mm) are placed in the right lower quadrant, right upper quadrant, and left lower quadrant under laparoscopic guidance as demonstrated in Fig. 2.1. All ports are generally placed lateral to the rectal sheath (see Tip 2.2).

> **Tip 2.2 Addressing Reach in Obese Patients**
> In obese patients, more medial placement may be beneficial to facilitate reach across the abdomen or to the upper abdomen. This may require a port to be placed through the rectus sheath, and care should be taken to avoid the inferior epigastric artery.

> **Tip 2.1 Communication**
> The surgeon should notify the anesthetist prior to insufflation. Hemodynamic compromise can occur while establishing pneumoperitoneum. Communication with the anesthetist helps to prepare for any instability.

The inferior ports should be a minimum of two fingerbreadths lateral and superior to the anterior superior iliac spine to prevent limitation of movement by the patient.

A 10 mm 30-degree camera is placed in the supraumbilical port. The assistant stands between the patient legs with the right hand controlling the camera. The assistant's left hand assists through the 5 mm left lower quadrant port. The surgeon stands on the patient's left side and will use the right upper and lower quadrants for operating.

Step 2: Laparoscopic Staging (if Indicated) and Restoration of Normal Anatomy

A laparoscopic staging is performed at the beginning of the surgery in cases of neoplasia or cancer. The surgeon evaluates the liver, abdominal wall, and adnexa for any signs of metastatic disease. The small bowel is evaluated to ensure that disease is localized. Biopsies are taken of any suspicious lesions.

In Crohn's disease, staging of active disease is useful for intraoperative and postoperative planning. The small bowel is run from ligament of Treitz to the ileocecal valve. The extent and location of diseased segments are noted and included in operative dictation. Pathologic strictures and obstruction will be addressed during the operation (see Tip 2.3).

> 💡 **Tip 2.3 Running the Small Bowel**
> Start running the small bowel proximally by lifting the transverse mesocolon and identifying the ligament of Treitz as it crosses under the mesocolon. As the bowel is inspected, it should be placed in left upper quadrant. By moving the colon out of the right lower quadrant operative field, the surgeon facilitates set up for the next phase of the operation.

For patients with significant adhesions or omentum stuck to the pelvis, restoration of normal anatomy is appropriate at this time. Until the terminal ileum and the right colon have been restored to their normal location, it may be difficult to proceed with laparoscopic surgery. The most common adhesions are anterior wall adhesions from prior surgery, omental adhesions to the pelvis or prior appendectomy incision, and small bowel adhesions to the right side of the pelvis, tethering the small bowel to the ovary and fallopian tube. Sharp lysis of adhesions, with care to preserve anatomic planes, may be required (See Chap. 10).

Step 3: Identification of Pathology

In neoplastic disease, the surgeon identifies the location of pathology. If not clearly visualized on CT scan, the pathology is marked preoperatively with an endoscopic tattoo (see Chap. 1). The location of the tumor will determine resection margins and vessel ligation. If there is any concern about the extent or location of pathology, an intraoperative CO_2 endoscopy may be performed (see Tip 2.4).

> 💡 **Tip 2.4 Tattooing the Colon**
> Endoscopic marking of a polyp in three quadrants of the colon facilitates intraoperative identification of pathology. A single quadrant marking may not be visible externally through a thick mesentery or prominent epiploica.

For cancer of the right colon, oncologic margins should be 10 cm proximal and distal to the cancer. High (proximal) transection of all vessels is performed to ensure appropriate lymphadenectomy. For a cecal lesion, this includes high ligation of the ileocolic and right branch of the middle colic artery. For a hepatic flexure lesion, the ileocolic and the entire middle colic vessels should be transected.

The patient is placed in Trendelenberg position with left side down. The surgeon inserts bowel

Fig. 2.2 Identification of pathology: The patient is in Trendelenburg position, with left side down, exposing the right colon and terminal ileum. The small bowel is moved from the right lower quadrant, allowing visualization of the right colon mesentery to begin the operation

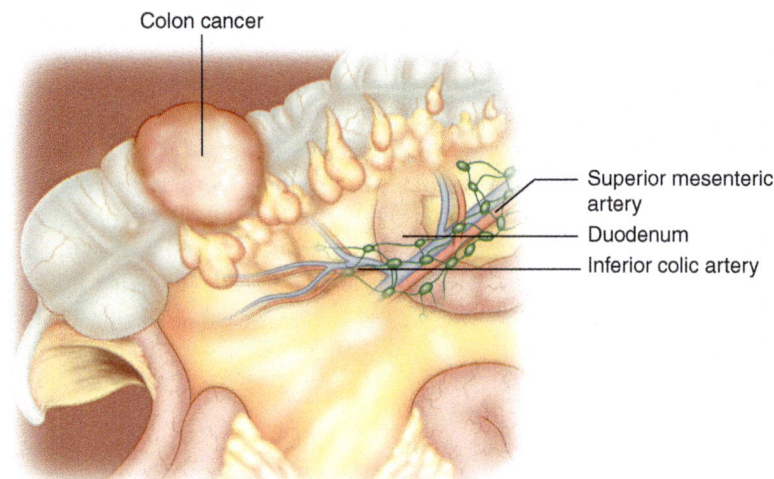

Colon cancer

Superior mesenteric artery

Duodenum

Inferior colic artery

graspers through the left upper and lower quadrant trocars. The omentum is freed from any distal attachments and the omentum elevated over the transverse colon. Attachments to the omentum are ligated using either an energy instrument or scissors with electrocautery. It is important to mobilize the omentum adequately to expose the right colon, transverse colon, and colon mesentery. The omentum is lifted above the transverse colon and tucked between the colon and the liver. A gentle shake or tug on the transverse colon epiploicae, after moving the omentum, is helpful in keeping the omentum out of the operative field. If not done previously, the small bowel is displaced from the right lower quadrant by running the bowel out of the field of vision (Fig. 2.2).

Step 4: Identification and Transection of the Ileocolic Pedicle

The assistant places a bowel grasper through the left lower quadrant port to elevate the cecum just distal to the ileocecal valve. Direction of gentle traction is anterior toward the abdominal wall and lateral toward the right sidewall. Even in heavy patients, this exposes the ileocolic pedicle at its origin from the superior mesenteric artery.

Occasionally, attachments from the transverse colon to the right colon will obliterate the plane between these two structures. The surgeon

should either carefully dissect the transverse colon off the right colon, finding a clear plane between epiploicae and mesentery, or vary approach to a lateral to medial dissection (see Special Considerations).

The peritoneum is scored superficially below the ileocolic artery (ICA), distal to the superior mesenteric artery using electrocautery. The direction of incision is parallel to the ICA (Pitfall 2.1; Fig. 2.3).

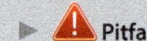 **Pitfall 2.1**
Scoring deeply into the peritoneum or proximally on ICA can result in electrocautery injury to the duodenum. Scoring the plane slightly distal to the bifurcation of the ileocolic and superior mesenteric artery will help prevent inadvertent injury to the duodenum.

A plane below the ICA is matured with blunt dissection. The surgeon's left hand is used to support the isolated ileocolic artery, while the right hand gently sweeps the retroperitoneal tissue down, away from the mesentery. A clear view of the duodenum is created without using electrocautery. The surgeon's left hand and the assistant's left hand can be relocated into the window to create greater upward tension on the mesenteric tissue.

Fig. 2.3 The cecum is retracted anterior and lateral, demonstrating the ileocolic artery and the plane directly below the vessel. Scoring this plane with electrocautery parallel to the artery facilitates entry into the retroperitoneal plane

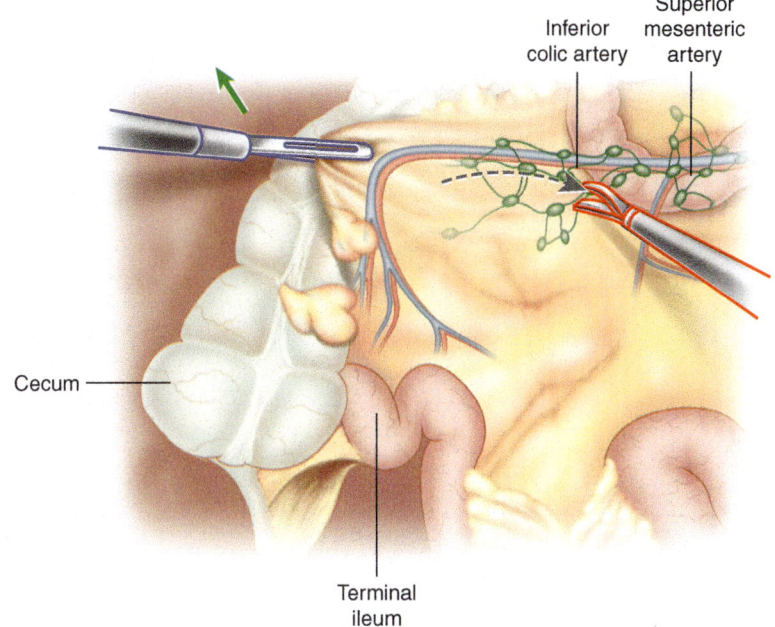

Fig. 2.4 After isolating the ileocolic artery, the retroperitoneal layers are swept downwards, revealing an avascular plane between the mesentery and retroperitoneum. The surgeon's nonoperating hand and assistant's hands are used to elevate the mesentery to demonstrate the white line of the retroperitoneum

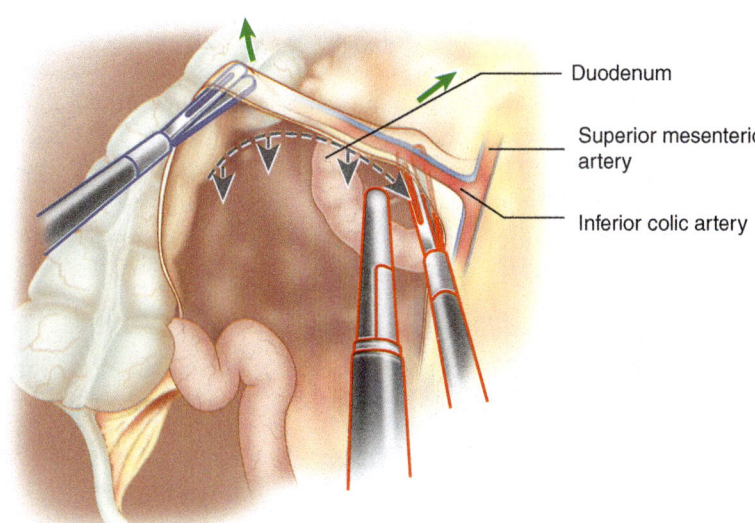

The surgeon's right hand is used for "sweeping" perpendicular to the plane of tension (Fig. 2.4).

The ICA is transected after the retroperitoneum is freed from the right colon mesentery. A "bare" area is seen just cephalad to the ICA artery once the retroperitoneal window has been established, and the duodenum is identified. This window is opened, creating a full 360-degree exposure of the ICA (Pitfall 2.2)

 ⚠ **Pitfall 2.2**

In patients with coronary artery disease, gently palpate the artery prior to transection. If the artery is calcified, consider alternate transection techniques such as stapling or endovascular vessel loop.

Fig. 2.5 Transection of the ileocolic artery is performed as a high ligation in cancer cases. Isolation of the duodenum is vital prior to ligation

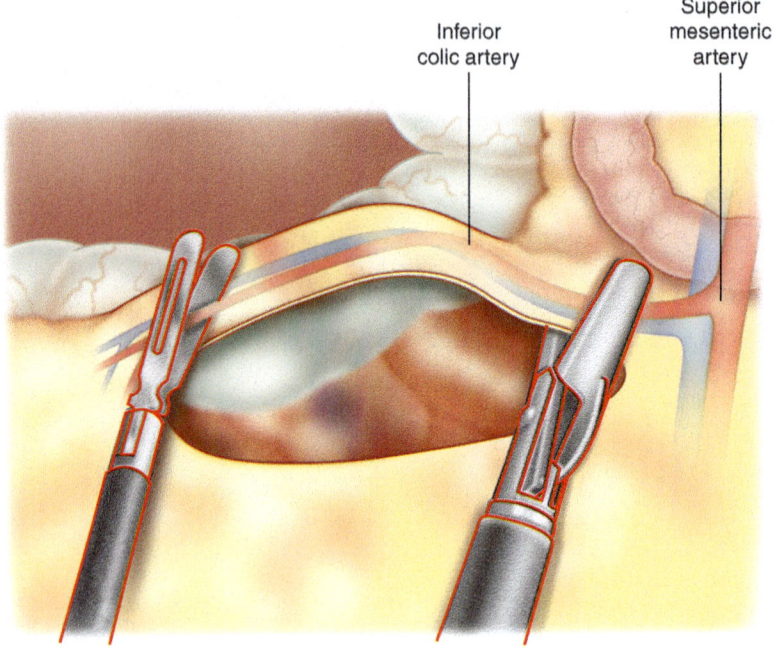

The ICA may be taken with energy, clips, or staples per surgeon preference (see Chap. 1). The location of the duodenum is verified prior to ligation to ensure it is clear of plane of transection. If using bipolar or ultrasonic energy, tension on the vessel should be released prior to transection. The surgeon's left hand generally holds the instrument of transection, while a grasper in the right hand releases tension as demonstrated in Fig. 2.5. The right hand instrument is available to occlude a vessel and prevent blood loss in case of bleeding from the superior mesenteric artery/ICA stump. (Fig. 2.5) (Tip 2.5).

edge of the retroperitoneum that should be preserved. The white edge should be gently pushed down with the retroperitoneum against tension. Without good tension on the mesocolon, the planes will not separate.

Occasionally, small vessels may require cauterization to prevent bleeding. Vessels from the mesentery run perpendicular to the colon; vessels parallel to the colon are swept down with the retroperitoneum. Bleeding or poor visualization indicate the surgeon is too deep in the retroperitoneal plane and should relocate more superficially. The correct plane is avascular and clear (Tip 2.6).

> 💡 **Tip 2.5 Anatomic Variation**
> The right colic artery is often noted as a branch off the ileocolic artery or middle colic artery, if it is present at all. Only 30% of patients have a separate right colic artery off the superior mesenteric artery that must be ligated.

Step 5: Dissection of the Retroperitoneal Plane

A faint white edge is noted at the margin of retroperitoneal and mesenteric tissue; this is the folded

> 💡 **Tip 2.6 Delayed ICA Transection**
> Delaying transection of the ICA until after the retroperitoneal dissection has been completed helps maintain countertension. This is a delicate balance, as care must be taken to prevent excessive tension on the pedicle.

A hand-over-hand technique is useful. The surgeon's operating instrument is moved further into the plane to create additional tension upwards on the mesocolon and is then replaced by the assistant's instrument, freeing the surgeon's hand for further dissection. Varying left and right hands as dissector may make dissection easier (Tip 2.7).

> 💡 **Tip 2.7 Maximizing Traction**
> Using blunt graspers as an open "V" rather than grasping or pulling tissue, allows greater tension and prevents inadvertent avulsion of the tissues.

Dissection in the retroperitoneal plane should continue superiorly and laterally. Superiorly, a plane below the transverse colon is realized when a purple/dark space is found deep to the transverse colon. This represents the space below the liver, into the lesser sac. Laterally, the retroperitoneal plane continues below the ascending colon to the line of Toldt, and the sidewall is revealed. In the medial aspect, the duodenum should be clearly seen and preserved. Dissection in the area of the duodenum and the pancreas should be exceedingly gentle to prevent bleeding, pancreatitis, and injury.

Step 6: Identification and Transection of the Middle Colic Arteries (MCA)

After the ileocolic artery is transected and the retroperitoneal plane is established, the assistant's left hand holds the free edge of the colon mesentery. The surgeon moves the right hand to place tension on the mesocolon, distal to the middle colic vessels. A subtle plane above the pancreas and duodenum just below the transverse mesocolon can be created to identify the branches of the middle colic vessel. Blunt dissection is performed, sweeping the duodenum and pancreas down with the surgeon's left hand. Once isolated, the middle colic vessels may be ligated en bloc or individually. There are usually 3–5 middle colic artery branches.

The extent of middle colic artery (MCA) transection will vary depending on indication for surgery. In Crohn's disease, the entire middle colic vessels may be preserved. In cecal cancer, the right branch is taken. For more distal tumors of the ascending colon or hepatic flexure, the entire MCA may be transected at its branch from the superior mesenteric artery.

The right branch of the MCA is ligated proximally, close to the superior mesenteric artery for complete lymphadenectomy. A window around the MCA is established by lifting the transverse mesocolon away from the lesser sac with the surgeon's right hand. Using an energy device, Maryland dissector, or bowel grasper, the vessel is identified and isolated. If the vessels are close together, a Maryland dissector may help with the fine dissection needed to separate the branches. Either stapler or energy device can be used to transect the vessel securely (Pitfall 2.3) (Fig. 2.6).

> **Pitfall 2.3**
> Branches of the gastroepiploic vein communicate with the middle colic veins. These vessels may be hard to see as they come from the lesser sac, behind the surgeons' view of the vessel. Care must be taken to prevent avulsing these crossing vessels when dissecting between the middle colic vessels and duodenum or pancreas.

Step 7: Transverse Colon Mesenteric Transection

After ligation of the right branch of the MCA, the distal extent of dissection is identified, and the mesentery leading to the transverse colon is transected with an energy device. Although this step may be done extracorporeally after extraction, intracorporeal transection of the mesentery prevents pulling or tearing of the mesentery during extraction. As the transverse colon mesentery is the least mobile part of the colon during this operation, this step facilitates a small incision and extraction site.

Fig. 2.6 The mesentery to the transverse colon can be transected perpendicular to the plane of the colon, from the free edge. Care is taken to ensure that the colon is not injured as the mesentery is resected

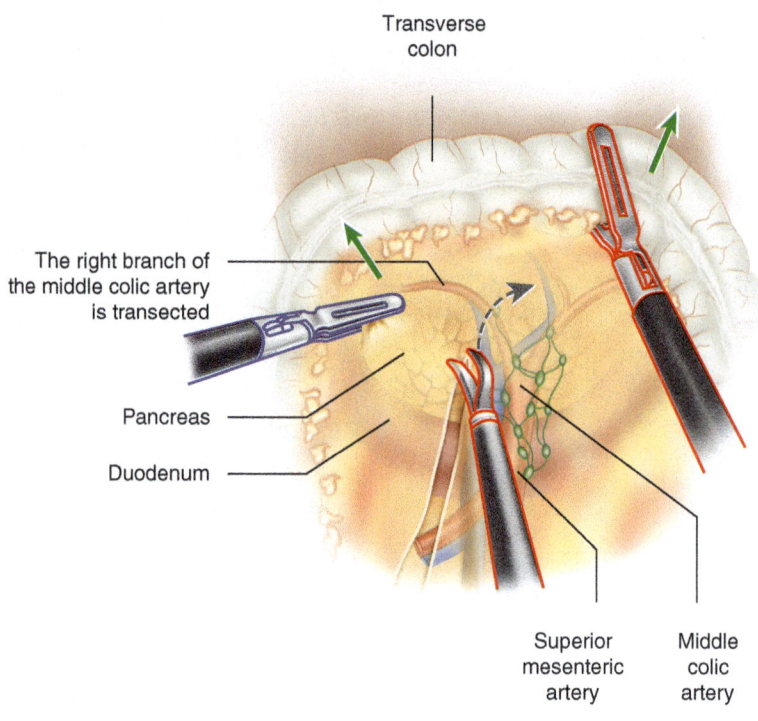

Fig. 2.7 Transection of the transverse Mesocolon. After identifying the distal extent of colon resection, the surgeon can transect the mesentery of the transverse colon to the colon wall with a bipolar instrument

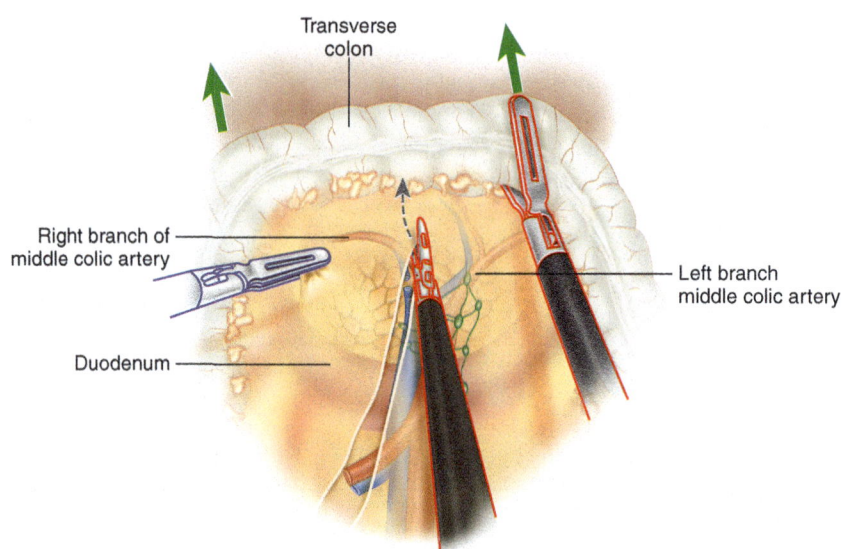

The mesentery is taken perpendicular to the colon. This retains blood supply to the mid or distal transverse colon. The assistant holds the proximal transverse colon, while the surgeon's right hand maintains tension on the distal transverse colon mesentery. An energy device is used in the left hand. Transection continues until the colon is exposed (Fig. 2.7).

Step 8: Entry into the Lesser Sac

The omentum is elevated with the surgeon's right hand, while the left hand is used for dissection into the lesser sac. The assistant holds the colon epiploicae caudal with the left hand. Either bipolar or electric scissors can be used during this step (Tip 2.8).

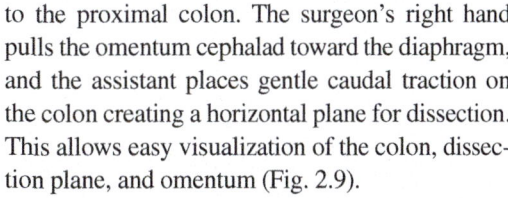

The plane is seen by differentiating subtle changes in color and quality of the transverse colon epiploicae and the omentum. An avascular plane exists, although it may be difficult to identify. There are two layers of the omentum; both must be freed superiorly to enter the lesser sac (Fig. 2.8). Definitive identification of the lesser sac is made when the posterior wall of the stomach with gastroepiploic vessels is visualized (Tip 2.9).

Once the plane is entered, rotating the plane horizontally allows for continued visualization of the transverse colon and prevents inadvertent injury

to the proximal colon. The surgeon's right hand pulls the omentum cephalad toward the diaphragm, and the assistant places gentle caudal traction on the colon creating a horizontal plane for dissection. This allows easy visualization of the colon, dissection plane, and omentum (Fig. 2.9).

The omentum should be mobilized off the transverse colon at least 10 cm distal to the transection margin. This prevents the omentum from limiting extraction of the specimen or creation of an anastomosis.

Step 9: Hepatic Flexure Mobilization

If proper retromesenteric dissection occurred during initial dissection under the ileocolic vessels, a subtle thin purple plane is noted after entering the lesser sac. This is the remaining attachment to the retroperitoneum. Entry into this plane frees the hepatic flexure completely from the retroperitoneum. The assistant pushes the hepatic flexure caudally, and a thin filmy plane is visualized. This can be transected with energy or electrocautery. The plane is below the colon and should not include any additional mesentery (Fig. 2.10).

Step 10: Lateral Mobilization

The dissection continues inferiorly down the line of Toldt in a top-down manner. Tension is created with the surgeon's left hand, displacing the colon

Fig. 2.8 Entry into the lesser sac holding the colon and omentum. The assistant holds the colon proximally to straighten the colon and provide counter tension. A subtle change in the fat plane can be identified and separated from the omentum

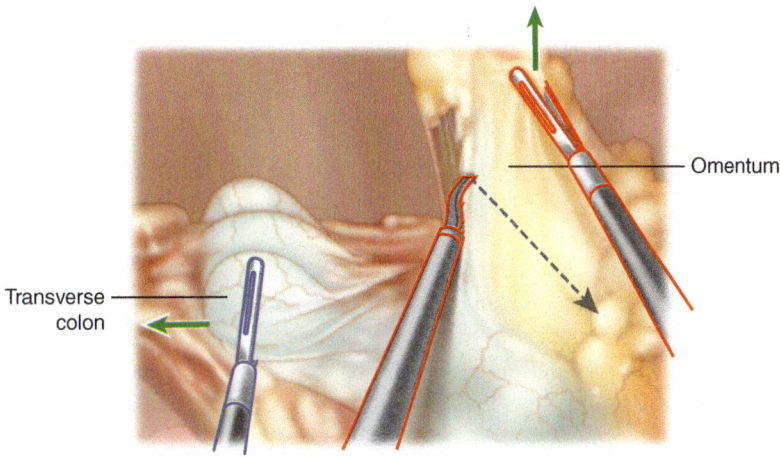

Omentum

Transverse colon

Fig. 2.9 Horizontal plane for lesser sac. By varying the perspective to a horizontal plane, the surgeon can easily visualize the omentum, epiploica, and the proximal colon. This prevents injury as the dissection proceeds proximally

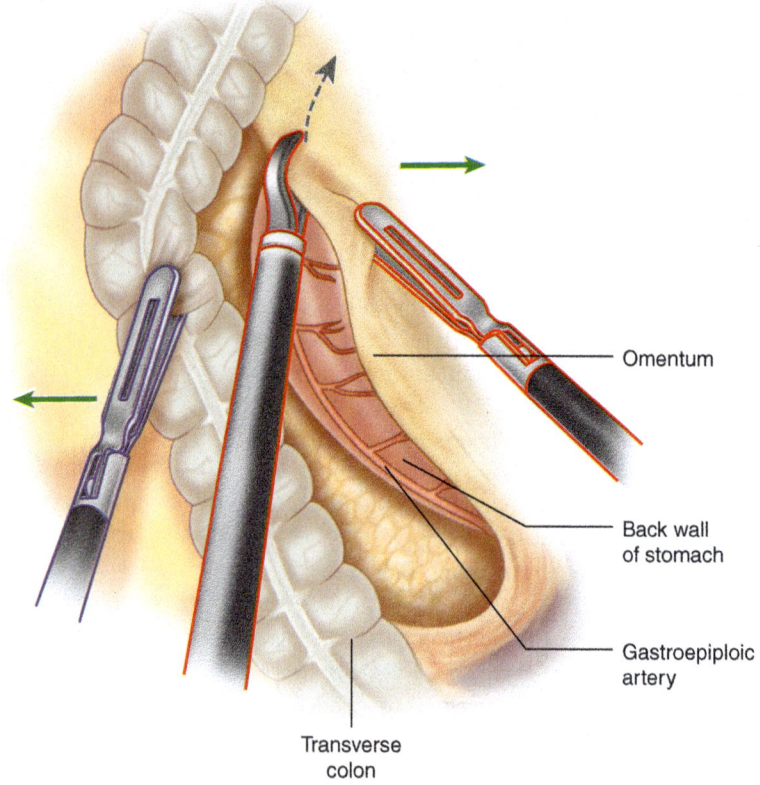

Omentum

Back wall of stomach

Gastroepiploic artery

Transverse colon

Fig. 2.10 Only filmy attachments should remain at the hepatic flexure. By pushing the colon inferiorly, attachments are clearly visualized and taken with an energy instrument

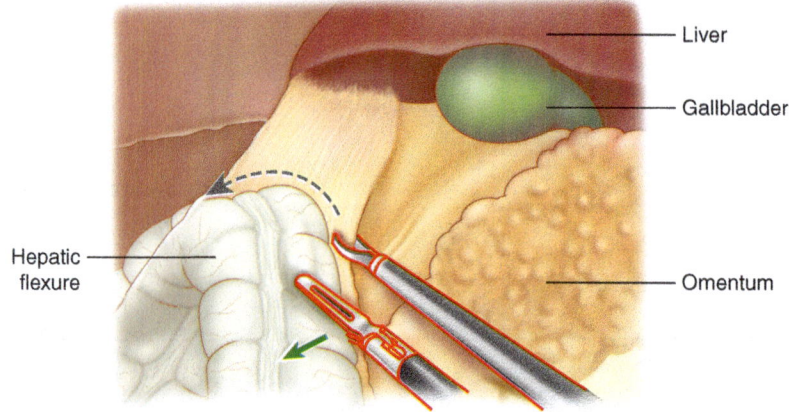

Liver

Gallbladder

Hepatic flexure

Omentum

medially away from the sidewall. Energy is used to separate the sidewall and line of Toldt from the colon, staying close to the colon unless extracolonic tumor extension is noted. The plane can generally be dissected using a scissors with cautery if tension is adequate (Tip 2.10).

> 💡 **Tip 2.10 White Line of Toldt**
> The white line of Toldt is actually a fold of retroperitoneum. The entire white line should be preserved and pushed laterally, keeping the retroperitoneum intact. Attachments should be taken just medially to this line for appropriate dissection.

Step 11: Attachments to the Terminal Ileum

Attachments to the terminal ileum, appendix, and cecum can be best seen by repositioning the patient to Trendelenburg position, left side down. The dissection can be started from the terminal ileum and proceed in a bottom-up fashion. The cecum can be retracted medially – putting the white line of Toldt under tension at the pelvic brim as demonstrated in Fig. 2.10. Generally, this is a convoluted line, rather than a straight line (Fig. 2.10).

At the inferior aspect of the cecum, the appendix and terminal ileum can be stuck to the pelvic brim. If the appendix is stuck, it can prevent adequate retraction to visualize planes and may need to be addressed prior to proceeding. The appendix is often stuck deep in the pelvis and at times may be covered by the ovary and tube. Placing the patient in steep Trendelenberg helps to isolate the right lower quadrant, moving the small bowel out of the pelvis. This allows for retraction of the ovary anteriorly. Use the scissors to identify the plane and carefully dissect any attachments to the appendix. The scissor can be placed in the surgeon's right hand, leaving the left hand free to create tension against the sidewall. The surgeon can either retract the cecum, if the port is placed sufficiently inferiorly, or pass the cecum to the assistant (Tip 2.11).

> **Tip 2.11 Operating Against the Camera**
> At times during a surgical procedure, it may be necessary for either the surgeon or assistant to operate "backwards" or the opposite direction from the camera. This should be minimized, as it is difficult to master. Thinking about the anatomy as superior, inferior, or lateral may be more helpful than using the camera view.

Alternatively, if patients have had a prior appendectomy, the cecum may be stuck to the anterior abdominal wall, necessitating careful dissection anteriorly to free and retract the cecum. An open bowel grasper can push up away from the attachments, to create tension and demonstrate the avascular adhesive plane.

Once the appendix and cecum are free laterally, the cecum should be lifted toward the anterior abdominal wall and cephalad, putting the tissues on tension. The peritoneum is scored below the mesentery of the terminal ileum. This plane will be thin and avascular plane. Unlike the medial plane, there is generally no white line demonstrating the separation of the retroperitoneum from the ileal mesentery. It is important to keep the retroperitoneum intact, preventing injury to the ureter, gonadals, or hypogastric nerves, all of which lay beneath the retroperitoneal fascia (Pitfall 2.4). By starting at the white line of Toldt laterally and using gentle blunt dissection above the retroperitoneum, the plane can be visualized.

> ⚠ **Pitfall 2.4**
> The gonadal vessels and ureters run close to the appendix and adhesions to the terminal ileum. Traction perpendicular to the retroperitoneum helps to prevent injury.

Consistent traction away from the right lower quadrant facilitates identification of the correct plane. The terminal ileum can be mobilized completely up to the duodenum for maximal reach.

The dissection is complete when the lateral attachments are free and join the medial mobilization under the colon. The entire right colon should be mobile and free from attachments. The abdomen is inspected to for any signs of bleeding prior to creation of an incision.

Step 12: Externalization of Specimen

A bowel grasper is placed on the cecum or appendix and closed to help facilitate extraction for anastomosis. This is left in place until secured extracorporeally through the extraction port.

The surgeon may choose from several extraction incision choices: most commonly a midline incision or Pfannenstiel incision. An upper midline incision optimizes reach from the transverse colon, where the middle colic vessels tether the colon and limit mobilization. However, a midline incision may have higher risks of incisional hernia. Cosmetically, a Pfannenstiel incision may be preferable. If this incision is chosen, adequate mobility of the transverse colon must be verified to ensure that the colon will reach to the Pfannenstiel incision. In the reoperative abdomen, using a prior incision may be appropriately.

The incision size depends on the size of the pathology. A large tumor or phlegmon may require a larger incision, even when well mobilized.

A wound protector is used to protect the skin and soft tissue from contamination during externalization and creation of anastomosis. Commercially available wound protectors also maximize the amount of exposure with respect to the size of the incision (see Chap. 1). Sterile towels are placed around the incision to prevent contamination. All instruments used for creation of the anastomosis should be passed off the sterile field at the conclusion of this portion of the case. Gloves are changed to prevent contamination and decrease the rate of wound infections.

The specimen is brought to the incision using the laparoscopic bowel grasper and then grasped with a Babcock. The colon is gently brought out through the incision until completely extricated. The colon is evaluated for adequate length, for resection margins, and for viability (Tip 2.12). Any remaining mesentery is transected using clamp and tie or energy

> 💡 **Tip 2.12 Transection Margins**
> In colon cancer, a 10 cm proximal and distal resection margin should be transected for appropriate oncologic margins. In Crohn's disease, normal-appearing bowel, without inflammation, stenosis, or creeping fat, should be selected. There is no advantage to taking additional margins in Crohn's disease.

devices until the bowel is completely clean of mesentery.

Step 13: Anastomosis

A double-stapled technique, described here, uses a longitudinal and then transverse staple line. Two 80 mm linear intestinal staplers are used.

The colon and small bowel are arranged to allow for a side-to-side longitudinal stapling. A full-thickness colotomy is created on the antimesenteric border of the colon, proximal to the transection line. A tonsil is used to ensure that the mucosa is visualized, and an Allis clamp is placed on the antimesenteric border of the colotomy. The larger arm of the stapler is then placed into the colon, ensuring that it is placed full thickness into the bowel lumen Fig. 2.11.

An enterotomy is made on the small bowel. Again, an Allis clamp is placed on the antimesenteric portion of the small bowel, and the smaller arm of the stapler is gently advanced into the lumen of the ileum.

The ileum is brought to the colon, the staple advanced fully into the lumen of the small and large bowel. The mesentery is then adjusted to ensure that there is no mesentery within the staple line, as any mesentery in the staple line is likely to cause bleeding. This stapler is then ready to be fired.

The staple line is evaluated with an empty sponge stick to ensure that there is no bleeding. If bleeding is noted, a 3–0 absorbable suture can be used to oversew the staple line.

The anterior and posterior staple lines are staggered to prevent overlap during transverse stapling. Allis clamps are used to ensure that the entire enterotomy is excluded from the staple line. A stapler is placed transversely below the Allis clamps. Any bleeding is oversewn with a 3–0 polyfilament absorbable suture. The specimen is passed off the field. Gloves are changed, and instruments are removed.

Step 14: Closure

The extraction sites and all port sites 10 mm or greater in size are closed. A Carter-Thompson may be used to close any port (see Chap. 1).

a   b

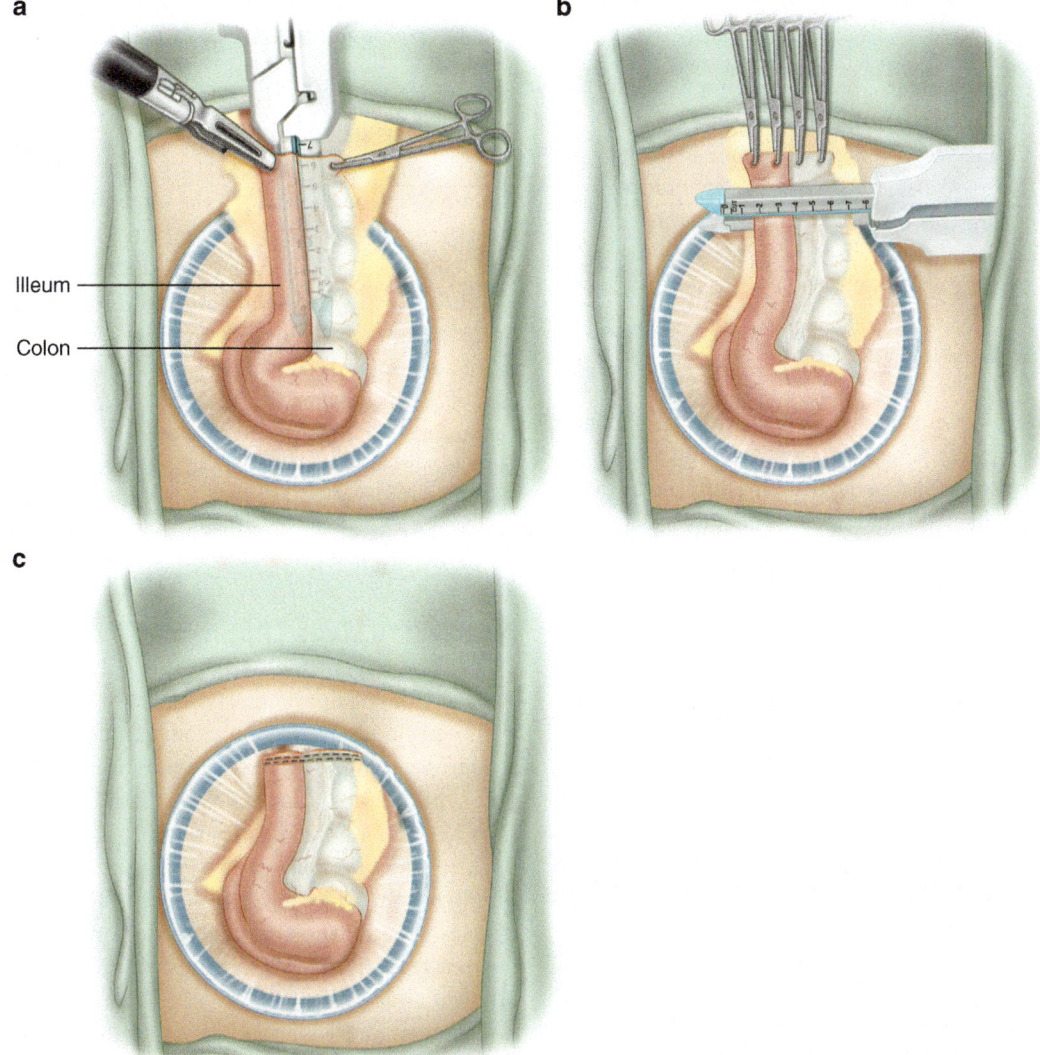

Illeum

Colon

c

Fig. 2.11 An extracorporeal anastomosis can be created with any number of techniques. Here a side-to-side, functional end-to-end anastomosis is demonstrated using the linear stapler. (**a**) Enterotomies are created in the terminal ileum and colon for stapler insertion. The stapler is inserted and fired. (**b**) A second linear stapler is used to transect the enterotomies, after the mesentery is cleaned from the edges of the stapler. (**c**) The completed anastomosis

Special Considerations

Varying the Approach

Depending on the disease process, patient anatomy, and surgeon comfort, the approach for a right colectomy may vary. In cases where inflammation or disease process is medial, a top-down or lateral to medial approach is helpful. This includes cases of Crohn's disease, obese patients, or perforated appendicitis with phlegmon. A patient who requires ileocectomy for volvulus, cecal arterial venous malformation, or Crohn's disease may not require a full take down of the hepatic flexure, so a limited lateral approach may be indicated. Knowledge and practice of all approaches help allow for variability in difficult cases where adhesions may obliterate the medial planes (Pitfall 2.5).

Pitfall 2.5

The key to varying approach is to understand the anatomy. When the medial dissection is not done early in the case, lateral dissection extending under the colon can easily put the duodenum in jeopardy, if the surgeon is not wary.

Top-Down Approach

A top-down approach begins with the patient in reverse Trendelenburg, left side down. The surgeon will stand on the patient's left, and the assistant will stand between the patient's legs with the camera in the assistant's right hand.

The omentum is lifted superiorly, and the transverse colon is identified. Entry into the lesser sac is facilitated lateral to the falciform ligament where the omental planes are fused. The surgeon's right hand is used to elevate the omentum, while the assistant retracts the transverse colon inferiorly. Electric scissors or energy device is used in the surgeons' left hand. The layers are carefully dissected on a broad plane until the posterior wall of the stomach is identified, signifying entry into the lesser sac.

As the plane is matured proximally, the surgeon's right hand instrument continues to move proximally toward the patient's right side. The assistant continues to apply countertension proximal to the plane of dissection on the transverse colon or colonic epiploicae. This straightens the colon to follow the plane of dissection. Care is taken to avoid injury to the gallbladder. The surgeon may elect to change hands, moving the energy instrument into the right hand and pushing the colon inferiorly and medially with the left. An open grasper, pushing medially and down, without actually grasping is used to displace the colon, to prevent injury to the colon.

The dissection is continued laterally at the white line of Toldt. The surgeon's left hand retracts the colon medially, while the right hand dissects just millimeters inside of the white line of Toldt. As the surgeon approaches the pelvic brim, the colon can be replaced into the right upper quadrant, and operative approach varied to bottom up along the white line of Toldt.

Bottom-Up Approach

A bottom-up approach allows the surgeon to visualize the planes around the pelvic brim ureter and gonadal vessels. The surgeon uses the right hand to lift the cecum and terminal ileum away from the pelvic brim as demonstrated in Fig. 2.8. Planes in this area may be redundant and thickened, so care is taken to ensure that the ureter and gonadal vessels are not injured, particularly in cases of medial inflammation. This is especially true when abscess or inflammation affects the deep portion of the mesentery, which may confuse planes.

A Lateral to Medial Approach

This approach is particularly useful when only a limited ileocectomy is needed, as in cases of a benign cecal polyp, cecal diverticulum, volvulus, or Crohn's disease. Depending on resection margins and indications for surgery, the hepatic flexure may not require complete mobilization. Adequate mobilization allows disease-specific resection and for creation of a tension-free anastomosis, either intracorporeally or extracorporeally.

The surgeon begins by retracting the cecum superiorly and medially as demonstrated in step 11 above. The key difference is that while dissecting from a lateral to medial approach, the retroperitoneum has not been separated from the duodenum. Care must be taken to ensure that the duodenum is not injured as the colon is lifted medially.

The plane starts inferiorly, then laterally, as the cecum is elevated and retracted anteriorly and medially. The dissected colon can be retracted medially, across the midline, demonstrating the duodenum, superior mesenteric artery, and the ileocolic pedicle. No vessels have been transected at this point in the operation. The dissection should continue medially and superiorly to the duodenum, pancreas, and root of the ileocolic artery.

Once the colon is completely mobilized superiorly, laterally, and inferiorly, the surgeon can choose to approach the vessels intracorporeally or to externalize the specimen and take the vessels through an open technique. For an intracorporeal technique, the surgeon will then replace the cecum and right colon on stretch laterally, demonstrating the ileocolic pedicle. As with the medial approach, care must be taken medially to ensure that the pedicle is freed from the duodenum prior to transection of the ileocolic pedicles.

Once isolated, the ileocolic pedicle can be isolated using scissors on an energy device and then transected using, clips, stapler, or energy device. The right branch of the middle colic vessels can be isolated and transected in a similar fashion.

Crohn's Disease

Patients with Crohn's disease may have multiple fistulas or abscess cavities. A Crohn's exploration starts with running of the small bowel from ligament of Treitz to the ileocecal valve. The bowel is measured, using the graspers as a guide to measure. Notes on length of normal and affected bowel are dictated into the operative report.

Areas of fistulas, adhesions, or severe disease can be approached laparoscopically. Combinations of blunt and sharp dissection are used to identify the location of fistulas and separate unaffected bowel from primary disease. Techniques are discussed further in Chap. 10.

The mesentery of the affected area may be significantly thickened in Crohn's disease. Lymphadenopathy and inflammation may make ligation of the vessels hazardous without substantial bleeding. Generally, prior to taking "major vessels" (ileocolic, middle colic, inferior mesenteric artery), the mesentery is assessed laparoscopically to determine whether an energy device or stapler can be safely used to transect the vessels. If the pedicle looks very thickened with prominent lymphadenopathy, laparoscopic energy devices may be unable to proper occlude and coagulate the vessels. A very proximal ligation can be used, as the vessels and surrounding lymph nodes tend to be less thickened at the bases. However, if bleeding does occur, this may be difficult to control.

In cases where significant lymphadenopathy is noted, a lateral approach is used, mobilizing the colon and terminal ileum entirely and then externalizing the terminal ileum and colon with the mesentery intact. This allows the mesentery to be transected using open technique of suture ligation through the extraction incision.

Intracorporeal Anastomosis

The advantages of an intracorporeal anastomosis are decreasing the extraction site size and moving the extraction site to a preferable location, such as a Pfannenstiel incision. This may decrease the rate of hernia formation. However, performing an intracorporeal anastomosis adds 20–30 min to the case when the surgeon is proficient (Tip 2.13).

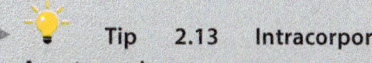

> 💡 **Tip 2.13 Intracorporeal Anastomosis**
> Intracorporeal anastomosis is facilitated by placement of a suprapubic port. This may be in addition to other ports or substituted for the right lower quadrant port. Additionally, the left lower quadrant port will be upsized to a 12 mm port to accommodate a laparoscopic stapler.

Steps of Intracorporeal Anastomosis

- *Preparation of the colon and small bowel*
- *Transection of the colon and small bowel*
- *Placement of stabilizing suture (stay suture)*
- *Creation of enterotomy*
- *Stapling of the anastomosis*
- *Suturing the common enterotomy*

Preparation of the Colon and Small Bowel (Fig. 2.12)

Once the dissection is completed, and the right colon is completely mobilized, an advanced bipolar device is used to divide the mesentery of the terminal ileum and the mesocolon, at the selected sites, circumferentially around the bowel. The omentum should be released from the transverse colon at least 15–12 cm distal to the staple line to facilitate creation of the anastomosis.

Transection of the Colon and Small Bowel

A laparoscopic stapler is introduced through the right lower quadrant port, and the bowel is divided. Usually, a 60 mm cartridge is required to transect the small bowel and the colon, respectively. The stapler should be deployed in a perpendicular fashion to minimize devascularized bowel and the number of stapler loads needed. The transected specimen is placed over the right lobe of the liver for later extraction (Tip 2.14).

> ### 💡 Tip 2.14 Multiple Staple Lines
> Multiple staple lines are a potential source of problems. Intersecting staple lines may cause areas of devascularization and staple malfunction and may increase risk of leaks. Stapling perpendicular to the bowel reduces the risk of requiring multiple staple loads.

The anastomosis should be formed in the right upper quadrant in order to optimize working room and space from operating ports. The terminal ileum and the transverse colon are then positioned in an isoperistaltic fashion next to each other, with at least 10 cm of overlapping bowel. The bowel should sit side by side without tension. In addition, prior to fixation, the mesentery should be checked to ensure that it is not twisted.

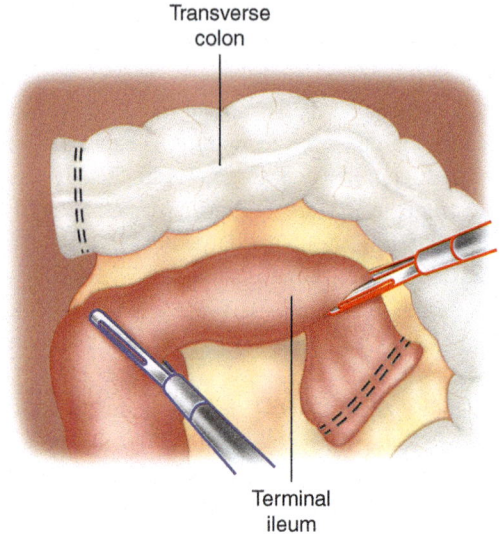

Fig. 2.12 Bowel overlapping for intracorporeal anastomosis. After stapling, the colon and small bowel are arranged to sit in an isoperistaltic fashion without twisting the mesentery and without tension. Approximately 12 cm of bowel should overlap between staple lines

Placement of Stabilizing Suture (Stay Suture)

A full-length 2–0 absorbable suture is introduced through the left lower quadrant port. The end of the suture should be secured outside the trocar with a hemostat. The surgeon uses the left upper quadrant port to place the stitch on the antimesenteric border of the small bowel, 15 cm proximal to the staple line. The stitch is then passed through the antimesenteric border of the colon approximately 3 cm from the colon staple line (Fig. 2.13). The needle is extracted through the trocar, and both ends are then held with a hemostat. This stay suture will generate countertraction when the stapler engages the bowel.

Creation of Enterotomy

A hook cautery is inserted through the left lower quadrant port, in the surgeon's dominant hand. A colotomy is made on the antimesenteric border just proximal to the proximal to the suture. The incision should be checked to ensure that mucosa is seen. The incision should be just large enough for the stapler to be admitted. An enterotomy will be made in the corresponding location on the small bowel. Tension from the assistant's grasper

Transverse
colon

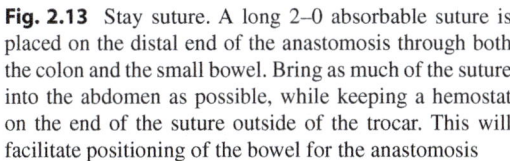

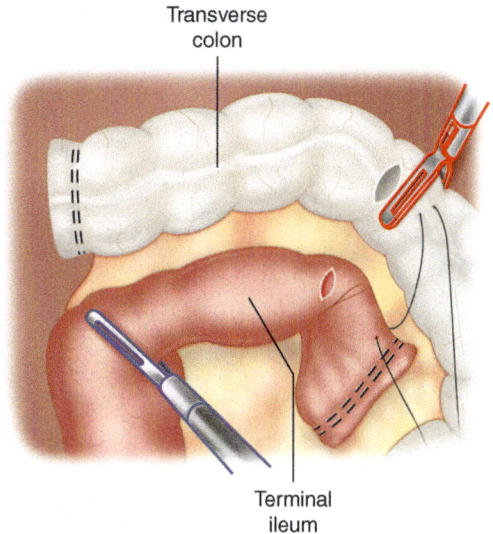

Terminal
ileum

Terminal
ileum

Fig. 2.13 Stay suture. A long 2–0 absorbable suture is placed on the distal end of the anastomosis through both the colon and the small bowel. Bring as much of the suture into the abdomen as possible, while keeping a hemostat on the end of the suture outside of the trocar. This will facilitate positioning of the bowel for the anastomosis

Fig. 2.14 Enterotomies. Enterotomies are made on the colon and small bowel with the hook cautery. In each case, the mucosa is fully visualized to ensure full-thickness entry into the bowel

facilitates creation of the enterotomies. The surgeon will lift the colon or small bowel toward the anterior abdominal wall with the left hand, while the assistant generates gentle countertraction with tension on the stay suture (Fig. 2.14).

Stapling of the Anastomosis

A laparoscopic stapler is introduced through the left lower quadrant port with a 60 mm load. The colon is lifted toward the anterior abdominal wall, using the bowel grasper through the suprapubic port and gentle countertraction from the 2–0 suture extracorporeally. This facilitates insertion of the stapler into the colon. As the stapler enters the colotomy, release the colon with the gasper and pull on the stay suture taut to facilitate entry into the colon. Once the tip of one side of the stapler is introduced to the colon, the stapler is rotated counterclockwise toward the small bowel. The small bowel is moved to the stapler, and a grasper is used to assist with entry in to the enterotomy. Countertension is maintained on the stay suture. The small bowel is released as the stapler is inserted. Tension is maintained on the stay suture to straighten the stapler, and the stay suture

is pulled to insert the stapler fully into the lumen without torquing the bowel (Fig. 2.15).

Once both limbs have been inserted, the stapler can be lifted toward the anterior abdominal wall. This allows the mesentery to fall away from the stapler prior to firing. Once placement is confirmed, the stapler is fired and then slowly withdrawn.

Suturing the Common Enterotomy

The common enterotomy is sutured laparoscopically. A 2–0 polyfilament, absorbable suture 20 cm in length, is used. A running first layer is performed. Tension is maintained on the suture to ensure a proper closure. The surgeon will use needle drivers through the left lower quadrant and suprapubic ports. The initial suture is placed and tied down on the proximal side of the common enterotomy. The suture is then placed full thickness through the bowel in a running fashion. At the end of each throw, the surgeon will grasp the suture a few centimeters away from the bowel wall and cinch it down. The bowel grasper is used to hold tension on the suture by pulling in the direction of the suture, while the needle driver is used to push against the bowel to tighten the suture (Tip 2.15).

> ▶ 💡 **Tip 2.15 Tension on Anastomosis**
> Tension must be maintained on the running anastomotic suture throughout the process to prevent gaps that might affect the integrity of the anastomosis. The assistant can help maintain tension by holding the suture between stitches.

The suture is then passed to the assistant, who uses a bowel grasper from the left upper quadrant port to maintain tension and lift the bowel toward the anterior abdominal wall. At the distal end of the enterotomy, the suture is again tied (Fig. 2.16).

A second layer of 2–0 polyfilament absorbable suture, cut to 12–14 cm, is used, and a Lapra-Ty® (Ethicon) is placed on the end of the suture. As the running suture progresses, Lapra-Ty® is placed after each suture. The Lapra-Tys create an interrupted Lambert suture, spreading the tension across multiple points and invaginating the entire staple line. After each stitch, the suture should be cinched down to maintain adequate tension and ensure a proper closure. Two Lapra-Tys are placed at the end of the suture.

Once the anastomosis is completed, irrigating the area decreases the risk of abscess formation. The specimen is then extracted, utilizing a wound protector, through a Pfannenstiel incision.

Fig. 2.15 Stapler placement. One end of the stapler is placed into the colon, and then the small bowel is moved to the other end of the stapler. Once both ends have been inserted, the stay suture is pulled to straighten the small bowel and colon. The surgeon's left hand assists by pulling on the proximal small bowel

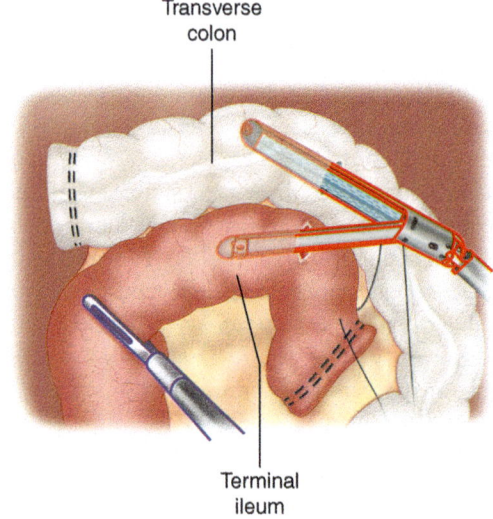

Transverse
colon

Terminal
ileum

Fig. 2.16 Suturing the common enterotomy. The common enterotomy is sewn from proximal to distal. The suture is placed and tied on the proximal end of the enterotomy. After each throw, pulling tension on the suture is crucial to prevent an anastomotic leak

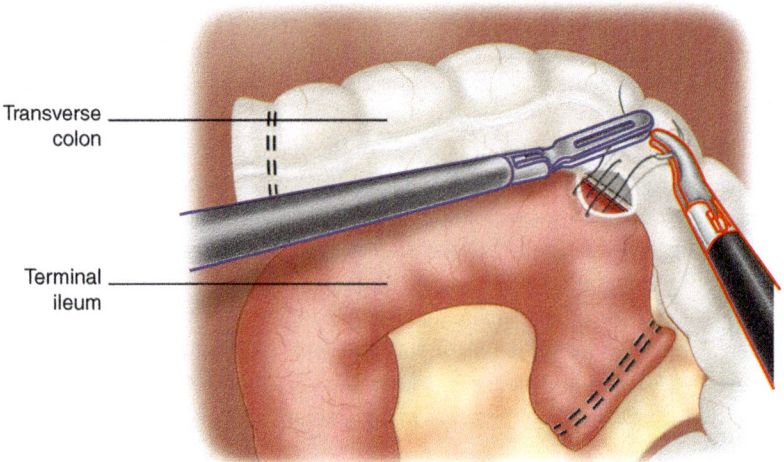

Transverse
colon

Terminal
ileum

Laparoscopic Transverse Colectomy

Govind Nandakumar and Tushar Samdani

Introduction

Transverse colectomy is performed for benign or malignant lesions of the transverse colon. If the lesion is located in close proximity to either flexures, then it is advisable to perform an extended right or extended left colectomy. A true laparoscopic transverse colectomy requires mobilization of both the hepatic and splenic flexures, with preservation of the blood supply to the rest of the colon.

This chapter will review additions to a right colectomy and left colectomy to accommodate a transverse colon lesion as well as steps for a true laparoscopic transverse colectomy. There are three methods of approaching the middle colic vessels:

1. Continuation of the right colectomy (proximal transverse colon lesion)
2. Continuation of the left colectomy (distal transverse colon lesion)
3. Direct resection (top-down or bottom-up approaches)

Each of these will be reviewed.

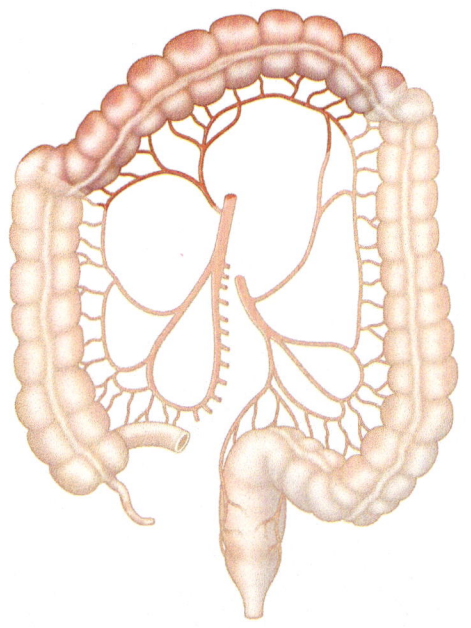

Indications
- Benign or malignant neoplasia of the transverse colon
- Diverticular disease of the transverse colon
- Inflammatory bowel disease (rarely)

G. Nandakumar (✉)
Department of Surgery, Weill Cornell Medical College New York, New York, NY, USA

T. Samdani
Department of Surgery, Medstar Saint Mary's Hospital, Leonardtown, MD, USA

© Springer Nature Switzerland AG 2020
S. L. Stein, R. R. Lawson (eds.), *Laparoscopic Colectomy*,
https://doi.org/10.1007/978-3-030-39559-9_3

Preoperative Planning
- Preoperative colonoscopic tattooing distal to the tumor and in three quadrants
- For malignant disease
  - Computed tomography (CT) of the chest, abdomen, and pelvis
  - Preoperative carcinoembryonic antigen
- Mechanical bowel preparation, per surgeon's preference
  - Advantages of bowel preparation
    Easier handling of the colon
    Ability to perform intraoperative colonoscopy
    Decreases intraperitoneal contamination if there is postoperative anastomotic leak

Steps of the Operation
Patient positioning
1. Step 1:Port placement
2. Step 2: Intraoperative staging
3. Step 3: Identification of pathology
4. Step 4: Extent of resection
5. Step 5: Continuation of right colectomy
6. Step 6: Medial middle colic vessel ligation

7. Step 7: Top-down approach – entering the lesser sac
8. Step 8: Omental resection
9. Step 9: Hepatic flexure mobilization
10. Step 10: Splenic flexure mobilization
11. Step 11: Transection of IMV and ascending branch of LCA for splenic flexure tumor
12. Step 12: Identification and transection of the middle colic pedicle, top-down approach
13. Step 13: Specimen extraction and anastomosis

Tools of the Operation
- 5 mm ports (5)
- 12 mm Hassan port (1)
- 10 mm 30-degree camera (1)
- Laparoscopic bowel graspers (3)
- Energy instrument for vessel ligation
- Wound protector
- Anastomosis: linear intestinal stapler

Patient Positioning for Laparoscopic Laparoscopic Transverse Colectomy

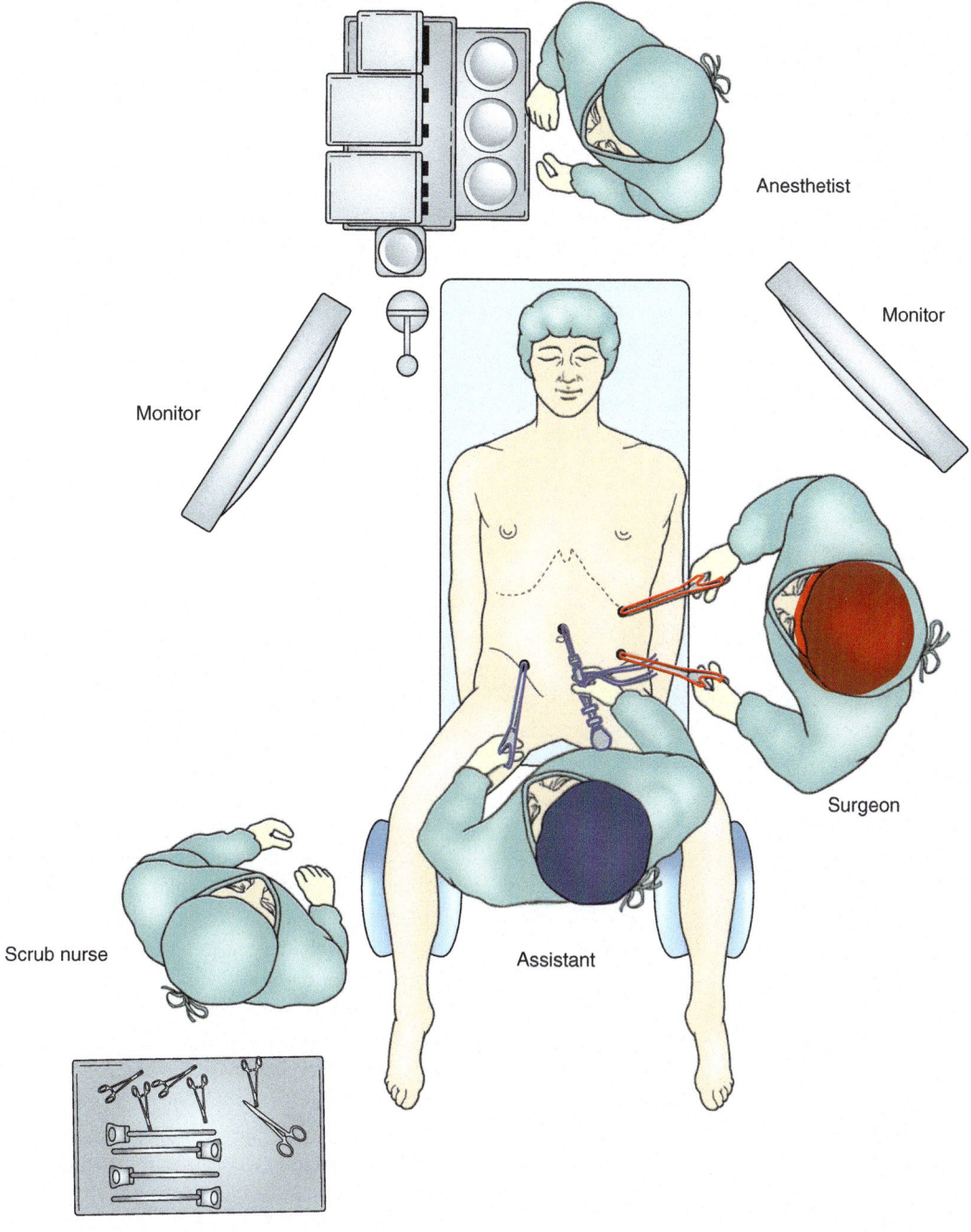

Room set up for a transverse colectomy. The surgeon stands on the patient's left, with the assistant between the patient's legs. Monitors are placed at the patient's heads to allow for visualization whether working towards the hepatic or splenic flexure

The patient is positioned in a modified lithotomy position with both arms tucked at the patient's side. Pressure points, fingers, and calves are padded adequately to avoid any peripheral nerve injury. Shoulder braces are avoided as they can cause brachial plexus injury. A beanbag and cloth tape across the torso can be used to prevent patient sliding during extreme tilting. It is advisable to check that the patient is secured well by tilting the operating table in steep Trendelenburg position prior to prepping. Most patients are offered and elect to have an epidural or intravenous catheter for patient-controlled anesthesia.

The abdomen is prepped from the nipples to the mid-thigh. Perineal access is maintained for possible intraoperative colonoscopy. Monitors are placed bilaterally above the patient's shoulders so that the surgeon, pathology, and monitors are appropriately triangulated.

Operative Strategy

Step 1: Port Placement (Fig. 3.1)

Open Hassan technique is used to achieve access to the abdomen for creating pneumoperitoneum. Once pneumoperitoneum is created, the perito-

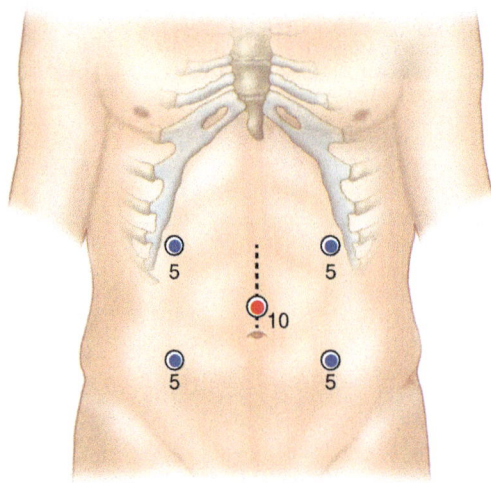

Fig. 3.1 A supraumbilical 10 mm port and 4–5 mm ports are placed in the right and left upper and lower quadrants. Extraction will generally be a supraumbilical incision, although this can be modified for surgeon preference

neal cavity is explored to rule out vascular or bowel injuries. Four 5 mm trocars are placed; two on either side of the abdomen lateral to the rectus with one handbreadth between the trocars. An optional trocar can be placed in the suprapubic area if required for retraction.

Step 2: Intraoperative Staging

The abdomen is explored in all four quadrants systematically to evaluate metastatic disease and/ or unexpected pathology. Biopsies are taken of any suspicious lesions.

Step 3: Identification of Pathology and Determination of Operative Plan

Initially on entry into the abdomen, identify the location of the tumor and determine operative plan. The location and nature of tumor (benign vs. malignant) will determine the extent of colon resection. For an oncologic resection, a segmental colectomy with transection of the vessels both proximal and distal to the tumor should be performed to ensure adequate lymphadenectomy. If the tumor is benign, a limited resection may be adequate.

Knowledge of the mesenteric anatomy is key to the successful resection of a transverse colon lesion, for both adequate lymphadenectomy and for preservation of adequate blood supply to the anastomosis. Figure 3.2 (Vascular anatomy of the colon) demonstrates the major vascular pedicles of the colon with the marginal artery. The marginal artery maintains collateral circulation when major pedicles are resected.

Surgeons should be familiar with the common variations in blood supply to the colon. The right colic vessel artery commonly originates from the ileocolic artery in 85% of patients. In addition, up to 55% of patients will have more than two branches of the middle colic arteries.

Step 4: Extent of Resection

For cancers that lie to the right of the middle colic vessels, an extended right colectomy is generally performed. Extended right colectomy will follow

Fig. 3.2 Most common anatomic arrangement of the vascular supply to the transverse colon. Understanding of marginal blood vessel anatomy is crucial in a transverse colectomy to ensuring a well-vascularized anastomosis

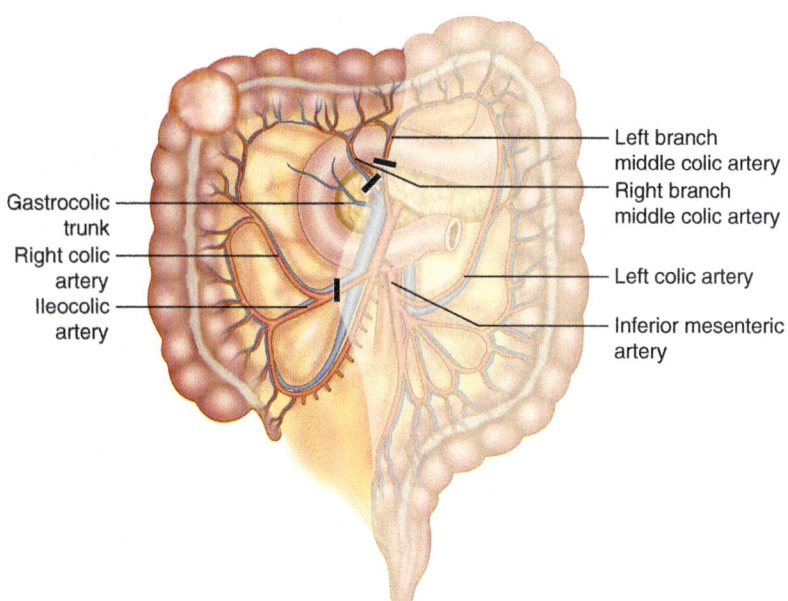

Left branch middle colic artery

Right branch middle colic artery

Gastrocolic trunk

Right colic artery

Ileocolic artery

Left colic artery

Inferior mesenteric artery

Fig. 3.3 Right-sided tumors are generally treated with extended right colectomy, with transection of the middle colic vessels and ileodistal transverse anastomosis. This anastomosis will require retrograde blood flow from the ascending branch of the left colic artery

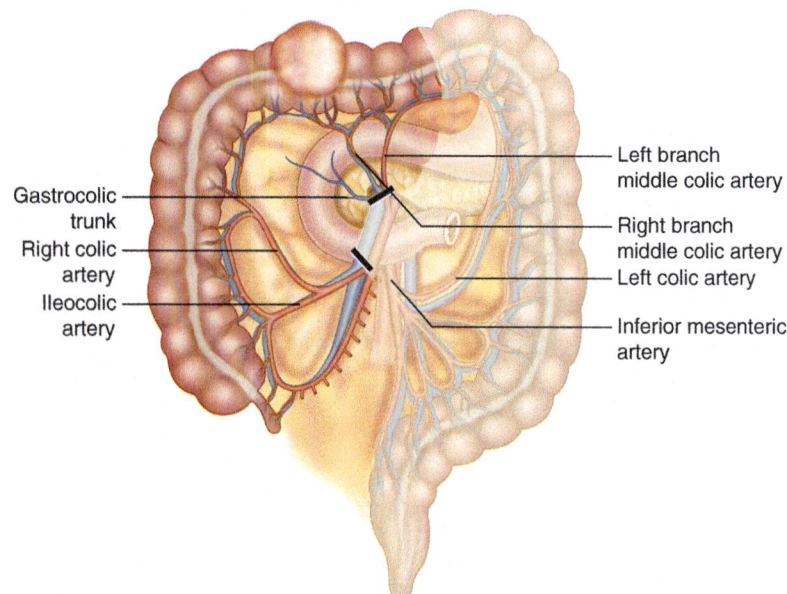

Left branch middle colic artery

Gastrocolic trunk

Right colic artery

Ileocolic artery

Right branch middle colic artery

Left colic artery

Inferior mesenteric artery

right colon resection (see Chap. 2) but requires ligation of the entire middle colic artery for a transverse colon lesion. For an extended right hemicolectomy, the anastomosis occurs between the terminal ileum and the distal transverse colon. This ileocolic anastomosis has a lower leak rate than a colo-colonic or colorectal anastomoses (Fig. 3.3).

If the tumor is at the splenic flexure, a formal left colectomy with resection of the left and middle branches of the middle colic vessels to the left colic artery should be performed (Fig. 3.4). This resection will require mobilization of the hepatic flexure and colo-colonic or colorectal anastomosis.

Fig. 3.4 Distal transverse colon cancers are generally treated with an extended left colectomy. The right branches of the middle colic artery are transected, along with the left colic artery. The major concern is reach from the transverse colon to the sigmoid or rectosigmoid

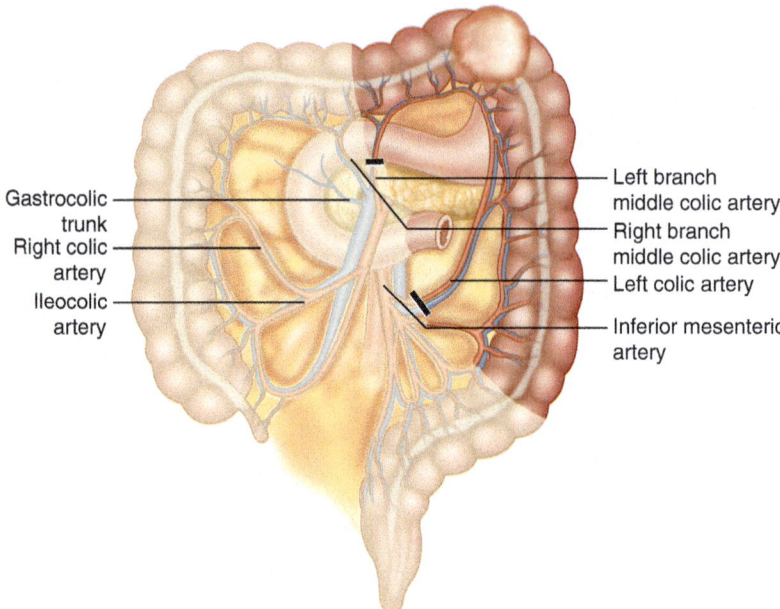

Gastrocolic trunk
Right colic artery
Ileocolic artery

Left branch middle colic artery
Right branch middle colic artery
Left colic artery
Inferior mesenteric artery

Fig. 3.5 Mid-transverse lesions are appropriate for a transverse colectomy with ileodescending anastomosis. The right colon generally has a vigorous blood supply from the ileocolic and right colon arteries. The left colon depends on the ascending branch of the left colic artery. Reach of the colon for colo-colonic anastomosis may be an issue

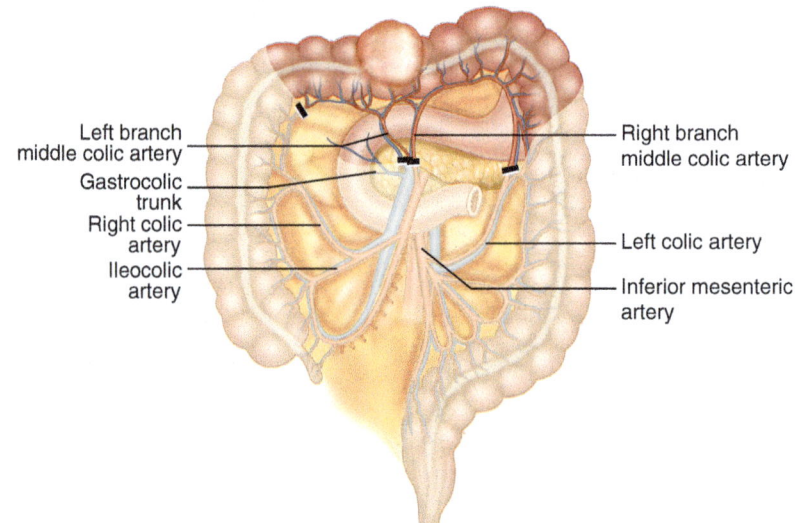

Left branch middle colic artery
Gastrocolic trunk
Right colic artery
Ileocolic artery

Right branch middle colic artery
Left colic artery
Inferior mesenteric artery

In cases where the tumor lies immediately above the middle colic vessels, a true transverse colectomy can be performed (Fig. 3.5).

If the tumor is not immediately obvious laparoscopically, and the tumor was not tattooed preoperatively, an intraoperative colonoscopy can be used to identify the location of the lesion (see Chap. 1). Distance from the anal verge is an unreliable marker of tumor location, particularly in the middle of the colon. Positive localization of the tumor is vital prior to resection (Tip 3.1).

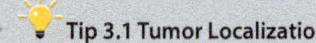

Tip 3.1 Tumor Localization

If the tumor cannot be definitively localized on endoscopy, imaging, or intraoperatively, no resection should be performed. The patient can be returned to the endoscopist for tattooing and marking, rather than resecting the wrong portion of the colon.

Step 5. Continuation of the Right Colectomy: Middle Colic Vessels

The middle colic vessels should be ligated high, close to the superior mesenteric artery, as this will be a primary lymph node drainage for transverse colon tumors. The assistant holds the transverse colon mesentery, giving cephalad and anterior traction. The surgeon also supports the mesentery, exposing the middle colic vessels that have been dissected away from the duodenum and pancreas during the right colectomy (Fig. 3.6; Tip 3.2).

> 💡 **Tip 3.2 High Middle Colic Ligation**
> In case of cancer of transverse colon, high ligation of middle colic artery is necessary for oncologic resection.

The surgeon's right hand will hold the middle colic vessels and transverse colon mesentery. With the left hand, the pancreas and duodenum should be gently pushed down, creating a plane behind the middle colic vessels. Extreme caution must be used here as there are often branches from the gastrocolic vessels that run through the lesser sac. Avulsion of these vessels can occur and will cause extreme bleeding, potentially requiring conversion to open surgery (Pitfall 3.1).

> ⚠️ **Pitfall 3.1**
> Meticulous retromesenteric dissection over the duodenum and head of pancreas is needed in order to prevent injury to gastrocolic venous trunk of Henley. Gentle blunt dissection can be used, but vessels should be identified and either preserved or transected with an energy instrument.

The middle colic vessels typically have between two and five branches. Each of these branches should be separately isolated and then

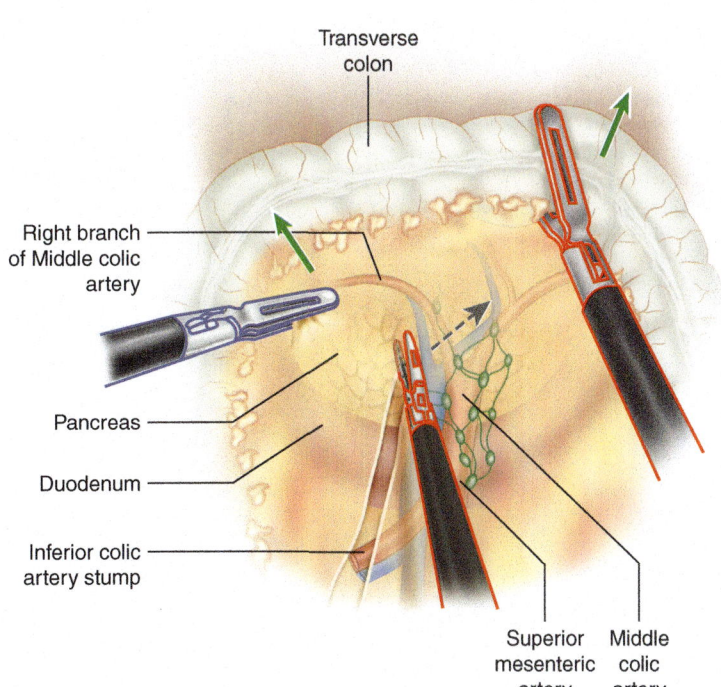

Fig. 3.6 For an extended right colectomy, the plane is continued over the duodenum and pancreas after transecting the ileocolic artery. This separates the middle colic vessels from the lesser sac, and the right, middle, and left branches of the middle colic artery may be transected

Transverse colon

Right branch of Middle colic artery

Pancreas

Duodenum

Inferior colic artery stump

Superior mesenteric artery

Middle colic artery

transected in turn. The peritoneum overlying the vessel is taken with electrocautery of bipolar energy. The vessel itself is then freed from the remaining mesentery and transected with multiple firings of the electrocautery or clips. Use of a stapler in this area is awkward, as the stapler can inadvertently damage the duodenum coursing through the transverse colon mesentery distal to the middle colic vessels at the ligament of Treitz.

As each vessel is sequentially scored, isolated, and transected, the surgeon works towards the ligament of Treitz, which must be clearly identified and preserved. This marks the left side of the middle colics and the extent of this dissection.

Step 6: Medial Middle Colic Vessel Ligation

If a right colectomy is not required, the dissection can begin at the bare area just above the ileocolic artery, lateral to the duodenum. This space is a consistent landmark, even in obese patients, marking entry into the mesocolic plane.

The middle colic vessels are identified by placing the colon on traction to tent the mesentery (Fig. 3.7). Adequate exposure is achieved by grasping the mesentery on either both sides of the vessels (surgeons' left hand and assistant right hand) and retracting superiorly and laterally (Tip 3.3).

> 💡 **Tip 3.3 Ole Procedure**
> Holding up and splaying out the middle colic vessels are also referred to as the "Ole procedure." The mesentery should be lifted and displayed from the left and right sided ports, while the surgeon carefully isolates each of the middle colic vessels.

After identifying the middle colic vessels, a window is created in the colon mesentery between the ileocolic and middle colic vessels (Fig. 3.8). With appropriate traction and counter-traction, the left hand elevates the mid-

Fig. 3.7 The "Ole" procedure. The assistant's hand and the surgeon's left hand elevated the mesentery on either side of the middle colic vessels, lifting them from the retroperitoneum and allowing for dissection away from the lesser sac

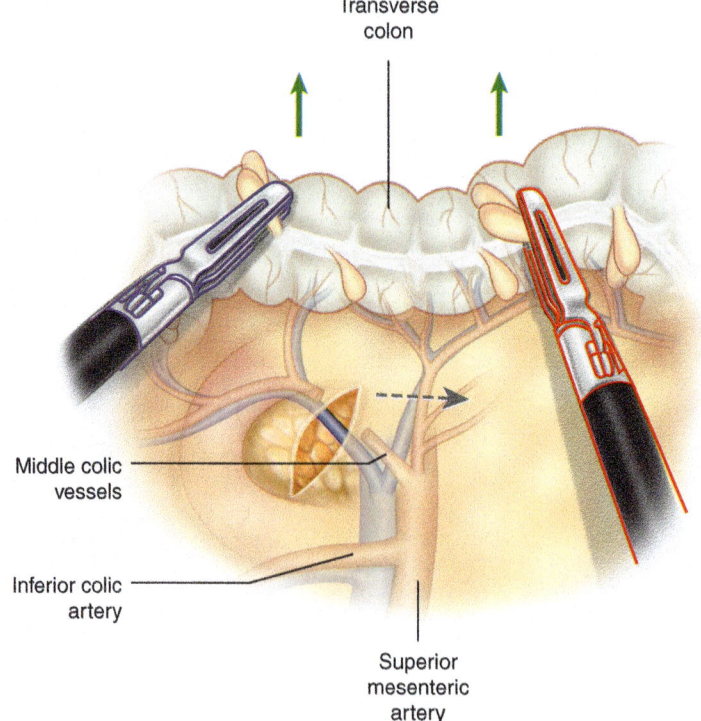

Transverse colon

Middle colic vessels

Inferior colic artery

Superior mesenteric artery

Fig. 3.8 The middle colic vessels are generally approached over the duodenum and pancreas

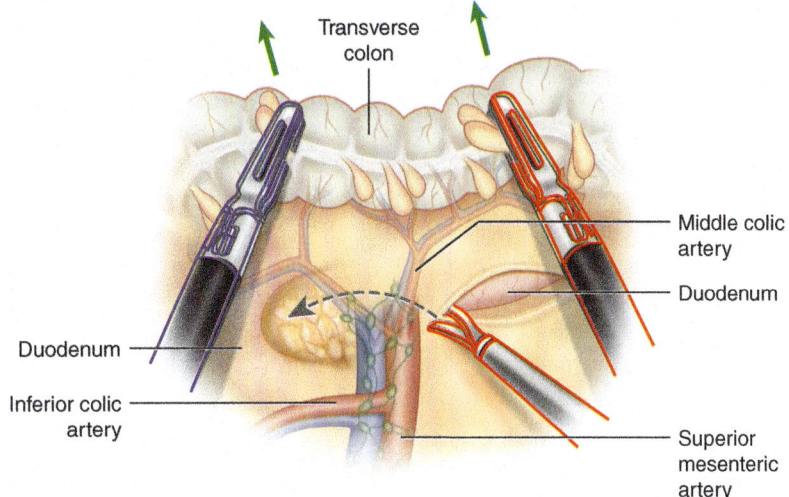

dle colic vessels, while the right hand carefully dissects in the lesser sac isolating the middle colic vessels. The middle colic vessels can be divided at the common trunk or divided individually after bifurcation depending on vascular variation. A bipolar vessel-sealing device is used to divide the pedicles. Strong anterior traction on the transverse colon mesentery optimizes middle colic dissection and decreases the likelihood of inadvertent injury to superior mesenteric artery (SMA).

The surgeon can continue in the mesocolic area to dissect towards the hepatic flexure. As in a right colectomy, the faint white line, representing the retroperitoneum, is carefully pushed down using tension and counter-tension. The surgeon will use one hand to elevate the mesocolon and one hand for dorsal displacement of the white line. The assistant will assist by elevating the mesocolon. Dissection should continue under the transverse colon up towards the liver, medially to the pancreas and duodenum.

Step 7: Top-Down Approach: Entering the Lesser Sac

Some surgeons are more comfortable with an alternative, top-down approach. This approach first enters the lesser sac, isolating the transverse

mesocolon prior to transection of the middle colic vessels. As the middle colic vessels are often short, close together, and multiple in nature, some surgeons find this method provides better visualization. Additionally, as transection will be the last step in the operation, if bleeding was to occur, conversion with extraction incision over the middle colic vessels would be possible, allowing for open vessel ligation.

Step 8: Omental Resection

For a transverse colon cancer, the omentum is generally resected with the specimen. The extent of omental resection can vary depending on the location of the tumor. Any omentum attached to the tumor should be transected with tumor. In addition, for bulky tumors with extra-lumenal extension, the omentum can harbor metastatic or lymph node deposits, and consideration of resection is appropriate.

Any distal omental attachments should be identified and freed. From the left side of the table, the surgeon can begin at the middle of the omentum, where the planes of the omentum are fused. Preserve the gastroepiploic artery for blood supply to the stomach. The assistant will elevate the omentum using the right lower quadrant port, standing between the patient's legs.

The surgeon will use the right hand to expose the omentum, identify the gastroepiploic artery, and lift the omentum anteriorly. The left hand holds a bipolar and begins transection just caudal to the gastroepiploic artery. As the omentum is transected, move the right hand closer to the transected edge while transecting the bipolar. Once the back wall of the stomach is exposed, the lesser sac has been entered. The right hand lifts the omentum enough to see the gastroepiploic artery and stomach, and the assistant's left hand can move to elevate the transected edge of the omentum, pulling to the right and caudally (Tip 3.4).

>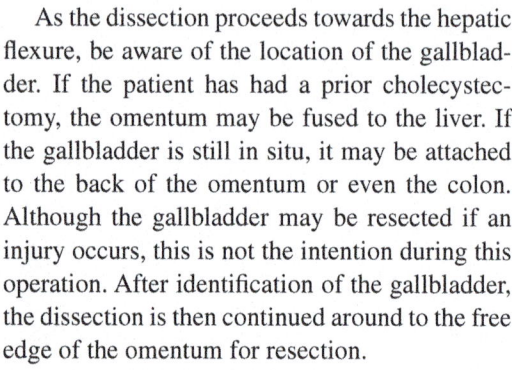
>
> ► 💡 **Tip 3.4 Efficient Dissection**
> Moving while the bipolar is firing provides efficiency of motion, elevates the plane, and provides ongoing traction. Switching hands with the surgeon's right hand retracting the colon, and the left hand using the energy instrument, may provide better exposure.

Care should be taken to ensure that the colon is well visualized during this transection. A redundant or tortuous colon can cause the colon to be fixated to the back of the omentum. If the colon is not well visualized under traction and straightened out with the assistant's hand, it can be inadvertently injured during this step.

As the dissection proceeds towards the hepatic flexure, be aware of the location of the gallbladder. If the patient has had a prior cholecystectomy, the omentum may be fused to the liver. If the gallbladder is still in situ, it may be attached to the back of the omentum or even the colon. Although the gallbladder may be resected if an injury occurs, this is not the intention during this operation. After identification of the gallbladder, the dissection is then continued around to the free edge of the omentum for resection.

Step 9: Hepatic Flexure Mobilization

The hepatic flexure can be lifted from the retroperitoneum and freed at this time. Under the colon, there should be an avascular plane lateral to the duodenum. The surgeon changes instruments so that the left hand will do the dissection and the right hand will have the bipolar or electrocautery (Fig. 3.9). The free edge of the mesocolon, lateral to the duodenum, is identified and carefully isolated using the left hand. The colon is then gently elevated with the surgeon's left hand and pulled caudally to expose the plane. The free edge of the mesentery is taken with the bipolar instrument until the hepatic flexure is completely free and anterior attachments to the white line of Toldt are isolated anterior and lateral to the colon.

In order to have adequate mobilization for a true transverse colectomy, the lateral attachments

Fig. 3.9 The colon is pushed inferiorly and deep to expose the plane between the colon and liver. The omentum will be resected with the specimen in the case of a full-thickness transverse colon tumor

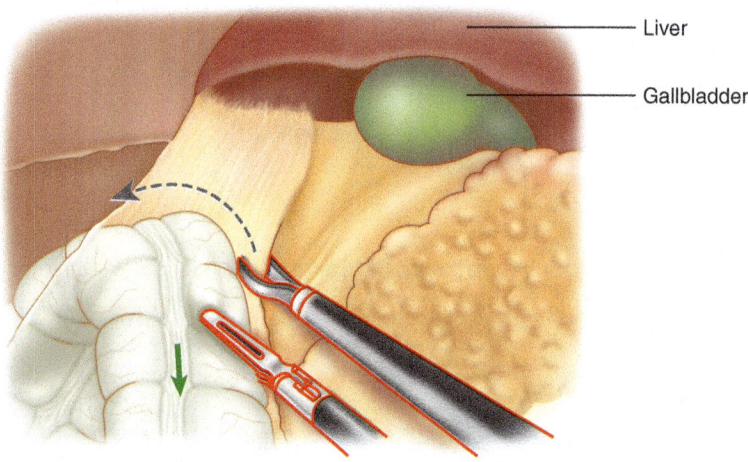

Liver

Gallbladder

of the right colon should be completely mobilized, all the way down to the cecum and terminal ileum. No medial mobilization is necessary if the right colon will be preserved. This is further described in Chap. 2.

Step 10: Splenic Flexure Mobilization

Following hepatic flexure mobilization, the surgeon moves to the patient's left side, for mobilization of the splenic flexure.

Dissection starts at the free edge of the omentum, where omental transection was previously dissected. The surgeon uses the left hand to identify and preserve the gastroepiploic artery and visualize the back wall of the stomach. The right hand transects the omentum using the bipolar. The assistant uses the right lower quadrant port and keeps tension on the omentum (Fig. 3.10).

This dissection is analogous to other splenic flexure mobilizations, except that the omentum may be taken with the specimen (see Chap. 4). As the dissection progresses, left hand elevating, right hand transecting, and assistant placing traction on the omentum, care should be taken to identify the back wall of the stomach. As the short gastric vessels are approached, veer away from the stomach, towards the colon. As with the right side, the assistant should provide visualization by straightening the distal portion of the transverse colon to ensure that there is no redundancy and that the colon is not inadvertently injured during dissection.

At the splenic flexure mobilization progresses, extreme care should be taken at the splenic flexure to ensure that tension is not placed on the spleen causing avulsion injuries to the splenic capsule. Stay close to the colon around the splenic flexure, to prevent veering off plane, while maintaining an appropriate oncologic margin. Careful anterior caudal retraction of the colon can provide adequate tension. Any mesenteric or omental tissue should be fully transected with the bipolar to prevent bleeding after transection. The transected tissue will retract into the left upper quadrant, making visualization poor. Any tissue with concern for back bleeding should be immediately treated with cauterization prior to transection.

As with the hepatic flexure, the entire lateral dissection, extending down towards the sigmoid colon at the white line of Toldt, should be performed in order to have adequate mobilization for true transverse colon resection (Fig. 3.11).

Once the omentum has been completely freed, the colon will be freed anteriorly and superiorly. Additional posterior attachments inferior to the pancreas and lateral to the ligament of Treitz will still require transection. Using the right hand to pull the colon towards the pelvis, the bipolar is gently used to separate the thin tissue inferior to the pancreas (Fig. 3.12). This will expose Gerota's fascia deep to the plane and roll the colon medially, providing optimal reach (Tip 3.5).

Fig. 3.10 Once entering the lesser sac, the plane is matured towards the splenic flexure for complete mobilization

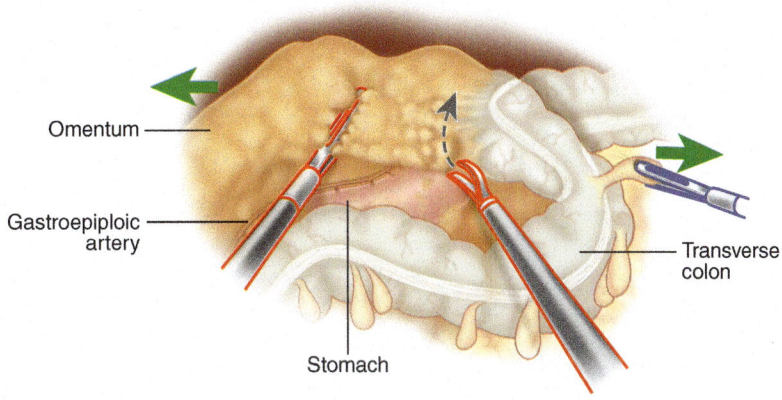

Omentum

Gastroepiploic artery

Transverse colon

Stomach

Step 11: Transection of the Inferior Mesenteric Vein (IMV) and Ascending Branch of the Left Colic Artery for Splenic Flexure Tumor

For a splenic flexure tumor, oncologic resection mandates that the inferior mesenteric vein is transected high, at the inferior pancreatic border. From a medial direction, the left colon mesentery is lifted laterally exposing the ligament of Treitz and inferior mesenteric vein. Often, there is a filmy attachment to the ligament of Treitz, which can be scored with electrocautery. Scoring this provides better separation between the ligament of Treitz and the mesentery just lateral to it. The ileocolic vein should be identified using elevation with the surgeon's left hand. The peritoneum is scored deep to the IMV, and the left hand can be used to lift the IMV, exposing it at the inferior border of the pancreas. Bipolar can then be used to transect the IMV with multiple firings. The plane should be continued to the middle colic arteries, just above the duodenum into the lesser sac, which has been approached from above. The mesentery should stay with the transected colon to ensure complete lymphadenectomy.

From this medial side, the dissection can be continued distally, exposing the bifurcation of the inferior mesenteric artery from the aorta. If a complete left colectomy will be performed, a high ligation of the inferior mesenteric artery will be performed (see Chap. 6). For a proximal transverse colon lesion,

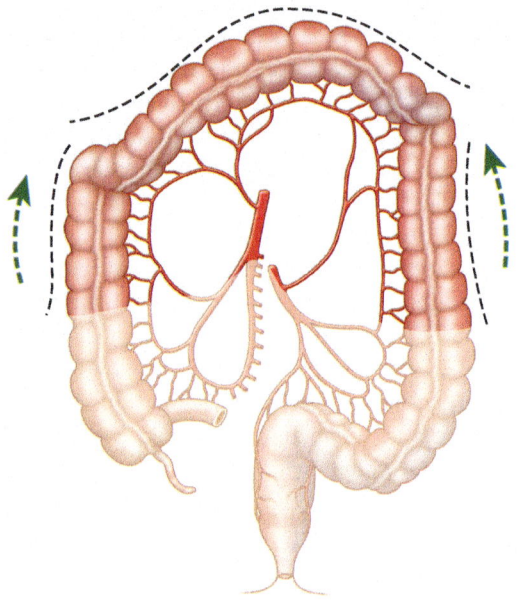

Fig. 3.11 The entire transverse colon, lateral attachments, and both flexures require mobilization for a true transverse colectomy

Fig. 3.12 Demonstration of the posterior attachments below the pancreas. These require transection for full mobilization of the splenic flexure

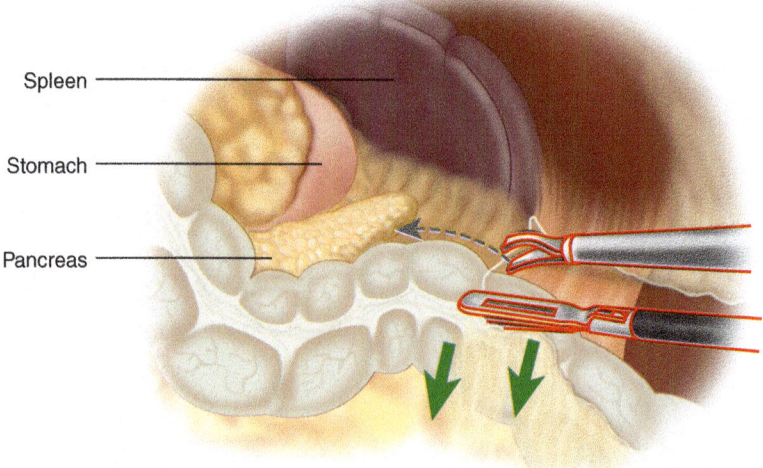

Spleen

Stomach

Pancreas

the entire left colic artery can be preserved, and for a mid-transverse colon lesion, the ascending branch of the left colic artery should be transected.

The peritoneum is scored below the inferior mesenteric vein. The mesocolon can be maintained anteriorly with the surgeon's left hand and the retroperitoneum swept downwards laterally towards the white line of Toldt. The inferior mesenteric artery is isolated from superior and inferior branches, and the left branch is evaluated. Prior to transection of the entire inferior mesenteric artery, it is imperative that the ureter be identified and preserved (see Chap. 6). Transection proceeds with bipolar, clips, or stapler, per surgeon preference.

middle colic vessels. Some surgeons prefer to transect the vessels from a top-down approach secondary to visualization of the vessels detached from underlying tissue. Alternatively, a right to left approach can be used, as discussed in Chap. 2.

In the top-down approach, the colon is stretched inferiorly, exposing the middle colic vessels (Tip 3.6). From the right side, elevate the retroperitoneum from the vessels. Identify the bare area proximal to the vessels at the second portion of the duodenum. Isolate the fourth portion of the duodenum, distal to the middle colic vessels. Isolation of the middle colic vessels is crucial in ensuring that the superior mesenteric artery, duodenum, and retroperitoneum are not injured.

Step 12: Identification and Transection of the Middle Colic Pedicle, Top-Down Approach

After the superior approach had been completed, only the middle colic vessels remain. The colon can be lifted anteriorly and superiorly, exposing the middle colic vessels (Fig. 3.13). The planes proximal and distal to the middle colic vessels have been established by the prior dissection, isolating the

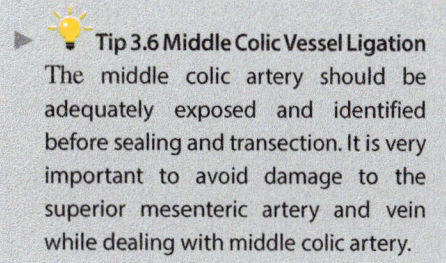

> 💡 **Tip 3.6 Middle Colic Vessel Ligation**
> The middle colic artery should be adequately exposed and identified before sealing and transection. It is very important to avoid damage to the superior mesenteric artery and vein while dealing with middle colic artery.

Fig. 3.13 The middle colic vessels are ligated after mobilization of the transverse colon is completed. This is the last remaining attachments to the colon

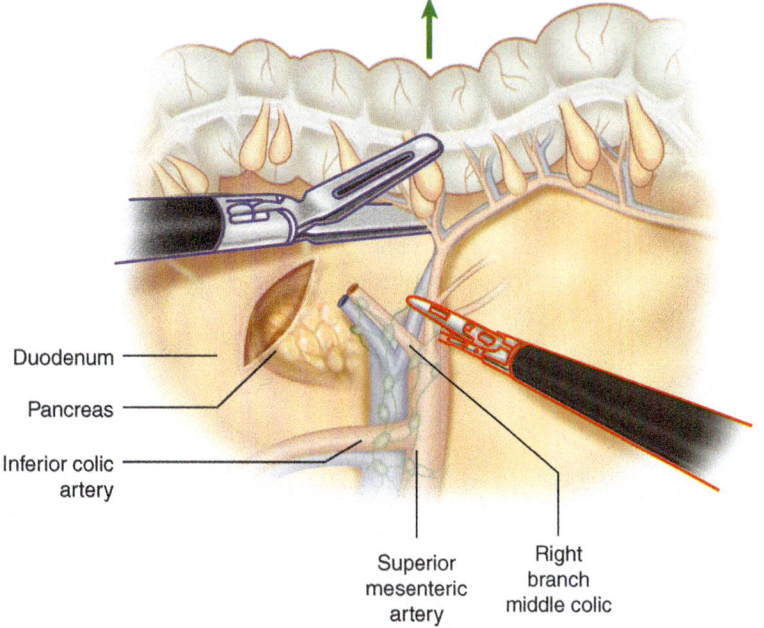

Duodenum

Pancreas

Inferior colic artery

Superior mesenteric artery

Right branch middle colic

The surgeon's right hand elevates the vessels away from the retroperitoneum. The left hand uses a bipolar to transect the middle colic vessels (Pitfall 3.2).

> **Pitfall 3.2**
> It is important to ensure that there is sufficient cuff of the superior mesenteric artery and vein to control bleeding should the vessel sealers fail.

Step 13: Specimen Exteriorization and Anastomosis

Creating an anastomosis is a challenging portion of the case. Generally, unless a formal left colectomy is performed, a circular stapler will not be used, as the resection margin is too proximal in the colon. The anastomosis is generally done extracorporeally through a midline supraumbilical incision.

A midline supraumbilical incision is made for the extraction of specimen and extracorporeal anastomosis. After the wound protector is placed (Fig. 3.14), mobilized transverse colon is exteriorized. Any remaining mesentery is divided and blood supply checked (Tip 3.7). A linear stapler is used to divide the colon 5–10 cm from the lesion.

A side-to-side, functional end-to-end, stapled anastomosis, or a hand-sewn, end-to-end anastomosis can be fashioned based on the preference of the surgeon. The specimen is either sent for gross examination or opened in the operating room to ensure that adequate margins (5 cm for cancer) are obtained. After the colon is replaced

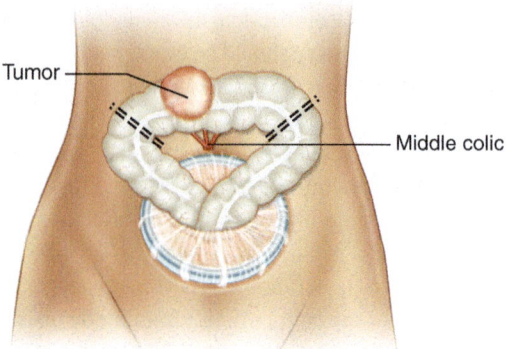

Fig. 3.14 Exteriorized transverse colon with full mobilization of the hepatic and splenic flexures. Colo-colonic anastomosis may be made extracorporeally using sutured or stapled techniques

> **Tip 3.7 Checking the Blood Supply**
> Prior to creating an anastomosis, check the blood supply to the conduit. Hemostats are applied proximally and distally, but only the resection side is clamped. Vessels are transected with a Metzenbaum scissors. If the blood supply is not vigorous and pulsatile, additional colon should be resected until a good blood supply is noted.

in the peritoneal cavity, reestablish pneumoperitoneum after clamping wound protector to check for hemostasis. Routine closure of mesenteric defect is not necessary.

Five millimeter trocars are removed under visualization. Midline fascial opening is closed with no. 1 delayed absorbable suture. Subcuticular stitches are placed to close the skin.

Splenic Flexure

4

Kevin R. Kniery, Michael J. Mulcahy, and Scott R. Steele

Introduction

Splenic flexure mobilization is a technique that allows for a tension-free bowel anastomosis during left colectomy or proctectomy and ensures adequate length of the descending or sigmoid colon to reach the skin when performing a colostomy.

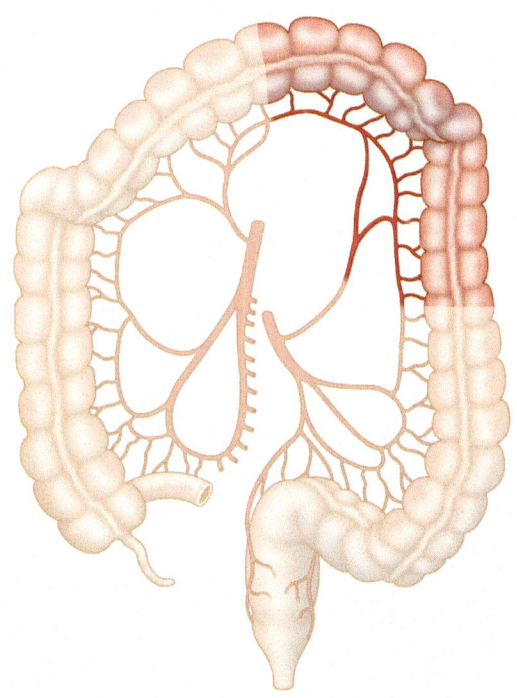

K. R. Kniery
Department of Surgery, Madigan Army Medical Center, Tacoma, WA, USA

M. J. Mulcahy
Tripler Army Medical Center, Honolulu, HI, USA

S. R. Steele (✉)
Department of Colorectal Surgery, Digestive Disease and Surgery Institute, Cleveland Clinic, Cleveland, OH, USA

Indications

Left-sided or pelvic anastomoses

Operative Approaches

Mobilizing the splenic flexure laparoscopically can be challenging even for experienced surgeons, given its close relationship to the spleen,

© Springer Nature Switzerland AG 2020
S. L. Stein, R. R. Lawson (eds.), *Laparoscopic Colectomy*,
https://doi.org/10.1007/978-3-030-39559-9_4

pancreas, stomach, ureter, and major vascular structures. Yet, as surgeons become more experienced with this approach, they often find it easier than an open approach, where limited visualization and individual body habitus can create their own set of difficulties.

This chapter will describe three of the most commonly used approaches to mobilize the splenic flexure. While some surgeons prefer one approach over another, having all three in your armamentarium is important as patient pathology may dictate an easier approach.

- Anterior (lesser sac) approach: Going through the gastrocolic ligament and using the lesser sac as your initial point of entry
- Lateral approach: Traditional "open" approach of mobilizing the lateral abdominal wall attachments first
- Medial/inferior mesenteric vein approach: Starting under the IMV at the ligament of Treitz or under the IMA at the sacral promontory and dissecting medial to lateral

Operative Steps

Unlike other chapters, this chapter is not a complete operation but highlights the various options for splenic flexure mobilization. This chapter reviews the pertinent anatomy, positioning, and surgical techniques to safely mobilize the splenic flexure in a variety of ways.

It should be noted that splenic flexure mobilization is not a necessity for all left-sided, or even pelvic, anastomoses. If the patient has a large redundant colon or they are undergoing a rectopexy, this step will likely be unnecessary. Small retrospective studies have compared routine splenic flexure mobilization versus no mobilization and have shown no difference in morbidity, anastomotic leak rates, and oncologic outcomes. Splenic flexure mobilization may be a necessity in many patients to provide adequate reach and prevent tension on the anastomosis. Surgeons need to be facile and familiar with several approaches (Fig. 4.1).

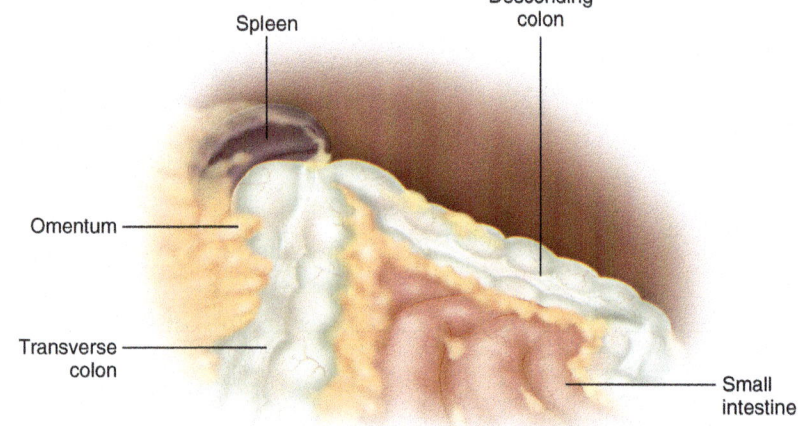

Fig. 4.1 Intraoperative view of the splenic flexure in situ. The spleen sits above the splenic flexure and may be intimately attached via the splenocolic ligaments. The small bowel fills the space between transverse and descending colon. A bulky omentum may also obscure the view and complicate dissection

Patient Positioning for Laparoscopic Splenic Flexure

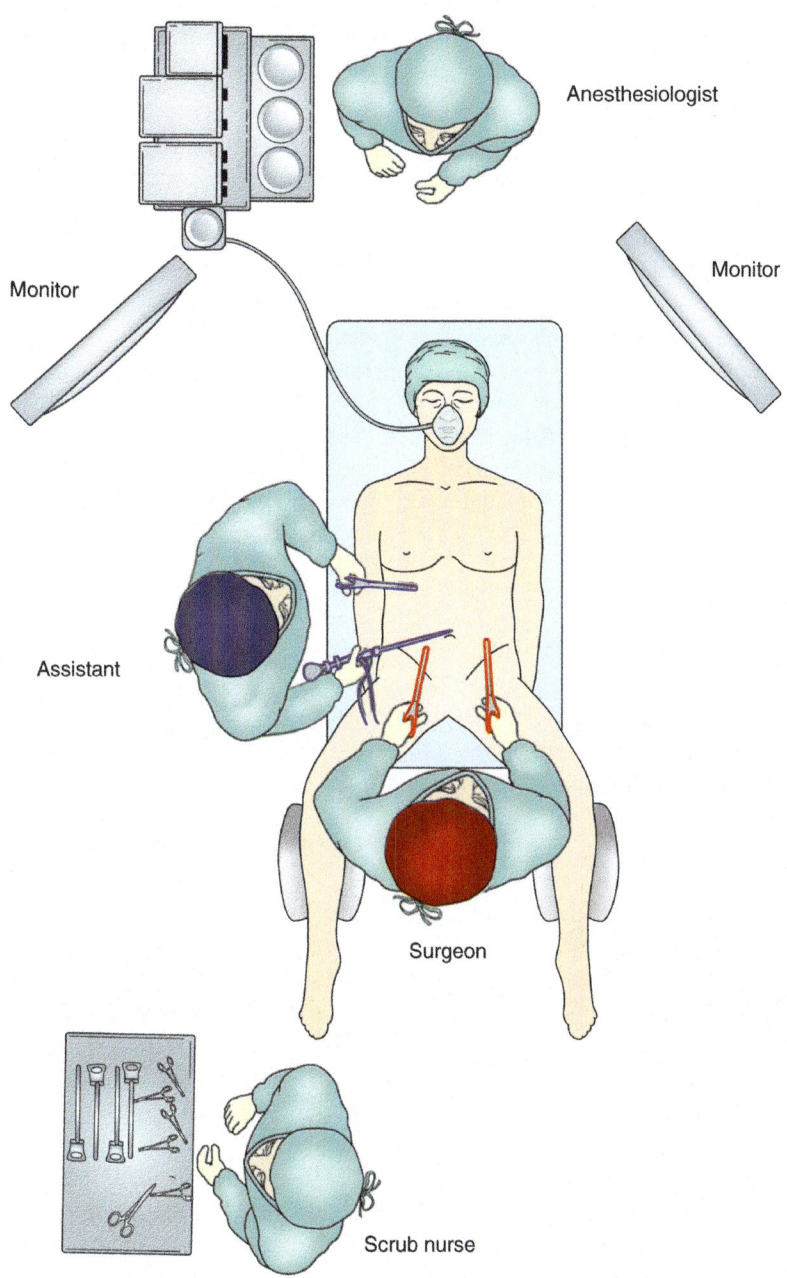

Patient positioning. The patient is placed in lithotomy position with right side down in reverse Trendelenburg. Both arms should be tucked at the patient's sides. Ports will be the same as used for the remainder of the case. Monitors should be off the patient's left shoulder for visualization by both the surgeon and the assistant

The patient is positioned in lithotomy with both arms tucked. The left arm may be kept on an arm board, if necessary; however, tucking both arms optimizes ergonomics and facilitates changing positions on the table.

Reverse Trendelenburg is preferred for the anterior approach to allow initial access to the gastrocolic ligament and lesser sac.

For the lateral-to-medial approach, the patient is initially placed in Trendelenburg position and then rolled to the right to allow the viscera to fall to the right upper quadrant. This maneuver exposes the base of the mesentery.

For the medial-to-lateral or sub-IMV approach, Trendelenburg with right side down is preferred to allow access to the forth portion of the duodenum-jejunal junction and medial side of the inferior mesenteric vein (Tip 4.1).

> **Tip 4.1 Port Placement in the Obese**
> For obese patients, move trocars slightly more medially to avoid losing the fulcrum required to lift the colon.

The surgeon will be primarily on the patient's right, looking at a monitor off the patient's left shoulder. Occasionally, it will be necessary for the surgeon to operate from between the patient's legs to fully mobilize the splenic flexure especially in tall or obese patients (Tip 4.2). The assistant will generally also be on the right or between the patient's legs.

> **Tip 4.2 Changing Surgeon Positions**
> Don't be afraid to change positions of the surgeon, assistant, or patient. Maintaining good ergonomics helps to minimize stress and optimizes concentration during stressful and long operations.

Operative Strategy

Anterior (Lesser Sac) Approach
(Fig. 4.2)

The anterior approach begins at the gastrocolic ligament with access into the lesser sac. This allows for identification of key anatomic structures and dissection of the colon under direct visualization. Once the colon is mobilized from the spleen and pancreas, the remainder of the dissection of the descending colon is performed from the lateral approach to complete the mobilization (Tip 4.3).

> **Tip 4.3 Move the Operation to the Surgeon**
> Rather than stretching to reach the anatomy of interest, if the omentum and colon are not under tension, bring them closer to the camera to facilitate reach. This helps facilitate a careful dissection.

Patient and Surgeon Positioning

Place the patient in reverse Trendelenburg and roll the patient to the right side. The surgeon stands between the patient's legs with the assistant on the right side of the patient.

Step 1: Gastrocolic Ligament
The surgeon frees any distal adhesions of the omentum to the abdominal wall or pelvis. The omentum is then placed above the colon, and the colon is retracted inferiorly to visualize the margin between the colon and omentum at the cephalad aspect of the colon wall.

The lesser sac is entered by separating the gastrocolic ligament near its midpoint just left of the falciform ligament. In this location, the two layers of the omentum are fused which facilitates entry into the lesser sac (Tip 4.4).

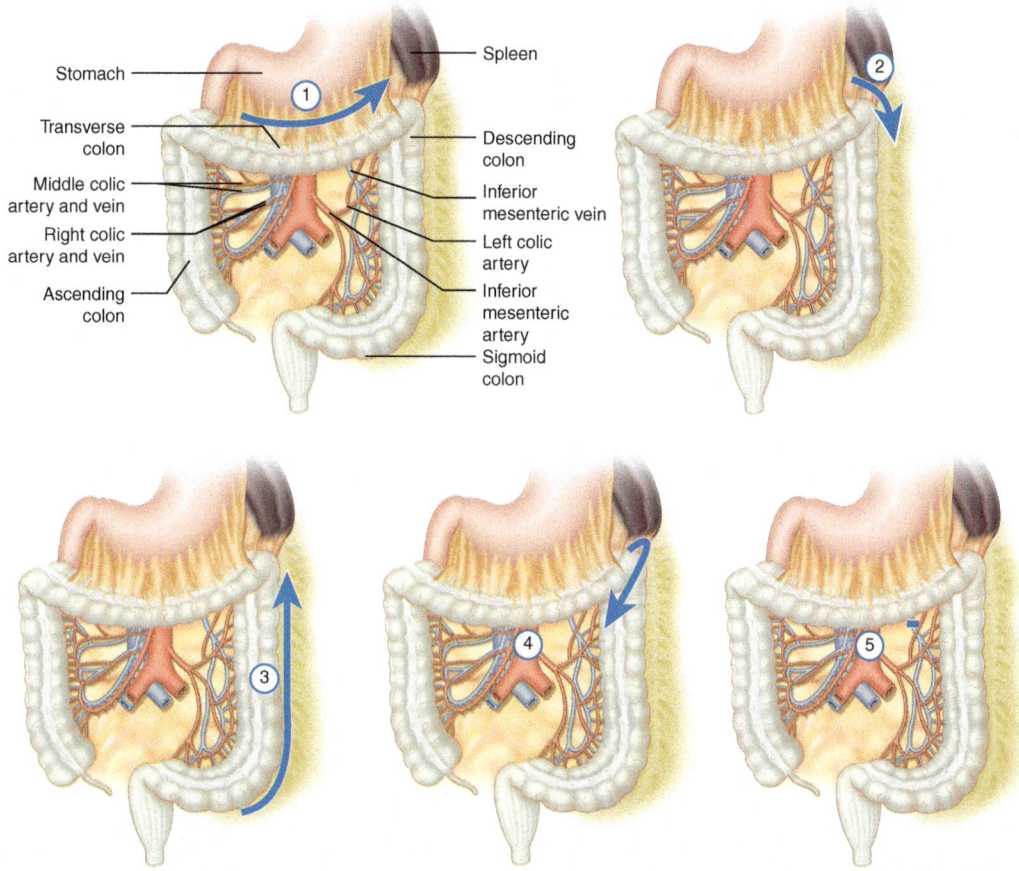

Fig. 4.2 Steps of the anterior approach. Anterior approach to splenic flexure mobilization. (1) Opening of gastrocolic ligament into the lesser sac (blue), (2) taking down of splenocolic ligament (green), (3) lateral mobili- zation at the white line of Toldt (orange), (4) retroperito- neal mobilization (red), (5) optional, inferior mesenteric vein ligation (pink)

> 💡 **Tip 4.4 Entering the Lesser Sac**
> Dissect over a wide plane, parallel to the colon, to prevent creating a narrow deep window into the omentum, which limits visualization of the plane. If the plane is difficult to open, reevaluation proximally towards the falciform ligament can be helpful.

Tension is needed on the omentum anteriorly and on the colon inferiorly. The assistant's left hand elevates the omentum, while the surgeon holds the colon caudally through the right lower quadrant port. Scissors or an energy device is used in the surgeon's right hand to enter the plane.

The correct plane is avascular, with a faint change in color or texture between the epiplo- ica of the colon and the omentum. The correct plane may be difficult to see, particularly in patients with truncal obesity. In this case, the anterior layer of the omentum may be dissected initially and then the second layer opened (Fig. 4.3).

Once the plane is established, the plane is rotated, to create a horizontal plane of dissection. The assistant holds the omentum cephalad, towards the patient's head, rather than anteriorly. The surgeon holds the colon slightly distal to the area of dissection. This creates a horizontal plane for the surgeon to dissect, with simultaneous visualization of the omentum and colon. This approach straightens the colon and prevents inadvertent injury to the colon during the dissection (Fig. 4.4).

Entry into the lesser sac is established when the posterior wall of the stomach, with gastroepiploic vessels, is visualized clearly (Pitfall 4.1). The omentum is free superiorly, and the colon

> **⚠ Pitfall 4.1**
> The stomach is often closer than expected and may have adhesions to the retroperitoneum. Dissect carefully until the adhesions are freed and the stomach is completely mobilized in a cephalad direction.

Fig. 4.3 In situ plane between colon and omentum. The surgeon retracts the colon caudally, while the assistant gently retracts the omentum anterior and cephalad. Subtle changes in the fat between the omentum and the colonic epiploica signal the correct plane into the lesser sac

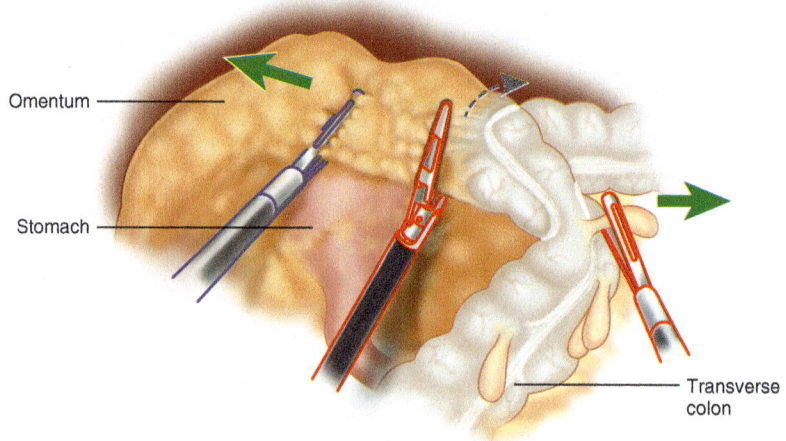

Fig. 4.4 Creation of horizontal plane. Gastrocolic ligament is incised to gain access to the lesser sac. The lesser sac is confirmed by visualization of the back wall of the stomach. The assistant now holds the omentum cephalad, while the surgeon holds the colon distal to dissection region. The horizontal plane created allows for dissection with visualization of both the omentum and colon

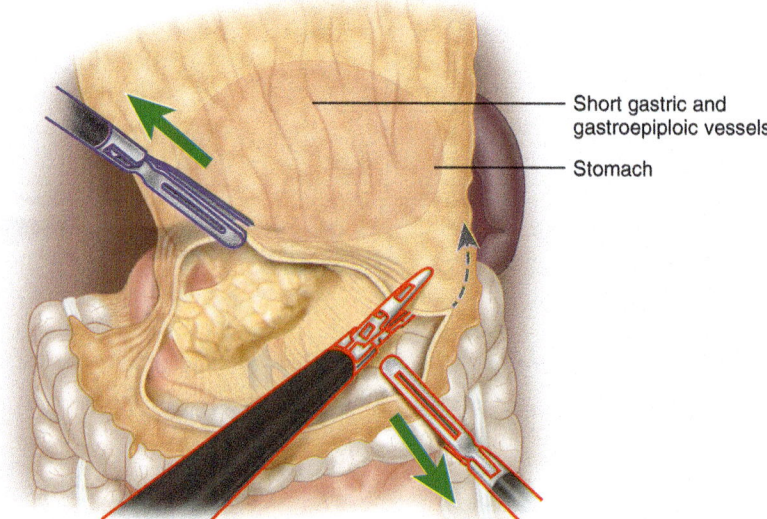

and colonic mesentery are preserved at the inferior aspect of the dissection. There are often avascular wispy connections to the posterior stomach, or the pancreas, that will require transection.

Step 2: Splenocolic Ligament

Once the plane between colon and omentum is established, continue separating the colon from omentum distally, until the inferior splenic pole is exposed. It is important to prevent excessive tension on the spleen, which can result in avulsion injury. The colon is retracted inferiorly to clearly visualize the colon wall. Dissection stays close to the colon, following the tortuosity of the colon around the splenic flexure. Minimal to no traction should be placed on the splenocolic ligament to prevent injury to the spleen (Pitfall 4.2). A bipolar energy instrument helps to prevent lateral spread of cautery, excessive tension, and bleeding into the retroperitoneum (Fig. 4.5).

> **Pitfall 4.2**
> If an avulsion injury occurs to the spleen during dissection, several treatment options exist to abate bleeding: cauterization with high settings, pressure with a gauze pad, placement of coagulation products, splenectomy, or conversion to open surgery can be performed.

Step 3: Lateral Attachments/Line of Toldt

Once the splenocolic ligament is dissected and the colon at the splenic flexure is released, the distal transverse colon will descend towards the pelvis. This dissection follows the white line of Toldt lateral to the descending colon towards the pelvis. This portion can be performed in a top-

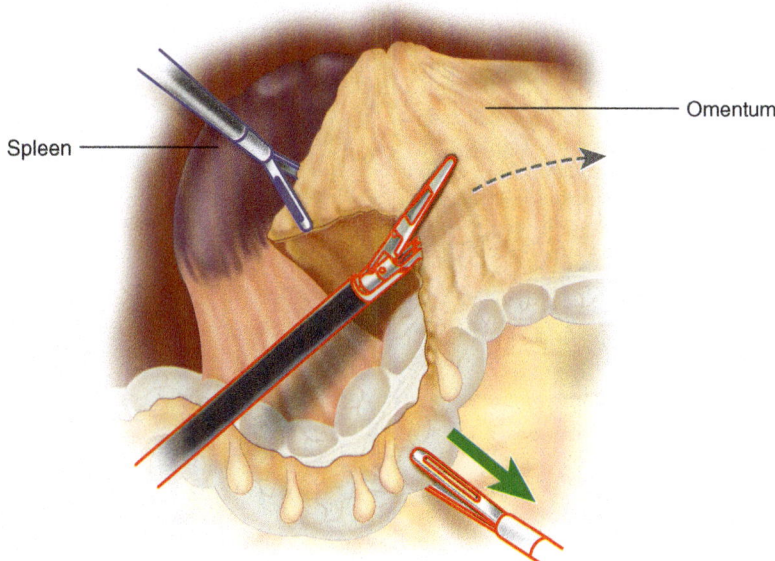

Fig. 4.5 Entry into the lesser sac. At the splenic flexure, care must be taken to prevent inadvertent avulsion injury to the splenic capsule. The dissection plane is just off the colon, to prevent injuring the colon due to lateral spread from bipolar coagulation. The omentum is freed superi-orly, with the assistant providing minimal to no traction on the splenocolic ligament. The surgeon provides traction on the colon to ensure preservation of the colon and colonic mesentery inferiorly

down or bottom-up approach. Staying just medial to the white line will prevent dissection into the retroperitoneum. As the dissection continues, medial traction on the colon helps facilitate dissection (Fig. 4.6).

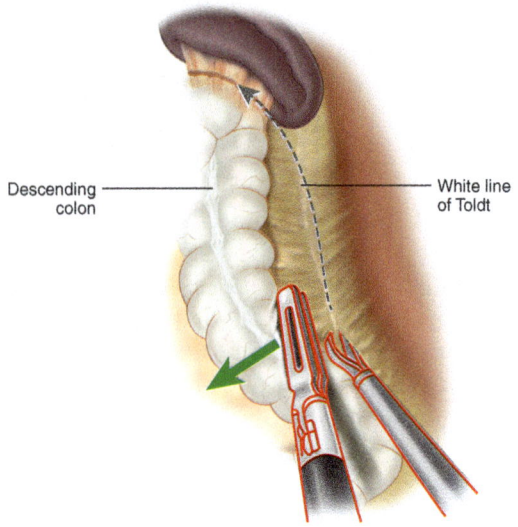

Fig. 4.6 White line of Toldt. The colon is retracted medially demonstrating the white line of Toldt. The dissection plane is just medial to the white line, to prevent injuring the colon due to lateral spread from bipolar coagulation from. The surgeon retracts the colon inferiorly, dissecting close to the colon. The assistant facilitates dissection at the omentum, being sure to provide minimal to no traction on the splenocolic ligament

Step 4: Retroperitoneal Attachments

Full mobilization of the splenic flexure is not complete until the posterior dissection is performed. The freed colon is retracted inferiorly and medially, exposing the pancreaticomesocolic attachment along the inferior border of the pancreas (Tip 4.5). Filmy attachments from the anterior aspect of Gerota's fascia, and from the retroperitoneum, may prevent optimal tension-free reach to the pelvis. These attachments may bleed during transection, so bipolar or ultrasonic dissection is used. Care should be taken to ensure that the pancreas is left in situ and not retracted in a cephalad direction. All attachments lateral and superior to the inferior mesenteric vein are freed, and the colon can be straightened towards the pelvis (Fig. 4.7).

> 💡 **Tip 4.5 Retroperitoneal Attachments**
> Place graspers on the transverse and descending colon and pull caudally, to better visualize the retroperitoneal attachments. By putting the retroperitoneum on stretch, the fibers will be better visualized and more easily divided.

Fig. 4.7 Resection of remaining retroperitoneal attachments. The freed colon is retracted inferiorly and medially, exposing the pancreaticomesocolic attachment. The tail of the pancreas lies just beyond the attachments, and care must be taken not to dissect under the pancreas

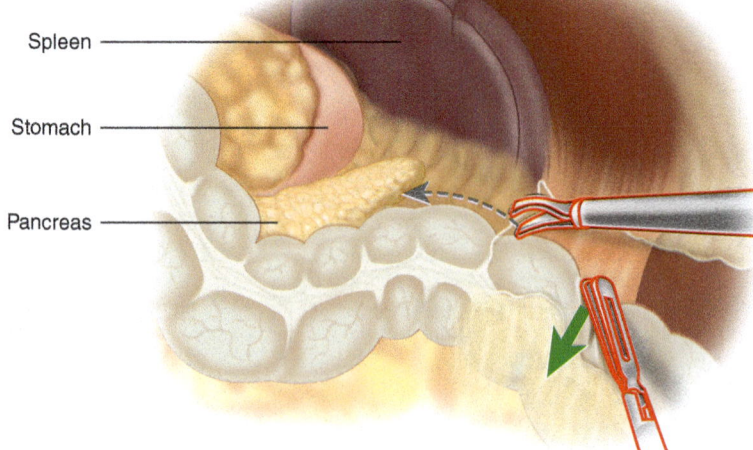

Fig. 4.8 Inferior mesenteric vein transection. For maximal reach from the splenic flexure, the inferior mesenteric vein should be ligated high, just below the inferior border of the pancreas. The small bowel is retracted by the assistant with bowel graspers, while the surgeon's left hand elevates the ligament of Treitz to identify the IMV proximal to the jejunum. Elevation of the IMV facilitates transection of the IMV with an energy instrument, clips, or staplers

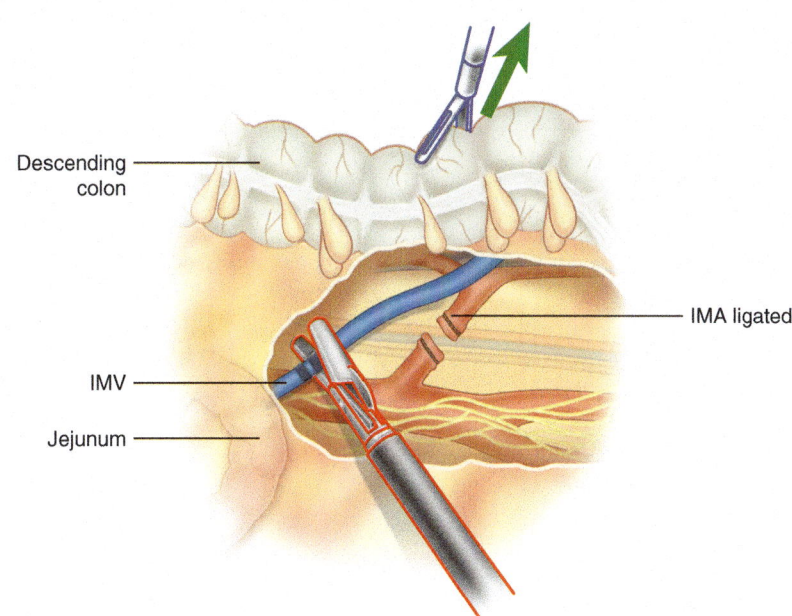

Descending colon

IMV

Jejunum

IMA ligated

Step 5: Inferior Mesenteric Vein (Optional)

The inferior mesenteric vein (IMV) is a consistent landmark running just lateral to the fourth portion of the duodenum/ligament of Treitz in a superior-inferior fashion. Division of the IMV at the inferior border of the pancreas provides additional length for the colon to reach the pelvis. If adequate reach is established without transection of the IMV, and transection is not necessary for oncologic reasons, the IMV may be left in situ (Fig. 4.8).

To proceed with an IMV transection, the colon is replaced in the left gutter. The small bowel is run out of the left upper quadrant with bowel graspers, to identify the ligament of Treitz. The surgeon's left hand is used to elevate the ligament of Treitz, identifying the IMV lateral to the proximal jejunum.

There is an avascular plane adjacent to the duodenum/jejunal junction that provides a window into the retroperitoneum, under the IMV. Avascular windows are established inferior and superior to the IMV, allowing complete access to the vessel. By gently elevating the IMV, this plane can be extended proximally to the inferior border of the pancreas. The IMV is then transected with an energy instrument, clips, or staplers, inferior to the pancreatic border and providing several inches of additional length.

Lateral-to-Medial Approach (Fig. 4.9)

In patients with a thickened mesentery from Crohn's disease or a mesenteric abscess, the lateral-to-medial approach is preferred due to the difficulty of dividing the mesenteric attachments in the avascular plane as well as the risk for bleeding and mesenteric hematomas. This approach is essentially a continuous dissection from inferior to superior in a counterclockwise manner around the bend of the splenic flexure. The surgeon will medialize the colon by keeping the avascular attachments under appropriate tension throughout the dissection.

Dissection begins in the left lower quadrant in Trendelenburg position. The surgeon stands between the legs, and the assistant stands on the right side of the patient.

Step 1: Lateral Attachments/Line of Toldt

The surgeon gently retracts the descending colon medially with the left hand, exposing the line of Toldt. Using scissors with electrocautery in the right hand, this plane is carefully dissected cranially towards the splenic flexure. The correct plan is just a cell layer medial to the white line. As the surgeon dissects, air may be seen entering the

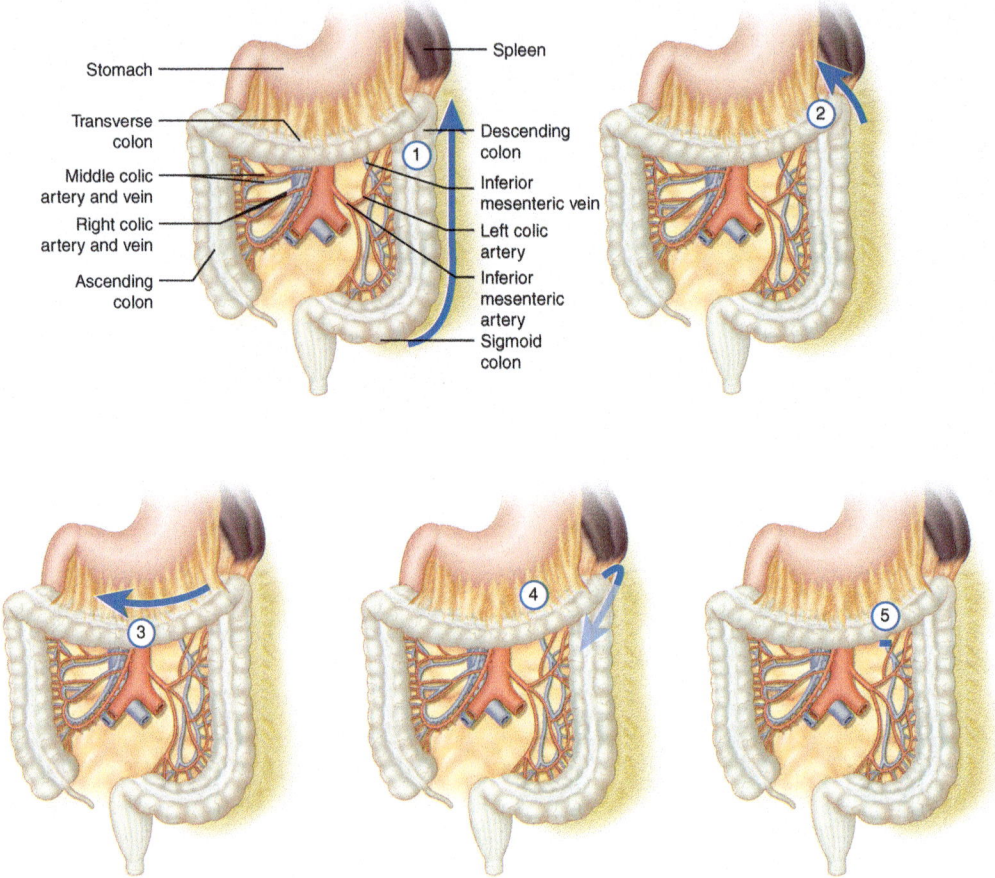

Fig. 4.9 Steps of the lateral approach. (1) Dissection at white line of Toldt up the lateral aspect of the colon (red), (2) around the splenic flexure (green), (3) into the lesser sac and opening the gastrocolic ligament (yellow), (4) retroperitoneal dissection (orange), and (5) optional, IMV transection (pink)

correct plane facilitating the dissection. This plane should be completely avascular.

Develop the avascular plane across a broad front, slowly medializing the entire left colon. Beginning the dissection with attachments to the pelvic brim at the sigmoid provides full medialization of the entire left colon and clear visualization of the line of Toldt. At the distal extent of the dissection, the ureter and gonadal vessels will be visualized and preserved in the retroperitoneum. As the dissection progresses superiorly, dissection stays close to the colon to prevent migration into the retroperitoneum behind Gerota's fascia (Fig. 4.10).

As the mobilization continues superiorly, reaching the splenic flexure with bowel graspers can be difficult (Tip 4.6). Options to prevent tension include having the surgeon relocate between the patients' legs or obtaining longer bowel graspers.

> 💡 **Tip 4.6 Inadequate Reach**
> Longer bowel graspers can help prevent excessive tension or inadvertent injury at the splenic flexure. Bariatric graspers work well when reach is compromised.

Step 2: Splenocolic Ligament

Care is taken to avoid excessive retraction on the spleen at the splenocolic ligament.

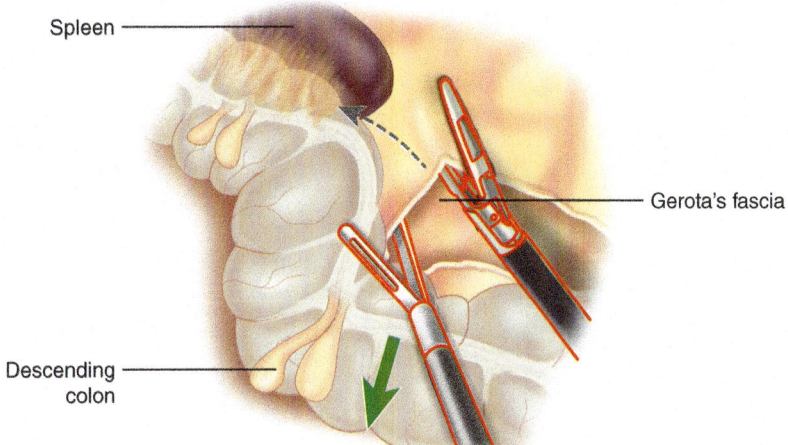

Spleen

Gerota's fascia

Descending
colon

Fig. 4.10 The white line of Toldt and Gerota's fascia. The surgeon's left hand retracts the descending colon, while the right hand dissects using scissors with electrocautery. The correct plane is just medial to the white line. A second lateral white line will connect with the retroperitoneum, behind Gerota's fascia. Care must be taken to prevent dissection under the kidney

Tortuosity of the splenic flexure, high splenic flexure, or deep splenic flexure makes following the redundant colon difficult, increasing the risk of injuring the colon or stomach during the dissection (Pitfall 4.3). Lifting the freed portion of the descending colon anteriorly towards the abdominal wall with the surgeon's left hand helps to identify the planes and prevent tension on the spleen.

> ⚠️ **Pitfall 4.3**
> It is critical to avoid too much medial tension on the splenic flexure. Think of gently retracting the colon from the spleen, rather than pulling too hard and causing a tear (and subsequent bleeding) from the splenic capsule.

It is difficult to balance adequate visualization of the colon wall to prevent injury, while staying close to the colon to ensure the correct plane. Using a bipolar or ultrasonic instrument may help reduce the risk of incomplete small vessel ligation, which may help in reducing bleeding and improve visualization.

The colon is followed closely around the splenocolic ligament, until the colon straightens towards the transverse colon. Often, there are anterior attachments towards the anterior abdominal wall just lateral to the splenocolic ligament. Dissection of these attachments does not affect the release of the splenic flexure but may assist with visualization.

Step 3: Gastrocolic Ligament

As the splenocolic ligament is released, progress can reorient to an anterior approach or continue from a lateral to medial approach (Tip 4.7).

> 💡 **Tip 4.7 Alternate Techniques**
> Don't hesitate to alternate between the transverse colon side and descending colon/lateral attachments if the dissection becomes more difficult.

The stomach is close to the colon and spleen in the left upper quadrant. Care should be taken to ensure that the stomach is clear from the plane of dissection when approaching from the lateral aspect.

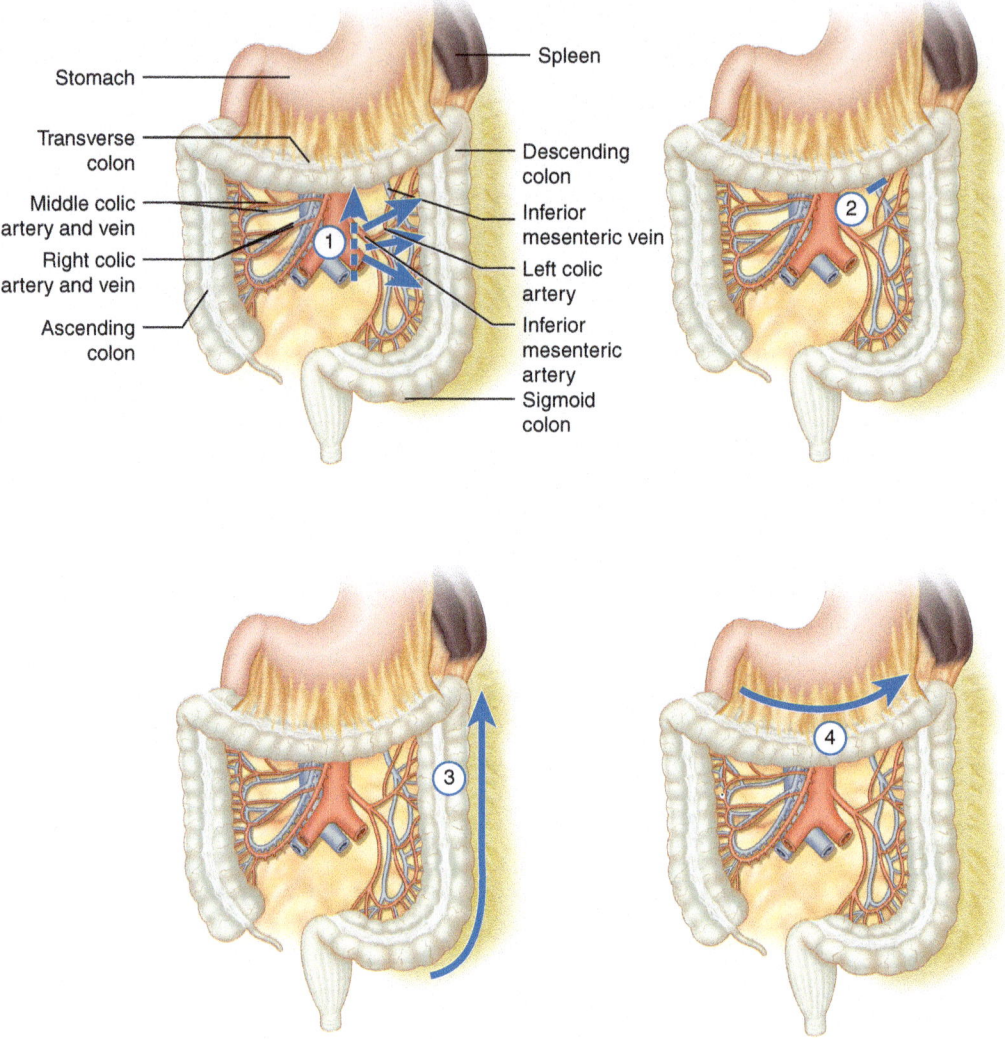

Fig. 4.11 Steps of the medial to lateral or inferior mesenteric vein approach. Step 1: Medial dissection (blue arrows). Step 2: transection of inferior mesenteric vein (green). Step 3: lateral dissection (orange). Step 4: gastrocolic dissection (yellow)

Steps for retroperitoneal dissection and optional transection of IMV are included in the anterior approach to splenic flexure mobilization.

Medial-to-Lateral Approach (Fig. 4.11)

The medial-to-lateral approach is a continuation of the medial-to-lateral approach under the inferior mesenteric artery starting at the sacral promontory. This approach allows for initial transection of vessels (inferior mesenteric artery, left colic artery, and inferior mesenteric vein), identification of key structures medially, and preservation of lateral attachments for retraction. This is generally considered a more difficult approach to the splenic flexure, as inadvertent dissection below the pancreas is possible (Tip 4.8).

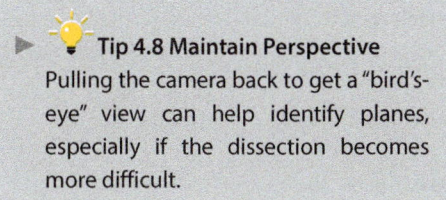

▶ 💡 **Tip 4.8 Maintain Perspective**
Pulling the camera back to get a "bird's-eye" view can help identify planes, especially if the dissection becomes more difficult.

The patient is placed in Trendelenburg, with right side down. The small bowel is relocated to the right upper quadrant to exposes the root of the mesentery. The surgeon stands on the patient's right side.

Step 1: Medial Dissection

After transection of the inferior mesenteric artery, and creation of the medial planes at the sacral promontory, the surgeon continues in this plane, in a cephalad direction. The dissection continues anterior to Toldt's fascia, preserving the ureter, gonadal vessels, and retroperitoneum below the plane of dissection. The shiny surface of the retroperitoneal fascia is visualized below the dissection (Fig. 4.12).

The dissection continues bluntly both laterally to the sidewall of the abdomen and superiorly. The mesentery should be tented towards the abdominal wall with blunt graspers in the surgeon's left hand, as the plane is dissected from retroperitoneal structures. Using an open bowel grasper as a retractor helps to increase the tension on the mesentery, so that blunt dissection can separate the retroperitoneum from the mesentery. This plane is anterior to Gerota's fascia and the perinephric fat. A purple hue is noted to the retroperitoneum, which is dissected down throughout the dissection (Fig. 4.13).

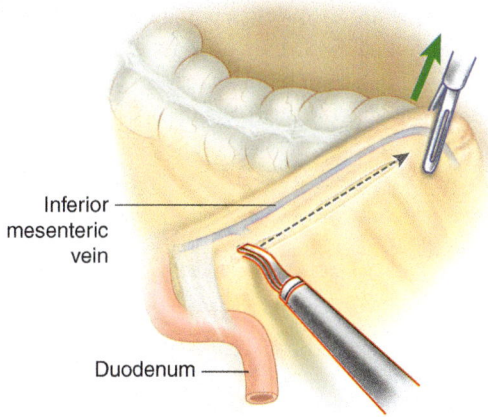

Fig. 4.12 Dissecting under the IMV. The assistant provides tension by pulling up on the IMV, facilitating dissection under the IMV. The peritoneum is scored from the left colic artery up to the ligament of Treitz, parallel and deep to the inferior mesenteric vein

Fig. 4.13 Retromesenteric dissection. The surgeon and assistant elevate the colon and mesocolon, exposing the retroperitoneum below the IMV. The white line is swept dorsally, away from the mesocolon

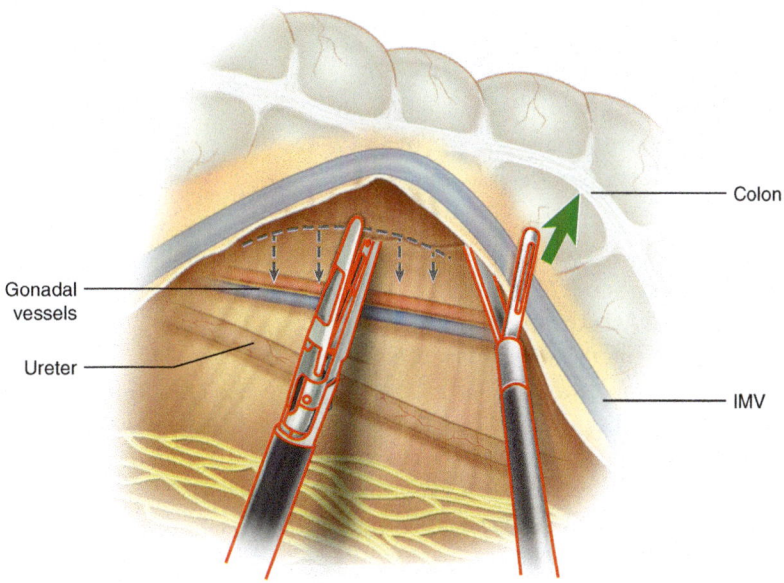

A key step is to identify the inferior border of the pancreas and to ensure proper dissection anterior to the surface of the pancreas. The anterior plane is avascular, and the subtle change from the mesocolon and retroperitoneal adipose tissue to pancreas is noted (Pitfall 4.4).

Pitfall 4.4
Avoid the urge to make a small window and dissect in a hole. Keep the plane very broad to help let in light and better visualize the correct avascular plane.

As the dissection continues cephalad, the inferior mesenteric vein is noted and tented up with the mesentery. Depending on reach, and oncologic margins, this may be transected using clips, staplers, or energy.

After transitioning above the pancreas, a filmy layer of peritoneum is opened, and the dissection continues into a clear space, which is the lesser sac (Pitfall 4.5). Within the lesser sac, the posterior surface of the greater curvature of the body of the stomach is visualized.

Pitfall 4.5
It is easy to dissect under the pancreas potentially causing damage to the splenic vein. If a large vein is visualized, reorientation should be done to ensure that this is not the splenic vein coursing posterior to the pancreas.

Step 2: Gastrocolic/Omental and Lateral Attachments

The benefits of the medial dissection include expeditious transection of the gastrocolic ligament and lateral attachments, as all the retroperitoneum has already been dissected from the medial side. Allowing air into the planes facilitates easy creation of the planes from an anterior approach.

Dissection can proceed as in anterior or medial approaches.

Variation: Sub-IMV Approach

A variation to the medial-to-lateral approach is the "sub-IMV" approach. With this technique, the surgeon begins the dissection at the ligament of Treitz. The surgeon's left hand is used to lift the IMV, while the peritoneum is opened medial and inferior to the IMV with electrocautery. The IMV is transected with an energy instrument after it is clear from the ligament of Treitz. Using the left hand to raise the mesentery, the surgeon's right hand is used to gently and bluntly dissect laterally towards the spleen and the left sidewall (Tip 4.9).

Tip 4.9 Bowel Retraction
A sponge may be placed through the umbilical port to aid in retracting the bowel. We have a nurse mark it on the board and only remove the notation when it is removed.

Identification of the inferior border of the pancreas will help ensure that the dissection remains anterior to the pancreas. Dissection posterior to the pancreas puts the splenic vein at risk.

The surgeon works in a broad plane to avoid tunneling into a long, narrow hole. The dissection from this plane can run from run superiorly to the lesser sac, laterally to the abdominal wall and white line of Toldt, and inferiorly to the inferior mesenteric artery.

How to Tell When the Splenic Flexure Is Completely Mobilized

Complete mobilization of the splenic flexure is confirmed once there are no omental, lateral colon, and retroperitoneal attachments (Tip 4.10).

The splenic flexure and descending colon can be pulled straight towards the pelvis from the middle colic vessels. The inferior border of the pancreas will be easily visualized. When the splenic flexure is completely mobilized with high ligation of the IMV, approximately 30 cm of length can be obtained.

> **Tip 4.10 Mistaking Visualization of the Spleen for Mobilization**
> Simply seeing the spleen and releasing attachments to the spleen is not a complete splenic flexure mobilization and does not free the splenic flexure for optimal reach to the pelvis.

Lengthening Procedures

If additional length is needed after a splenic flexure mobilization, several steps can be taken:

1. Verify that no further attachments (omental, lateral, or retroperitoneal) are restricting the splenic flexure. The omental and retroperitoneal attachments to the transverse colon can often be mobilized proximally (i.e., towards the hepatic flexure) to provide a few additional centimeters of length.
2. If the IMV has not been divided, divide the IMV distal to the convergence of the left colic vein. This will provide an extra 5 cm of additional length.
3. In certain cases, the base of the middle colic artery needs to be divided to further free up the transverse colon and allow the colon to reach the pelvis.
4. Finally, the rectum can be circumferentially dissected in the avascular plane, pulling the rectum cephalad, which will add a few more centimeters of length.

If needed, division of the left branch of the middle colic artery can garner additional length. Prior to transection, determine if there is adequate collateral circulation to avoid any additional devascularization of the descending colon bowel (Pitfall 4.6). To divide the left branch of the middle colic artery, develop avascular windows on either side of the left branch middle colic artery. The left branch of the middle colic artery will be divided just caudal to inferior border of pancreas.

> ⚠️ **Pitfall 4.6**
> Prior to division of the middle colic vessels, place a bulldog atraumatic clamp on the middle colic artery, or grasp the base of the pedicle with a laparoscopic grasper. Wait a few minutes after occluding to ensure adequate collateral blood flow.

Laparoscopic Sigmoid/Left Colectomy

5

Todd D. Francone and Ron G. Landmann

Introduction

Left colectomy is the resection of the descending colon and/or splenic flexure with anastomosis of the distal transverse colon to the sigmoid colon. A sigmoid resection is the removal of the sigmoid colon with restoration of intestinal continuity between the descending colon and the rectum. Both can be done for malignancy, ischemia, stenosis, and inflammatory bowel disease. Sigmoid colectomies are also frequently performed for diverticulitis and occasionally for sigmoid volvulus.

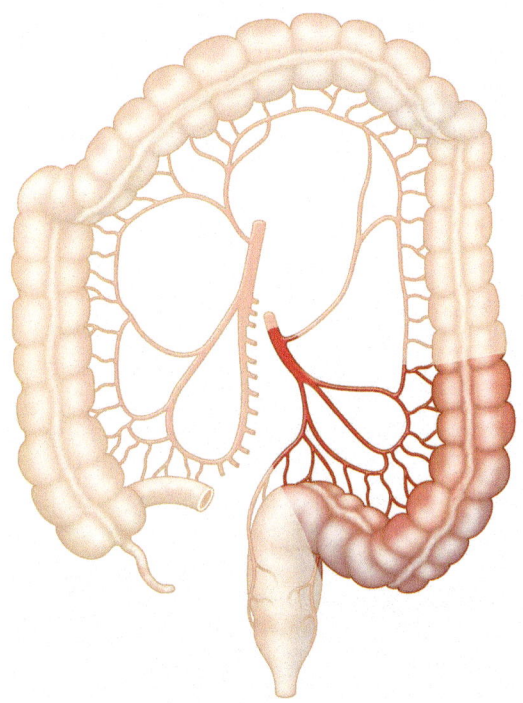

T. D. Francone (✉)
Division of Colon & Rectal Surgery at Newton-Wellesley Hospital, Newton, MA, USA
e-mail: tfrancone@partners.org

R. G. Landmann
MD Anderson Cancer Center - Baptist Medical Center, Jacksonville, FL, USA
e-mail: ron.landmann@bmcjax.com

> **Indications**
> - Neoplasia (benign or malignant) of the descending or sigmoid colon
> - Inflammatory bowel disease (i.e., Crohn's disease) of the descending or sigmoid colon
> - Diverticular disease and associated complications (diverticulitis, perforation, stricture, hemorrhage)

© Springer Nature Switzerland AG 2020
S. L. Stein, R. R. Lawson (eds.), *Laparoscopic Colectomy*,
https://doi.org/10.1007/978-3-030-39559-9_5

- Ischemia
- Sigmoid volvulus

Preoperative Planning
- Colonoscopy to confirm diagnosis, confirm relevant anatomy, and evaluate for synchronous lesion and localization with tattooing (Tip 5.1)
- Preoperative evaluation
  - Carcinoembryonic antigen (CEA) for colorectal cancer
  - Evaluation for familial/genetic colorectal cancer syndromes
    Hereditary nonpolyposis colorectal cancer (HNPCC) or familial adenomatous polyposis (FAP)
- Preoperative diagnostic imaging
  - Computed tomography (CT scan)
    Cancer staging for metastatic disease
    Evaluation of the extent of diverticular disease and potential abscess/fistula
    Enterography for the evaluation for IBD
  - Magnetic resonance imaging (MRI)
    Enterography for the evaluation for IBD
- Deep venous thrombosis prophylaxis
- Preoperative antibiotics prophylaxis
- Mechanical bowel preparation
- Enhanced recovery protocol

> 💡 **Tip 5.1 Preoperative Localization of Neoplasia** While estimates of the location of neoplasia can be very accurate in the distal and proximal colon, they are notoriously inaccurate in the rest of the colon. Placing a tattoo in 3–4 quadrants distal to the lesion is recommended to ensure laparoscopic identification of correct colon segment.

Steps of the Operation
Patient positioning
1. Step 1: Port placement
2. Step 2: Diagnostic laparoscopy
3. Step 3: Identification of pathology
4. Step 4: Identification of the vascular anatomy (inferior mesenteric artery and vein)
5. Step 5: Identification of the proper retroperitoneal plane
6. Step 6: Identification of the ureter and other vital structures
7. Step 7: Transection of the inferior mesenteric artery (IMA) pedicle
8. Step 8: Development of the retroperitoneal plane medial-to-lateral dissection
9. Step 9: Transection of the inferior mesenteric vein (IMV) pedicle (if needed)
10. Step 10: Lateral mobilization
11. Step 11: Splenic flexure mobilization (if needed)
12. Step 12: Distal transection and extraction
13. Step 13: Extraction and proximal transection
14. Step 14: Anastomosis and intraoperative leak testing
15. Step 15: Closure

Tools of the Operation
- 5-mm ports (1–2)
- 10-mm port (1) – for camera
- 12-mm port (1) – for endoscopic stapling devices
- 10-mm 30-degree camera (1) (can be substituted with 5-mm 30-degree camera)
- Laparoscopic atraumatic (bowel) graspers (2–3)
- Laparoscopic scissors with electrocautery
- Devices for vessel ligation and division (surgeon preference)
  - Energy devices
    Ultrasonic
    Bipolar cautery
  - Endoscopic staplers
  - Endoclips
  - Endoloop

- Endoscopic GIA stapler (1) with reloads
- Wound protector
- Circular end-to-end anastomosis (EEA) stapler
- Rigid proctoscope or CO_2 flexible sigmoidoscope

Hand-Assisted Technique

All of the same tools as above, with the addition/substitution of

- TA stapler
- Hand insertion port device

Patient Positioning for Laparoscopic Laparoscopic Sigmoid/Left Colectomy

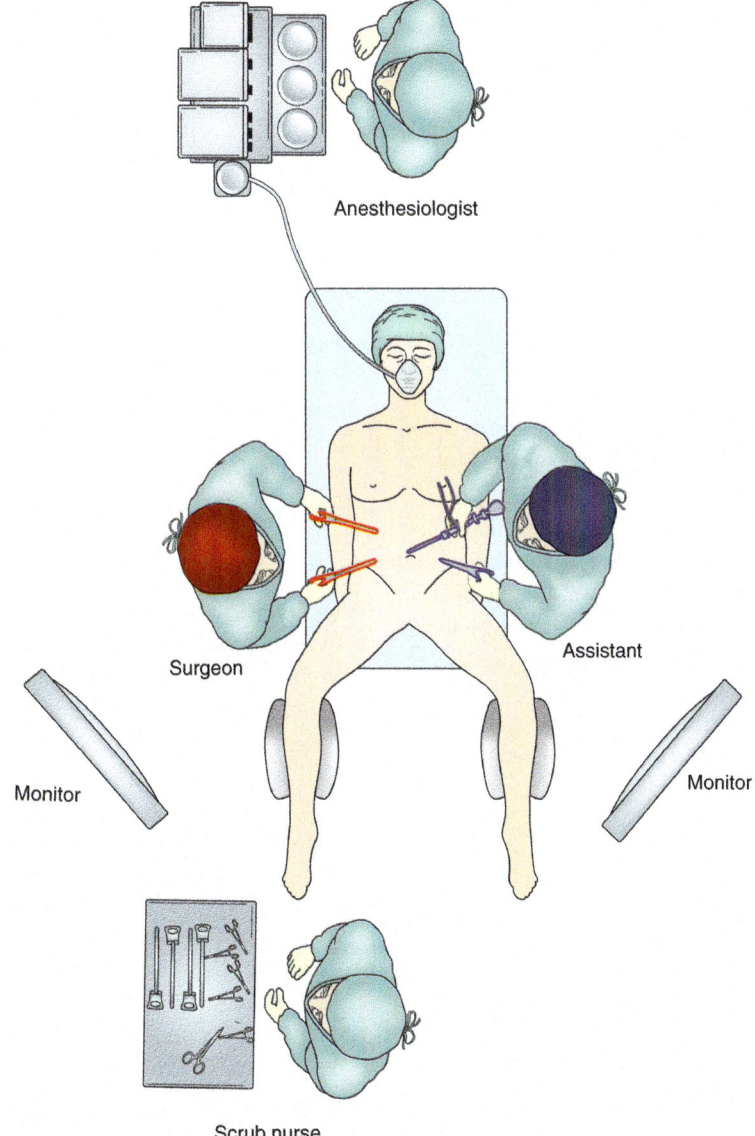

Room setup for sigmoid colectomy: the surgeon will stand on the patient's right side. The assistant can stand on the left or right above the surgeon. Placement on the left facilitates the use of the left lower quadrant port. The monitor must be able to move from the patient's head to thigh during different parts of the case

Position the patient on foam, gel pads, or beanbags with safety straps and/or tape to minimize movement during extremes of positioning (Trendelenburg and reverse-Trendelenburg, right or left side tilt). Place the patient in modified lithotomy (legs in slight hip flexion) or split-leg position with both arms tucked at the sides. Prior to prepping the patient, verify that the patient is appropriately secured to the bed and there is no patient slippage by moving the bed in various extreme positions. Positioning in this manner affords the surgeons numerous advantages:

1. Insertion of transanal anastomotic stapling device
2. Exposure to the anus/rectum for intraoperative colonoscopy if needed (Chap. 1)
3. Surgeon positioning between the legs during mobilization

The surgeon stands on the patient's right hand side utilizing the right upper quadrant (RUQ) and right lower quadrant (RLQ) ports for retraction and dissection. The assistant stands on the patient's right or on the left and operates the camera through the supraumbilical port site. Standing on the left affords easier access to the left lower quadrant (LLQ) port site and the ability to help in retraction and mobilization. The monitor should be able to swing from the patient's left upper quadrant down to the foot of the bed.

Operative Strategy

Step 1: Port Placement

Appropriate port placement is critical in facilitating exposure and anatomic definition. For a left colectomy, four "working" ports are utilized (umbilical, 12-mm RLQ, 5-mm RUQ, 5-mm LLQ) (Fig. 5.1). Use an open cut-down technique (Hassan technique) to place a supraumbilical port and introduce the 10-mm laparoscope into the abdomen.

In a left colectomy, a 12-mm port will be required for intracorporeal stapling of the colon

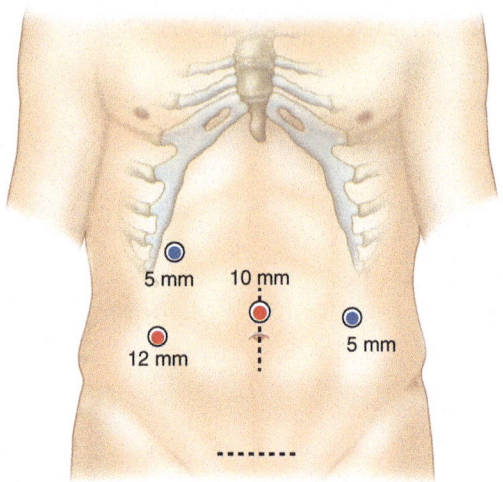

Fig. 5.1 Port placement for sigmoid colectomy: A 10-mm port is placed supraumbilically, with 5-mm ports placed in the right upper quadrant and left side of the abdomen. A 5/12 port may be placed in the right lower quadrant for stapler

and potentially stapling of the vascular structures. For this reason, at least one 12-mm port is placed in the right lower quadrant (RLQ) for left-sided resections. Ideal placement is 2 cm medial and 2 cm superior to the anterior superior iliac spine (Tip 5.2). Place the third port right upper quadrant (RUQ, 5 mm) subcostally and parallel to the RLQ 12-mm port along the same cranial-caudal line. Attention to allow for at least 10–12 cm of space between these two ports to allow for appropriate triangulation and minimize intraperitoneal collision of instruments. A fourth port may be helpful for retraction. This port is placed in the LLQ with similar localization to the anatomic landmarks as the RLQ port or more medially in the planned stoma site if one will be required.

>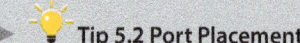
> 💡 **Tip 5.2 Port Placement**
> For obese or tall patients, the port placement may be modified. After the abdomen is insufflated, place the ports just lateral to the rectus muscle as visualized laparoscopically. More medial placement may assist with better reach in a high splenic flexure or deep pelvis.

Step 2: Diagnostic Laparoscopy

In oncologic procedures, inspect the liver on both anterior and posterior surfaces and examine the peritoneum, omentum, and mesentery for metastatic studding. If the latter is identified, biopsy and surgical judgment dictate whether to proceed with resection.

During diagnostic laparoscopy, attempt to identify the pathology. In the setting of a colonic neoplasm, the pathology's location may be marked with an endoscopic tattoo (Tip 5.3). If the tumor is not identified, intraoperative CO_2 endoscopy should be performed for localization (see Chap. 1).

> 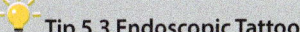 **Tip 5.3 Endoscopic Tattoo**
> Ideally, the endoscopic tattoo is placed in 3–4 quadrants, distal to the lesion and clearly visible on the antimesenteric surface. Marking the lesion in only one quadrant may pose difficulty if the tattoo lies on the mesenteric border or is in a difficult location such as the splenic or hepatic flexures.

Once the pathology is localized, adjust the preoperative surgical plan as required. In the setting of malignancy, the location of the tumor determines resection margins and vessel ligation. For cancers in the left colon, oncologic margins should be 5 cm proximal and 5 cm distal to the tumor. A high ligation of the inferior mesenteric artery (IMA) pedicle is performed to ensure adequate mobilization and appropriate lymph node harvesting. Pathology in the proximal sigmoid colon or distal descending colon may necessitate mobilization of the splenic flexure for tension-free anastomosis. For lesions in the proximal descending colon, a high ligation of the inferior mesenteric vein (IMV) may be necessary to allow mobilization and approximation of the transverse colon to the upper rectum to create a tension free anastomosis.

Orient the patient in the Trendelenburg position with the left side tilted up, which displaces the small intestine into the upper abdomen. This provides an opportunity to appreciate the pelvic anatomy in its entirety before starting the dissection (Tip 5.4).

> **Tip 5.4 Pelvic Anatomy**
> Prior to any mobilization or resection, inspect the abdominal and pelvic cavity to evaluate for any altered anatomy (phlegmon or occult metastatic processes) not previously appreciated or identified on preoperative imaging, as well as anatomical relationships.

Step 3: Identification of the Inferior Mesenteric Artery

Knowledge of the vascular anatomy is paramount to understanding both the vascular supply to the colon and rectum for creation of a healthy and viable anastomosis and ability to perform appropriate lymphadenectomy for cancer. The inferior mesenteric artery (IMA) is the last branch of the aorta prior to its bifurcation into the iliac vessels. The takeoff of the IMA occurs roughly at the level of L3 vertebrae. The IMA and its branches are the vascular supply to the hindgut structures including the distal transverse, descending, sigmoid colon, and the rectum. The left colic artery is the first branch off the IMA and is typically located 2 cm distal to the origin of the IMA. The distal transverse colon and descending colon are perfused via the ascending branch of the left colic artery, while the descending colon and proximal sigmoid colon are supplied by the descending branches of the left colic artery. Distally, the IMA gives off various sigmoid branches, courses over the left common iliac artery, and then gives rise to the superior rectal arteries. The superior rectal arteries supply the distal sigmoid and upper rectum.

The initial dissection for a left colectomy develops the avascular plane between the parietal peritoneum overlying the retroperitoneum and the visceral peritoneum encompassing the mesentery of the left colon. There are multiple approaches including medial to lateral and lateral to medial. The medial approach is preferred for several reasons:

1. Lateral abdominal wall attachments of the colon function as a fulcrum, exerting counter-traction to the uplifted mesocolon and aid the initial mesenteric dissection.
2. Manipulation of the diseased segment of colon is minimized.
3. Early identification of the ureter and gonadal vessels reduces the risk of damage to these retroperitoneal structures.
4. Early division of vascular pedicles reduces subsequent bleeding from dissection.

The medial-to-lateral approach will be covered in this chapter. In the setting of inflammatory disease or circumferential malignancy, this approach generally allows for exposure to virgin, disease-free planes of dissection without adhesions to other vital structures. In some cases, a combination of medial-to-lateral and lateral-to-medial dissection may be necessary or beneficial to avoid injury of vital structures by obtaining various anatomic exposures and allow forward progression during the operation.

For a medial approach, identify the IMA pedicle. Next, find the mesenteric fold containing the IMA overlying and cephalad to the sacral promontory. The assistant then retracts the sigmoid and left colon mesentery anteriorly, through the LLQ port, which bowstrings the IMA pedicle as it enters the pelvis to form the superior rectal artery (Fig. 5.2).

Adhesions to the left pelvic sidewall may prevent adequate ventral retraction of the colon and visualization of the IMA in benign inflammatory diseases such as diverticulitis. If this occurs, retract the colon towards the patient's right side with the left hand and use electrocautery to carefully dissect the filmy tissues between colon and epiploica on the medial side and the retroperitoneum on the left. Start with the most obvious adhesions, continuing proximally and distally, preserving the shiny retroperitoneum on the sidewall (Pitfall 5.1). If a clear bowstring of the IMA is not visualized after division of these adhesions, the surgeon can consider an alternative approach such as the lateral approach to successfully mobilize the left colon (see Step 11*).

> ⚠️ **Pitfall 5.1**
> When dissecting adhesions from the left colon to the pelvic brim and left sidewall, the ureter and iliac vessels have not yet been identified. Care should be taken not to score deeply. A light touch with the cautery or cold laparoscopic scissors are used to carefully dissect just the adhesions, without entering the retroperitoneum.

Fig. 5.2 Identification of the IMA pedicle. Ventral retraction of the sigmoid colon out of the pelvis will highlight the IMA pedicle in relation to the sacral promontory and underlying common iliac vessels

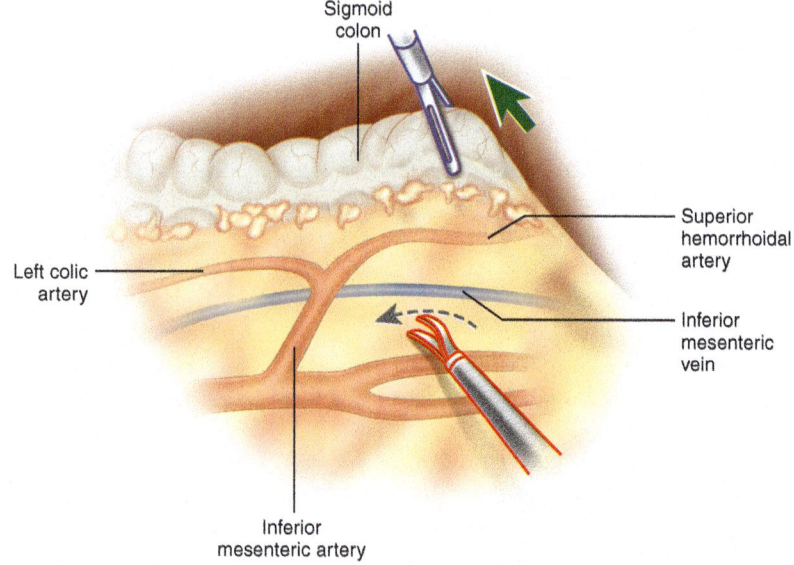

Sigmoid colon

Superior hemorrhoidal artery

Left colic artery

Inferior mesenteric vein

Inferior mesenteric artery

Once the IMA has been clearly identified, score the mesentery with electrocautery parallel to the posterior aspect of the IMA pedicle to enter into the avascular plane. The fenestration of the mesentery overlying the sacral promontory creates a ballooning pillow-type effect as air enters the avascular plane and expands the mesentery away from the presacral fascia, aorta, iliac vessels, and autonomic nerves. Extend this incision proximally towards the origin of the IMA and distally into the pelvis. Opening the window widely allows visualization under the IMA to the left sidewall. Use electrocautery to open the peritoneum. The tissues deep to the IMA can be bluntly swept towards the retroperitoneum.

The dissection can be continued to the IMA origin, but transection of the IMA is not performed until retroperitoneal structures, such as the ureter and hypogastric nerves, have been isolated and preserved out of harm's way (Fig. 5.3) (see Steps 5–7 below).

Step 4: Identification of the Proper Retroperitoneal Plane

The ureters lay under the parietal peritoneum along the pelvic sidewall on the anterior surface of the psoas muscle. They follow a straight path from the renal pelvis to the pelvic brim, 4–5 cm laterally to the IVC and the aorta, respectively, and run medial and parallel to the gonadal vessels above the pelvic brim. The ureters cross the iliac vessels to enter the pelvic brim. The right ureter classically traverses the external iliac artery, whereas the left ureter lies slightly more medial and typically crosses the common iliac artery. The ureters run posterior and inferior along the lateral pelvic sidewall before entering the posterolateral surface of the bladder to form the trigone (Pitfall 5.2).

> ⚠ **Pitfall 5.2**
> When performing a laparoscopic left colectomy or pelvic dissection, the ureters may be encountered in two locations: (1) where they cross over the common iliac vessels and (2) the lateral walls of the pouch of Douglas as they course beneath either vas deferens or the uterine arteries. They must be identified and preserved at both locations to ensure a safe complication free operation.

Step 5: Identification of the Ureter and Other Vital Structures

At times, the ureter may not be easily identified, due to a surrounding fat pad, or if the ureter has been mobilized ventrally with the inferior mesenteric

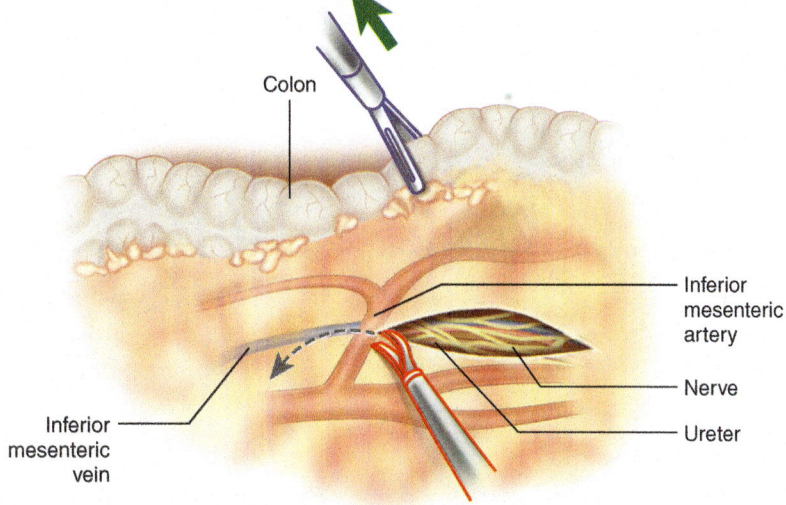

Fig. 5.3 Identification of ureter and retroperitoneal structures. Prior to ligation of the IMA, the ureter and gonadal vessels should be clearly identified

Colon

Inferior mesenteric artery

Nerve

Ureter

Inferior mesenteric vein

artery. In cases where the ureter has not initially been identified, back up, reidentify the inferior mesenteric artery, and release any additional tissue laterally that may have been swept up with the vessel. If the ureter is still not identified, vary the approach to a lateral-to-medial approach by taking the attachments on the left sidewall and white line of Toldt. This will allow identification of the ureter from the lateral side, ensuring that it is mobilized away from the IMA prior to transection (Tip 5.5).

> 💡 **Tip 5.5 Use of Ureteral Stents**
> Occasionally, in the setting of inflammatory disease, prior radiation therapy, or reoperative pelvic surgery, placement of preoperative ureteral catheters/stents may aid in visualization of the ureters. Though these stents do not minimize the risk for transection or injury, they do permit for earlier identification of these events and facilitate correction.

The sympathetic and parasympathetic nerves can also be injured during dissection of the inferior mesenteric artery and rectum. High ligation of the IMA may lead to injury of the sympathetic preaortic nerves, high on the nerve root. The hypogastric nerves can be injured at the sacral promontory where the hypogastric plexus gives rise to two main hypogastric nerve trunks which travel along the lateral sacrum and pelvic sidewalls. Deeper in the pelvis, the pelvic plexus is located lateral to the lower rectum in the lateral stalks of the mesorectum.

Develop the avascular plane between the mesorectum and presacral fascia at the level of the sacral promontory or the concavity of the sacrum to expose the superior hypogastric plexus and the hypogastric nerves (Fig. 5.4). Refrain from the use of electrocautery until the planes are defined, using blunt sweeping for all of the nerve roots that do not travel directly into the colon and rectum to prevent injury. As dissection proceeds, the correct plane will be medial and anterior to the nerves (Pitfall 5.3).

> ⚠️ **Pitfall 5.3**
> Nerve injury leads to functional issues: sympathetic denervation with intact parasympathetic innervation leads to bladder dysfunction and retrograde ejaculation. Damage to the sympathetic and parasympathetics at the pelvic plexus can lead to rectal, urinary, erectile dysfunction, vaginal dryness, and dyspareunia.

Step 6: Transection of the IMA Pedicle

Once the key retroperitoneal structures have been identified, the inferior mesenteric artery is ligated to

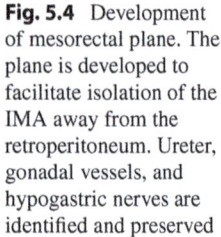

Fig. 5.4 Development of mesorectal plane. The plane is developed to facilitate isolation of the IMA away from the retroperitoneum. Ureter, gonadal vessels, and hypogastric nerves are identified and preserved

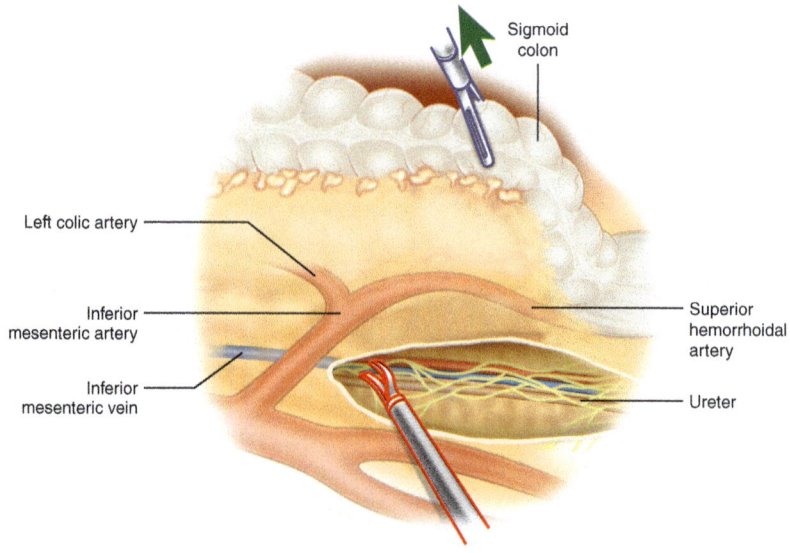

Sigmoid colon

Left colic artery

Inferior mesenteric artery

Inferior mesenteric vein

Superior hemorrhoidal artery

Ureter

facilitate the pelvic dissection (Fig. 5.5). There are several methods to securely divide the IMA. Options include utilization of energy devices (bipolar or ultrasonic-type devices), endomechanical stapling, endoloops, and clips. The choice of which ligation and division method utilized is dependent upon patient and anatomic features (calcification, inflammatory disease, vessel size) as well as cost. When the surgeon is using an energy device throughout the procedure, it may be most cost-effective to continue using this modality for vessel ligation/division. If calcification is noted, mechanical ligation and division with a stapler or clips can facilitate a more secure closure. During transection, release tension on the vessel to allow the device to fully ligate and divide the vessel. The transection device is held in one hand, while an atraumatic grasper provides appropriate exposure on the vessel. An assistant's instrument is available to occlude a vessel and prevent blood loss in case of bleeding from the stump (Tip 5.6).

colon and proximal sigmoid colon. Typically, this is not a limiting factor in achieving adequate mobilization of the colon into the deep pelvis.

Step 7: Development of the Retroperitoneal Plane via Medial-to-Lateral Dissection

After transection of the IMA, elevate the newly dissected pedicle and mesocolon with the left hand. This exposes the faint white line of the retroperitoneum. Sweep the shiny surface of the retroperitoneum down with the right hand, using a bipolar or blunt bowel grasper, above the plane that contains the nerves, ureters, and gonadal vessels. By adjusting tension with the left hand, the plane can continue laterally to the white line of Toldt (Tip 5.7).

> 💡 **Tip 5.6 Preservation of the Left Colic Artery in Benign Disease**
> In benign disease, the left colic artery can often be preserved by dividing the superior rectal artery (branch of the IMA as it crosses over the left common iliac artery), thereby maintaining collateral flow to the distal descending

> 💡 **Tip 5.7 Tension and Counter-Tension**
> The critical maneuver in performing a medial-to-lateral dissection is to sustain proper tension and counter-tension. Only by doing so will surgeon be able to identify and maintain the correct plane allowing the procedure to continue along its natural progression.

Fig. 5.5 Ligation of the IMA. Mobilization cephalad and caudal to the takeoff of the IMA will give a "T" appearance; this allows proper identification of the IMA and left colic artery which may be preserved when appropriate

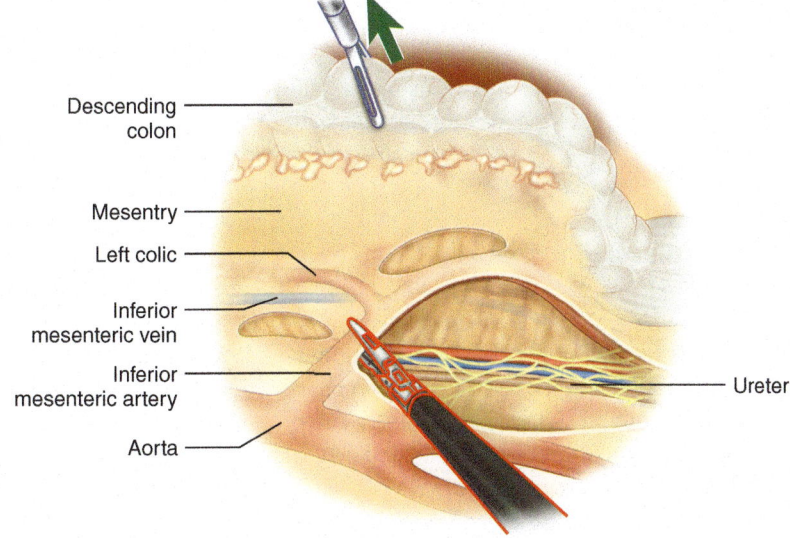

Fig. 5.6 Medial dissection. Optimizing the medial dissection helps to facilitate lateral dissection as well as entry into the lesser sac. The dissection can continue laterally under the colon, superiorly to the border of the pancreas, and inferiorly to the pelvic brim

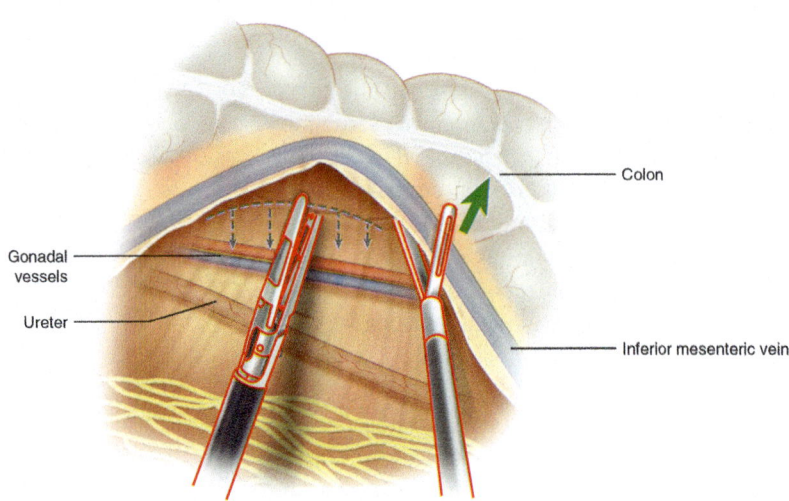

The plane is maintained cephalad to the level of the superior pole of the kidney and inferior aspect of the spleen (Fig. 5.6). Care should be taken to not mobilize under the tail of the pancreas as the dissection proceeds cephalad in the region of the IMV; make sure the plane transitions anterior to the pancreas. The pancreas can be identified by its typical salmon color.

Inferiorly, the plane can continue to the pelvic brim. Occasionally, small vessels may require electrocautery or bipolar/ultrasonic energy to prevent bleeding. Mesenteric vessels run perpendicular to the colon; retroperitoneal vessels run parallel to the colon and may be swept down with the retroperitoneum. Bleeding or poor visualization generally indicates the surgeon is in the inappropriate retroperitoneal plane and should relocate more superficially (ventrally/closer to the mesentery). The correct plane is relatively avascular and clear.

At this point, the IMV may be identified, and mobilization of the splenic flexure may be performed.

Step 8: Transection of the IMV Pedicle (if Needed)

A proximal ligation of the IMV aids in optimizing mobilization for tension-free colorectal or coloanal anastomoses. With the colon mesentery retracted anteriorly, just distal to the ligament of Treitz, the inferior mesenteric vein (IMV) can be

identified with avascular areas surrounding the vessel (Fig. 5.7). Often, the fourth part of the duodenum or proximal jejunum will have some attachments to the descending colon mesentery in this area that will need to be divided for full mobilization. Use either cold scissors or electrocautery to prevent lateral spread of heat to the duodenum.

The IMV transection is performed at the inferior aspect of the pancreas. Ligation can generally be performed with an energy source such as ultrasonic shears or bipolar-type vessel sealing devices. Use care to avoid excess tension or inappropriate ligation that can cause injury to the IMV which can retract into the retroperitoneum and cause excessive bleeding which is difficult to control.

Once performed, the mesentery of the splenic flexure can then be retracted ventrally, and the retroperitoneal reflection line of Toldt mobilization can then be continued. Mobilization proceeds proximally and superiorly as cranial as possible towards the spleen.

Step 9: Lateral Attachment Release

Once medial-to-lateral mobilization is completed, the remaining avascular lateral attachments of the colon to the omentum, spleen, and abdominal and retroperitoneal sidewalls are divided (Fig. 5.8). Grasp the descending colon

Fig. 5.7 IMV identification and transection. The IMV is identified at the inferior tail of the pancreas near the splenic flexure

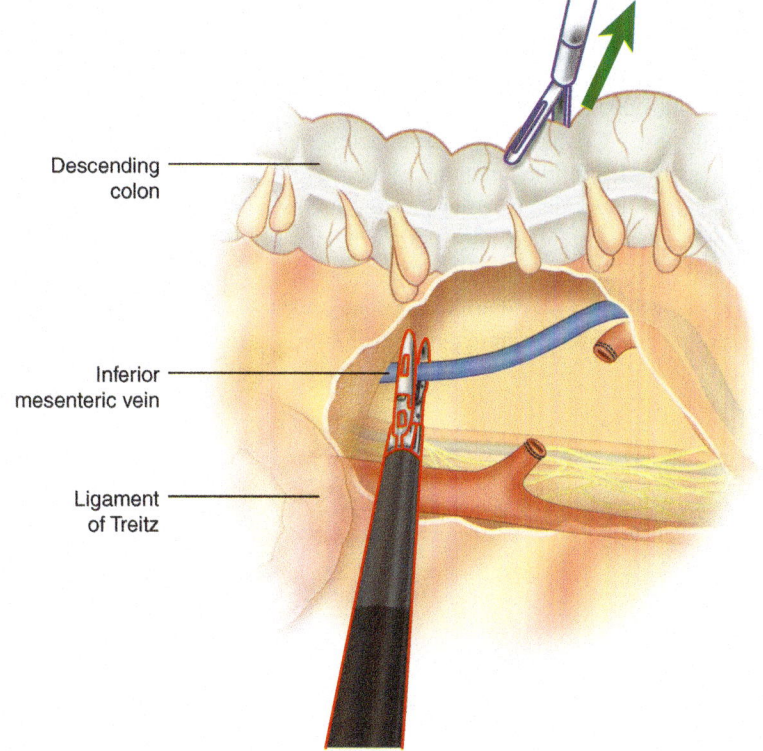

Descending colon

Inferior mesenteric vein

Ligament of Treitz

and retract medially with the right upper quadrant port. This provides appropriate tension and exposure of the lateral attachments at the white line Toldt. Frequently, there will be a bluish-purple hue visible beneath this tissue from the prior medial-to-lateral dissection/mobilization and CO_2 exposure.

Division of these attachments is performed using sharp non-energized scissors, electrocautery, or energy devices. This plane is mobilized cephalad to the splenic flexure with eventual entry into the lesser sac from the patient's left side.

Step 10: Splenic Flexure Mobilization (if Necessary)

Splenic flexure mobilization is generally performed using a combination of approaches. The patient is placed in a reverse Trendelenburg position with the table inclined towards the right. If an adequate medial-to-lateral mobilization was performed on the left colon, then the remaining

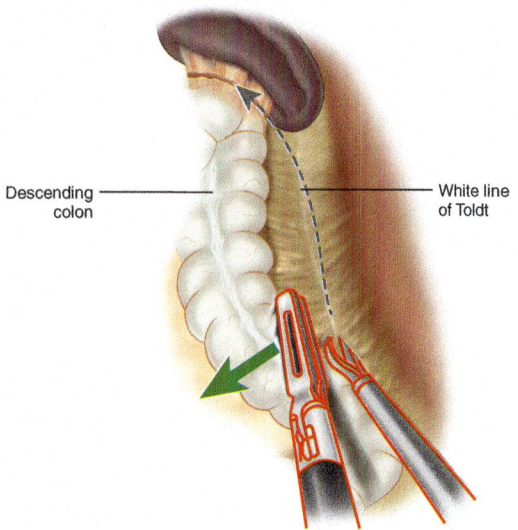

Descending colon

White line of Toldt

Fig. 5.8 Lateral dissection at white line of Toldt. When dividing the lateral attachments, dissection is carried from the pelvis towards the splenic flexure

splenic flexure attachments may only consist of the omentum and lateral attachments of the splenocolic ligaments.

Start at the falciform ligament to divide the gastrocolic attachments of the omentum. The surgeon's left hand will elevate the omentum, while the assistant, standing between the legs, pulls the colon inferiorly. Congenital fusion attachments of the posterior leaf of the omentum to the mesocolon need to be divided to enter into the lesser sac, which is verified by visualization of the posterior wall of the stomach (Fig. 5.9). The omental window is generally close to the colon; after entering the window, the omentum can be ele- vated and the colon stretched laterally to prevent inadvertent injury to a redundant colon, as the plane approaches the splenic flexure. As the plane approaches the colon, ensure that tension on attachments to the spleen is minimal. Often times, there will be close and dense adhesions of the colon to the spleen. Use an energy device or ultrasonic in the right hand to ensure hemostasis without significant tension (Fig. 5.10).

At this point, the previous dissection plane from the prior lateral attachment release (Step 10)

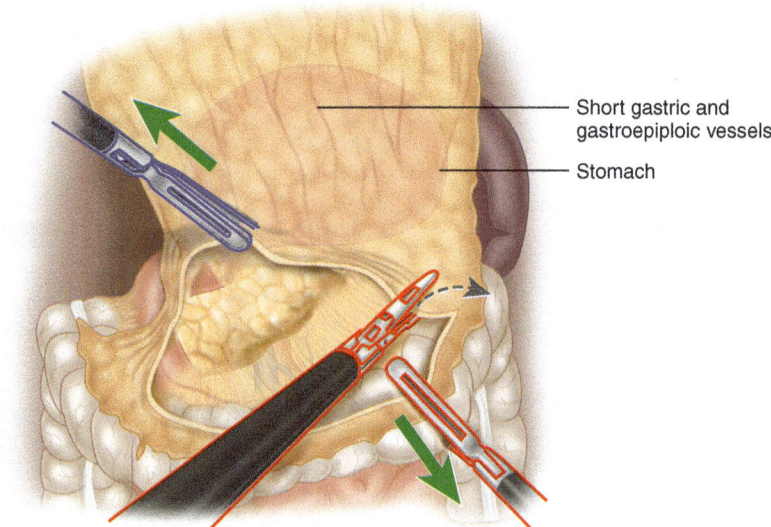

Fig. 5.9 Entry into the lesser sac. The lesser sac is identified by visualization of the posterior wall of the stomach. Often, congenital fusion attachments must be divided to enter the correct space, facilitating complete mobilization of the splenic flexure

Short gastric and gastroepiploic vessels

Stomach

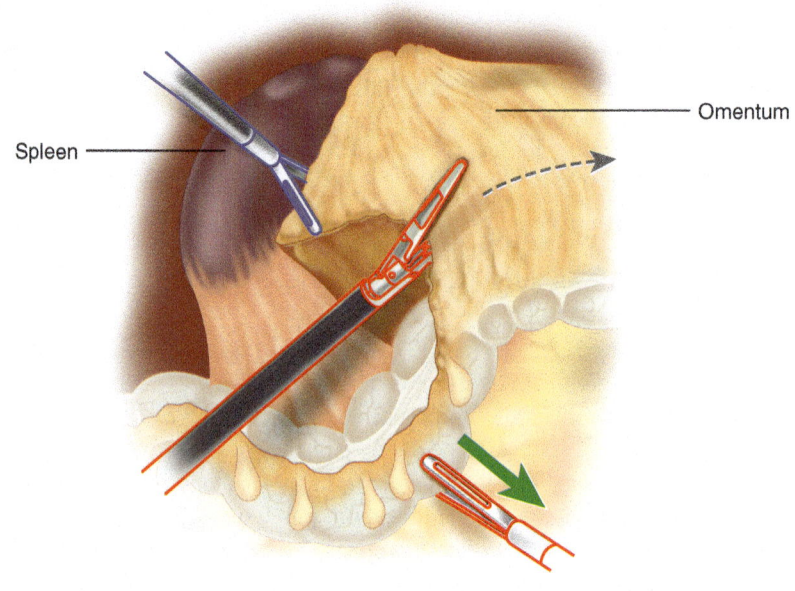

Fig. 5.10 Splenic flexure mobilization. The attachments to the sidewall and spleen are carefully divided while being mindful not to injure the splenic capsule

Spleen

Omentum

should be met. Attachments of the colonic mesentery to stomach may be encountered and safely divided, precluding inadvertent gastric injury. Roll the splenic flexure medially to determine if any posterior attachments exist which will limit mobilization and reach, transecting these attachments at this time. Check the reach into the pelvis by gently pulling the colon towards the pelvis; if additional adhesions exist, transect them at this time.

Step 11: Distal Transection

A critical step in left or anterior resection is identification of a distal transection point. Distal transection localization is dependent upon both anatomic and physiologic entities. Appropriate mesenteric vascular supply must be accounted for as well as distal resection margins in the setting of malignancy. For a sigmoid or distal left colectomy, division is generally performed at the level of the proximal rectum, distal to the splaying of the tenia coli on the antimesenteric surface (Tip 5.8).

Once the point of transection is selected, the assistant grasps the bowel at the location of tran-

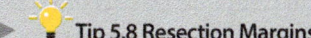

> 💡 **Tip 5.8 Resection Margins**
> For diverticular disease, transection typically occurs at the upper rectum where the tenia has already splayed. Resection of the high pressure zone encountered in the rectosigmoid colon minimizes recurrence of diverticular disease distal to the anastomosis. For malignant disease, distal dissection and transection may be required for appropriate oncologic margins. Generally, at least a 5-cm distal margin is required for colonic malignancies.

section, which frees the surgeon to use two hands to divide the mesentery. This can proceed in an antegrade fashion from the posterior fascia propria of the mesorectum and working through the mesorectum and towards the posterior wall of the rectum. An alternative retrograde method involves creation of a window between the posterior wall of the rectum and mesentery at the proposed transection site (Fig. 5.11). The fascia is

Fig. 5.11 Division of the mesorectum. Once the site of distal transection has been identified, the mesorectum is divided by creating a window between the posterior wall of the rectum and the mesorectal fat. The mesorectum is then divided with an energy device to maintain hemostasis and avoid troublesome bleeding

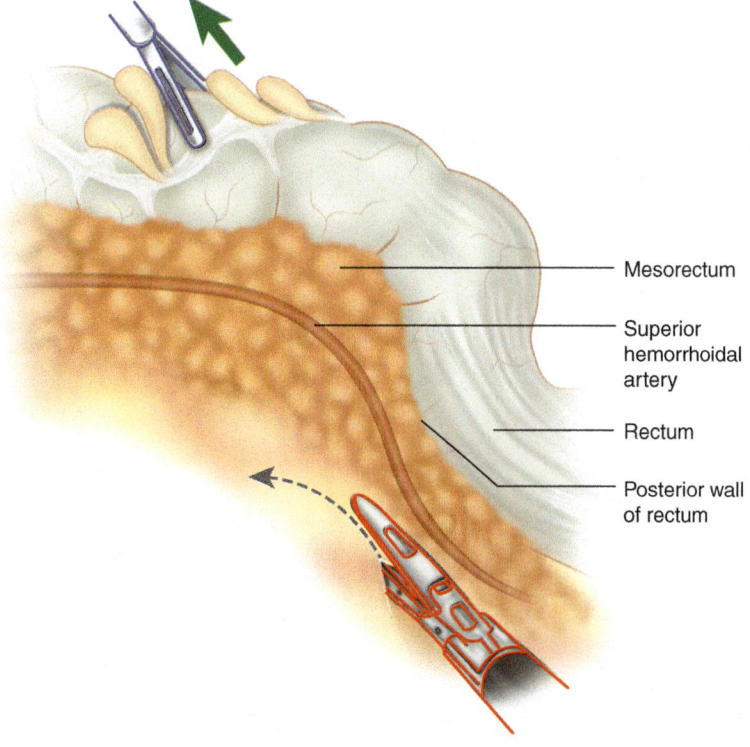

Mesorectum

Superior hemorrhoidal artery

Rectum

Posterior wall of rectum

scored with electrocautery. A bowel grasper is used to identify the posterior aspect of the rectum by spreading just below the rectum. Transect all the tissue lateral and posterior to the identified rectum with an energy instrument. Continue in this fashion of identification of the posterior rectal wall and dissection lateral and posterior until the rectum has been freed circumferentially. With both approaches, mesenteric division should remain perpendicular to rectal stump to maintain appropriate vascular supply to the anastomosis.

Once the mesentery has been dissected from the rectum, divide the rectum with an endomechanical stapling device through the RLQ port

(Fig. 5.12a). Choose the stapling load based on the thickness of the tissue to be divided. Additional loads may be required in some cases.

Security and completeness of the rectal stump staple line may be tested at this point. Submerge the rectal stump under sterile solution using a suction irrigator and gently insufflate per anus (Fig. 5.12b). This can be done using rigid proctoscopy, flexible sigmoidoscopy, or bulb syringe insufflation. Endoscopy allows for visualization of the mucosa and staple line as well as leak test. The leak test is performed by direct laparoscopic visualization during rectal insufflation. The rectal stump should be completely submerged, and the

Fig. 5.12 Transection and evaluation of rectal stump. (**a**) The rectum is divided with an endoscopic GIA stapler. Multiple loads may be required; careful attention should be taken to avoid a staggered staple line. (**b**) The security and completeness of the rectal stump staple line may be tested. The stump is submerged under sterile solution, and gentle insufflation per anus is performed

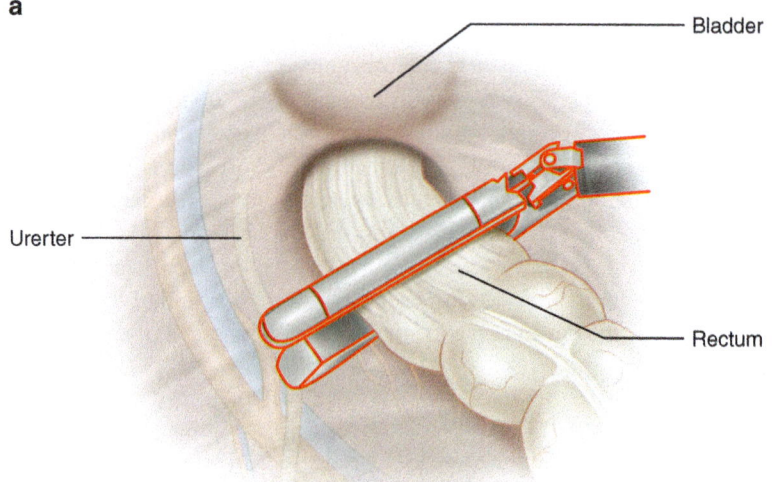

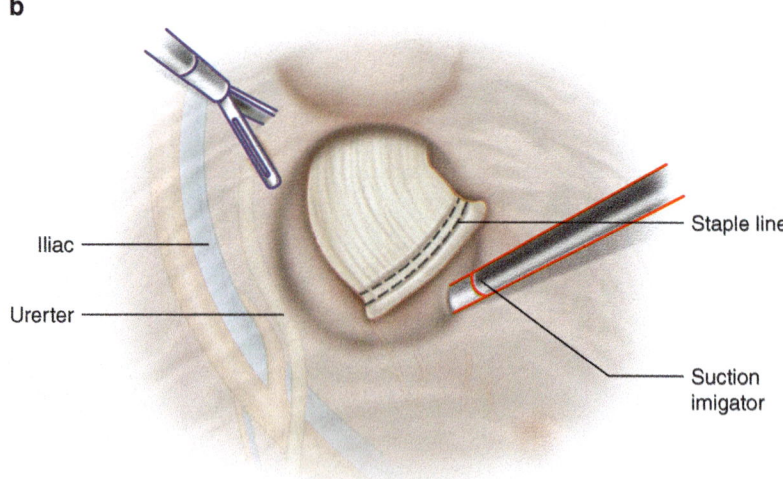

surgeon confirms appropriate distention of the stump without air leak (visualized bubbles). If an air leak is encountered at this point, two options are available. The first is to introduce the spike of the end-to-end anastomotic circular stapler through the defect. The second option is to resect an additional distal margin incorporating the prior staple line. Air testing may then be repeated.

Step 12: Extraction and Proximal Transection

Prior to extraction, grasp the distal end of the colon with a locking grasper and place the stapled colon under the location of the anticipated extraction site. A choice of extraction site exists. Options include extension of the periumbilical incision, creation of a Pfannenstiel incision, or extension of the RLQ incision (Tip 5.9). Once the abdominal wall is opened and the peritoneal cavity entered, insert a wound protector to protect the skin and soft tissue from contamination during externalization and creation of anastomosis. This also maximizes the exposure with respect to the size of the incision.

> **Tip 5.9 Pfannenstiel Incision**
> In a patient who has had prior abdominal operations, using a prior incision may be appropriate. Cosmetically, a Pfannenstiel incision may be preferable and may minimize hernia rates. The incision size will vary between 3 and 6 cm and is determined by the size of the pathology and the patient's body habitus.

Through the wound protector, the proximal colon and mesentery are externalized. The proximal dissection point is determined. In the setting of malignancy, at least a 5-cm margin is required. With Crohn's or inflammatory disease, the site should be chosen while assuring a soft, supple, disease-free area along the colon without evidence of disease. In all cases, appropriate maintenance of vascular supply is confirmed to minimize the risk of ischemia of the anastomosis. Sharp transection of the marginal artery with resultant pulsatile flow from the proximal end is one method to verify and document appropriate healthy vascular tissue. Newer methods including fluorescence imaging may also be utilized to identify well perfused, vascular tissue prior to transection.

Step 13: Anastomosis and Intraoperative Leak Testing

A double-stapled technique is often employed during a left or sigmoid colectomy. An end-to-end anastomotic (EEA) stapler height is chosen based on tissue thickness and compliance of the tissue. The diameter of the stapler will also vary between 28 and 33 mm and may be selected based on the diameter of the proximal and distal bowel as well as patient's anal tone. Too small of an aperture may lead to stenosis or stricture.

End to end The anvil of the circular stapler is secured in the proximal bowel at the distal end using a purse string. The purse string may be placed utilizing several techniques including manual placement of a monofilament suture (Fig. 5.13a), disposable purse-string device, or reusable clamp using a straight Keith needle.

When the point of transection is decided, the purse-string clamp is applied perpendicular to the bowel. The suture passed back and forth through the keyholes using the Keith needle and the distal colon divided flush with the clamp. The colotomy with purse string is opened and the anvil placed within it, with the spike extending through the colotomy. The purse string is then cinched and tied down, securing the anvil in place. Redundant tissue created by the closure of the purse string is trimmed to minimize the risk of additional tissue being incorporated into the stapler well and along the staple line, which can disrupt proper stapler closure and anastomosis integrity.

Side to end Proponents of this method (also called Baker anastomosis) (Tip 5.10) favor this due to the theoretical increased vascularity of the anastomosis as there is perfusion circumferentially to the anastomosis. In diverticular disease, it can avoid incorporation of diverticula at the

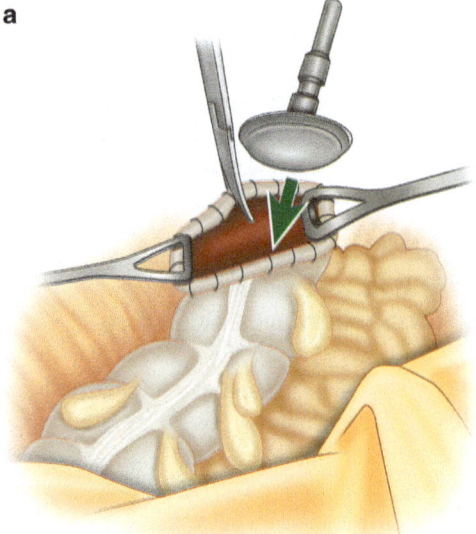

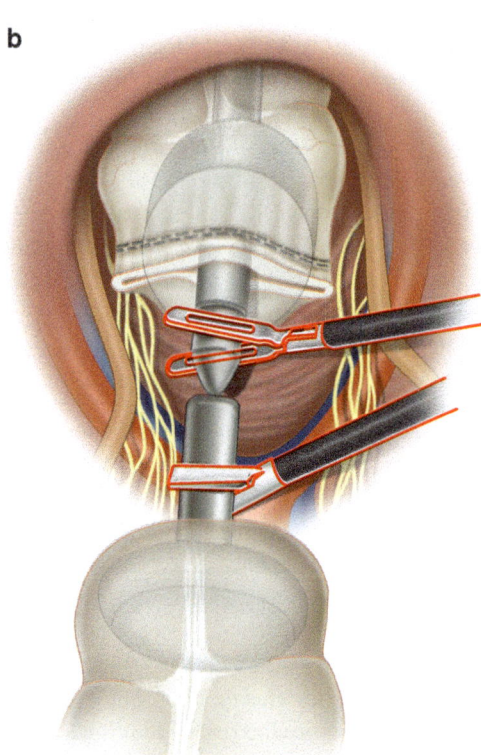

Fig. 5.13 Creation of anastomosis. The purse string may be placed utilizing several techniques including (**a**) manual placement with a monofilament, disposable purse-string device, or a reusable purse-string clamp. (**b**) The anvil is placed on the end of the stapler intralumenally

purse string by using the unaffected antimesenteric portion of the bowel. Also, when performed in the setting of a distal coloanal anastomosis, it provides for a fecal reservoir (or pouch) to minimize stool frequency.

> **Tip 5.10 Baker Anastomosis**
> Baker anastomosis: too short of a stump between the staple line and circular stapler may result in ischemia; too long of a distal end can lead to constipation and difficulty evacuating.

At the point of proximal colon transection, the bowel is divided between clamps. Any remaining distal mesentery attached to the specimen side is ligated and divided and the specimen subsequently passed off the field. The anvil of the EEA stapler is introduced via the colotomy and brought out 5 cm proximally along the antimesenteric wall between the two teniae coli. This is done by making a very small pinpoint colotomy in this location while tenting the wall of the colon with the plastic spike in the anvil. The anvil is secured in place with a monofilament purse-string suture around the base of the anvil. The plastic spike is taken off from within the anvil and discarded.

The colotomy is closed using another firing of the endoscopic (or open) linear anastomotic stapler. Based on surgeon preference, this staple line may be secured with Lembert imbricating sutures. The proximal colon is then placed back within the peritoneal cavity. Gloves are changed (Tip 5.11).

> **Tip 5.11 Preventing Wound Infections**
> The inside of the colon is colonized with bacteria that increase the rate of wound infections during colorectal procedures. By changing gloves and passing all instruments off the sterile field after manipulating the inside of the, the surgeon can minimize the rate of wound infections.

Anastomosis creation Once the anvil is secured in place, the proximal colon is placed back within the peritoneal cavity. The extraction site may be permanently closed with the appropriate suture or temporarily closed by twisting of the wound protector tightly and securing it with a clamp or a wet laparotomy pack. When pneumoperitoneum is reestablished, several spot checks should occur before proceeding with the anastomosis. First, confirm the colon and its mesentery are not twisted or kinked by following the free edge of the mesentery back to the retroperitoneal attachments. There should be a straight line appreciated. Second, ensure that the small intestine has not been entrapped by the mobilized left colonic mesentery which may result in immediate postoperative obstruction. Finally, confirmation of adequate mobilization and mesenteric length to create a tension-free anastomosis should be performed prior to completing the anastomosis. Attempting to achieve further mobilization after the anastomosis has been created can result in ischemia of the distal colon and possibly disruption of the anastomosis.

The assistant goes to the patient's perineum to perform the anastomosis. The circular stapler is introduced per anus and advanced until flush with the staple line. Under laparoscopic guidance, the middle of the stapler is placed appropriately at the end of the rectum. If the staple line is created in a longitudinal fashion, extrude the spike just posterior of the center of the bowel circumference. This may minimize the potential for inclusion of the vagina or other neurovascular structures in the anastomosis.

The stapler knob is turned counterclockwise to express the spike posterior to the transverse staple line. Once the spike is completely extended, a marking line is visible towards the base of the stapler. At this point, no movement should be made by the operator from below. The anvil is mated to the spike from above. Mating the anvil to the spike may be challenging especially in the morbidly obese or in the narrow male pelvis. Typically, the proximal colon with anvil is placed at the pelvic brim for easy retrieval when performing the anastomosis.

Once the spike is in the correct position, the anvil is grasped along its shaft away from the tip, to help maneuver the anvil over the spike (Fig. 5.13b). The assistant holding the EEA stapler should remain still throughout this maneuver but may need to adjust their hands slightly to assist sliding the anvil over the spike. A click is heard and/or palpated, and the reference line should no longer be visible once the anvil and spike are mated securely. Reconfirm orientation of the proximal bowel.

Close the stapler by turning the knob. Based on the stapler manufacturer, there is demarcation of an appropriate amount of tissue compression applied with either a green line or a range of green noted on the stapler. Once satisfied with the appearance of the closed stapler, the safety is released, and the stapler fired by squeezing the handle in one brisk movement, with appropriate force. Take care not to release or squeeze the handle repeatedly or part way with release and reapplication as this can result in firing of the cutting blade numerous times and creation of a potential leak. Maintain the stapler in position with minimal torquing movement during stapling to prevent too much sheering and traction on the anastomosis. Depending on the manufacturer, the anastomotic device should be released per instructions.

The stapler is withdrawn. Inspection of the anastomotic rings (or donuts) should verify two intact circumferential rings representing the proximal and distal ends of intestine. The proximal ring will have the purse-string suture in place.

Air leak testing
Testing of the anastomosis has been demonstrated to reduce the incidence of missed anastomotic leak (Tip 5.12). The anastomosis is submerged under sterile saline solution while the proximal colon is occluded using an atraumatic grasper (Fig. 5.14). The intestine is insufflated using a variety of modalities including rigid proctoscopy, flexible sigmoidoscopy, or bulb syringe. Flexible sigmoidoscopy is preferred to allow superior visualization of the mucosa and staple

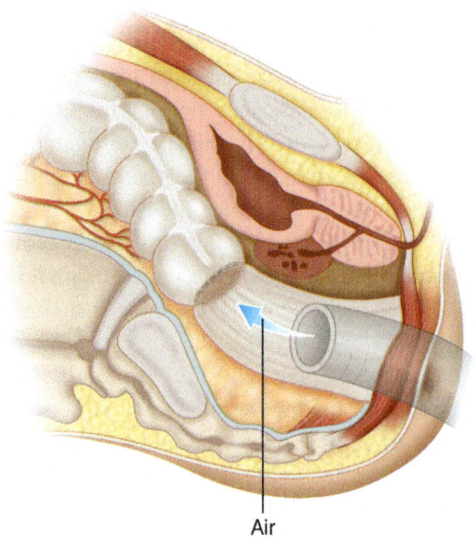

Air

Fig. 5.14 Hydropneumatic leak test. The proximal descending colon is occluded to prevent insufflation of the entire colon, and the anastomosis is submerged under saline to check for air leak

line as well as quick resolution of CO_2. If an air leak is encountered, several options exist including direct repair of the anastomotic leak point(s) with or without fecal diversion, takedown and creation of a new anastomosis, or creation of an end colostomy. Choosing the appropriate surgical management of a positive air leak test is dependent on multiple factors and is beyond the scope of this chapter.

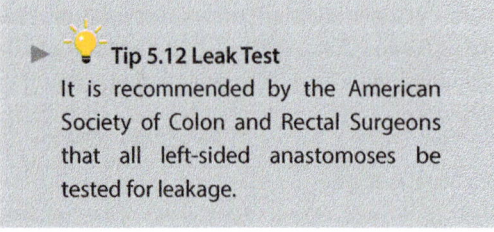

▶ 💡 **Tip 5.12 Leak Test**
It is recommended by the American Society of Colon and Rectal Surgeons that all left-sided anastomoses be tested for leakage.

Step 14: Closure

The extraction sites and all port sites 10 mm or greater in size are closed. A port site closure device may be used to close any port sites laparoscopically.

Special Considerations

Alternative Approaches

Lateral approach is often used in cases of diverticular disease or phlegmatous disease of the left sidewall. This method is preferred when the surgeon has trouble identifying the ureter at the inferior mesenteric artery.

Adhesions from the left sidewall and pelvic brim are performed as described above (Step 7). Lateral attachments at the white line of Toldt are opened as described in Step 11. The major difference is that with the lack of prior medial dissection, the purple hue and thin plane will not yet exist. The left hand is used to retract the colon medially, and scissors are generally used in the right hand to free the white line of Toldt cephalad. The plane is often closer to the colon, with a second white fold more laterally that will mistakenly lead the surgeon into the retroperitoneum and behind the kidney if pursued.

The shiny plane of the retroperitoneum should be maintained over the retroperitoneum, providing separation and protection from the gonadal vessels, ureters, and hypogastric nerves. The plane can be continued up to and around the splenic flexure from this lateral side. Continuous retraction with the left hand will provide much needed counter-tension to continue the dissection.

Distally, prior to freeing attachments over the pelvic brim, the ureter should be identified and maintained with retroperitoneum. Again, the plane will be medial, close to the colon and mesocolon. Once the ureter and retroperitoneum have been preserved from this lateral aspect, switching back to the medial aspect can provide good visualization and confirmation of safe plane for IMA ligation.

In addition, although medial-to-lateral and lateral-to-medial approaches have been discussed, neither of these is used exclusively. Indeed, it is common to need multiple methods to verify anatomy and attain appropriate exposure and dissection even within a single case. In certain cases, due to disease processes and variations in anatomy, it may be required to initiate distal entry along the presacral space and then proceed with a retrograde (bottom-up) dissection. Similarly, initial dissection of the splenic flexure may help attain entry into the appropriate plane for dissection distally (top-down). The steps and areas of concern remain the same, even if the order is changed.

Fistula/Phlegmon in Diverticular Disease

In the case of fistulae or phlegmons between the colon and other intraperitoneal structures, special care must be made to minimize concomitant injury/resection. Consideration of preoperative ureteral catheters (or stents) may help in identification of these structures during dissection. Placement of the stents after obtaining laparoscopic visualization and starting some of the lateral dissection may assist the surgeon to clearly visualize the course of the ureters, which may not be anatomically predictable in these situations.

Often, a combination of lateral-to-medial and medial-to-lateral dissection is required in these cases. The phlegmon is most frequently anterior and lateral, putting ureters, bladder, and uterus at risk for fistulization. Initiating the dissection with a medial-to-lateral mobilization in the posterior plane, close to the takeoff of the IMA, may help gain access to the retroperitoneal surface and uninvolved space between the colon and its mesentery. This can aid in identification of the ureter and other structures more easily than a primary lateral-to-medial dissection. Dissection can proceed laterally with anterior retraction of the colon and mesentery.

In some cases, it may be helpful to initiate the dissection proximal to the inflammation along the proximal descending colon at an area of decreased inflammatory reaction and proceed caudally. Similarly, rectal mobilization with retrograde dissection can be helpful to mobilize the colon from the pelvic sidewall and ureter.

In certain cases, this dissection and separation of the colon to the sidewall and ureter may require manual disruption with a finger-fracture technique. To maintain laparoscopic surgery, using the suction irrigator or laparoscopic peanuts may be a substitute to gently push on structures to separate. If significant inflammation and/or abscess is encountered, conversion to open or hand-assisted surgery may be necessary to maintain patient safety. Anastomosis may be precluded by inflammation, infection, or medical comorbidities, and consideration of an end colostomy or anastomosis protected with a diverting loop ileostomy may be prudent.

If there is a fistula to the bladder or vagina, and dissection from primary process is possible, the secondary organ can often be simply dissected free without requirement for repair. In the case of the bladder, if no visible defect noted, testing with blue dye may be performed. If no leak is noted, bladder catheter drainage for a few days (3–5) with removal after negative retrograde cystogram may be adequate for adequate healing. If the defect is noted, a two-layer closure of the bladder is advised. Drainage and removal are performed as above.

The vagina is rarely in need of repair and generally will heal spontaneously once the inciting phlegmatous or fistula organ is resected. In these instances, the defect may function as a drain.

In the setting of a prior fistula (colovesical or colovaginal), the anastomosis should be placed distal to and away from the inflammation and vaginal or bladder defect. By dissecting farther down the rectum, the colon anastomosis and vaginal or bladder defect will be staggered, decreasing the chance of re-fistulization. Furthermore, a pedicle of healthy, well-vascularized mobilized omentum should be interposed and secured between the anastomosis and the anterior fistula defect to prevent future contamination and fistulous communication with the new anastomosis.

If small bowel is noted to be fistulized with the diseased colon, after separation of the fistula, either primary repair or small bowel resection is indicated. The decision is predicated upon appearance and health of the small bowel and size of the fistula.

Volvulus

Volvulus of the sigmoid colon can be encountered in the chronically infirm patient or those on other psychotropic or other agents. Occasionally, patients with long-standing chronic constipation may present with sigmoid volvulus. The laparoscopic approach is particularly helpful in these patients due to the significant redundancy encountered. These patients frequently have a very long, narrow, fixed point of mesenteric torsion that can be identified and divided using techniques as above. Depending on excess length, anastomoses can be created in a side-to-side fashion of the descending to distal rectosigmoid colon (using linear staplers) or an end-to-end or end-to-side colorectal anastomosis as described above. Extensive proximal dissection is generally not required or recommended due to the redundancy encountered. Particular attention should be made to maintain the appropriate orientation during creation of the anastomosis and to prevent torsion or volvulus of the new anastomosis itself (particularly if creating a side-to-side anastomosis).

Laparoscopic Hartmann's

In certain cases, anatomic, physiologic, or disease processes preclude safe or appropriate anastomosis. In those cases, as above, the distal colon or proximal rectum should be transected and divided using an endoscopic stapling device. If there is any potential for future anastomosis, it is helpful to add tags at the distal staple line using permanent monofilament suture to ease future identification of the rectal stump. When mobilizing the proximal sigmoid and descending colon, all attempts should be made to minimize excess dissection, mobilizing only the colon necessary to bring out a tension-free colostomy. This will aid in future Hartmann's reversal. Similarly, it may be prudent to have localizing ureteral stents placed at the time of Hartmann's reversal.

Obese Patient

Obesity presents challenges to the surgeon, particularly centered on the increased mesenteric adiposity and patient weight. To prevent falls and slippage during extremes of positioning required in these cases, extra care must be taken to tape and securely strap the patient to the bed. Obesity can create challenges in identification of landmarks and typical planes that would otherwise be easily accessed (i.e., space over the sacral promontory, around the takeoff of the IMA, retroperitoneal reflections). Additionally, the additional weight of the colon and mesentery may make appropriate retraction and visualization difficult. In these instances, liberal use of additional ports with retracting devices may be utilized. It is helpful to carefully observe the differences in coloration of the visceral mesenteric fat and the retroperitoneal fat during dissection. Additionally, an appropriate fundamental understanding of typical anatomy and landmarks and prior experience in the nonobese patient will aid in progression of dissection and performing colectomy. In all instances, if the anatomy is not clear or safety becomes a concern, conversion to an open procedure is advised.

Laparoscopic Proctectomy

6

Jason S. Mizell

Introduction

Laparoscopic proctectomy (often referred to as a low anterior resection) involves the removal of the rectum with creation of a coloanal or low colorectal anastomosis. It is performed for pathology of the rectum such as neoplasia or isolated Crohn's disease.

Indications
- Neoplasia (benign or malignant) of the rectum
- Isolated Crohn's proctitis

Preoperative Planning
- Colonoscopy to confirm diagnosis, relevant anatomy, synchronous lesions, extent of disease, and tattooing if appropriate
- Clinical assessment of fecal continence and digital rectal exam for evaluation of sphincter tone
- Preoperative staging for malignancy
  - Digital rectal exam to confirm tumor margin and fixation
  - Rigid proctoscopy to determine distance from tumor to anal verge
  - CT scan of the chest, abdomen, and pelvis for distant staging
  - MRI or endorectal ultrasound to evaluate for local staging (depth of tumor invasion and lymph node involvement)

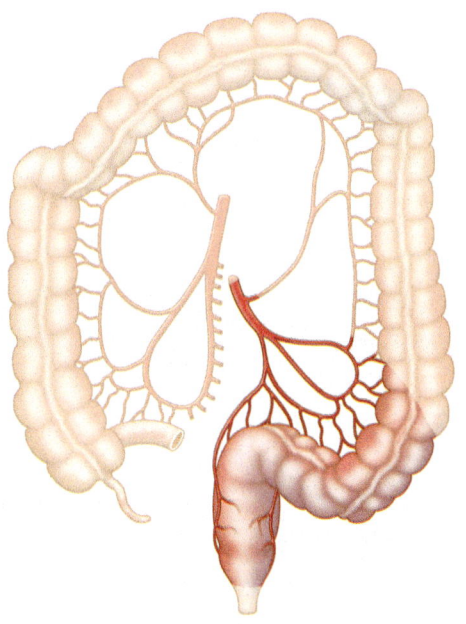

J. S. Mizell (✉)
University of Arkansas for Medical Sciences,
Division of Colon and Rectal Surgery,
Little Rock, AR, USA
e-mail: JSMizell@uams.edu

© Springer Nature Switzerland AG 2020
S. L. Stein, R. R. Lawson (eds.), *Laparoscopic Colectomy*,
https://doi.org/10.1007/978-3-030-39559-9_6

- Carcinoembryonic antigen serum level
- Consideration of neoadjuvant chemoradiation for advanced malignant disease
- Deep venous thrombosis prophylaxis
- Preoperative antibiotics
- Mechanical bowel preparation

Steps of the Operation

Patient positioning

1. Step 1: Port placement
2. Step 2: Staging laparoscopy (for neoplastic disease if indicated)
3. Step 3: Identification of pathology
4. Step 4: Creation of the retroperitoneal plane
5. Step 5: Identification of inferior mesenteric artery (IMA) and left ureter, with high ligation of IMA
6. Step 6: Ligation of the inferior mesenteric vein
7. Step 7: Mobilization of sigmoid and descending colon
8. Step 8: Splenic flexure mobilization (if indicated)
9. Step 9: Rectum mobilized for appropriate resection margins
10. Step 10: Rectal transection
11. Step 11: Colon exteriorized and specimen resected
12. Step 12: Anastomosis
13. Step 13: Formation of loop ileostomy (if indicated)
14. Step 14: Closure

Tools of the Operation

- 5 mm ports (3)
  - Fourth port occasionally needed
- 12 mm port (1)
- 5 mm 30-degree camera (1)
- 5 mm 0-degree camera if Visiport technique is to be used
- Laparoscopic bowel graspers (3)
- Laparoscopic extended cautery tip
- Laparoscopic scissors
- Energy instrument for vessel ligation (bipolar vs ultrasonic) (1)
  - Stapler for vessel ligation (optional)
- Wound protector
- Anastomosis
  - Laparoscopic linear stapling device
    1 firing if 60 mm staple load
    2 firings if 45 mm staple load
  - Circular stapling device
    Purse stringer (optional)

Patient Positioning for Laparoscopic Laparoscopic Proctectomy

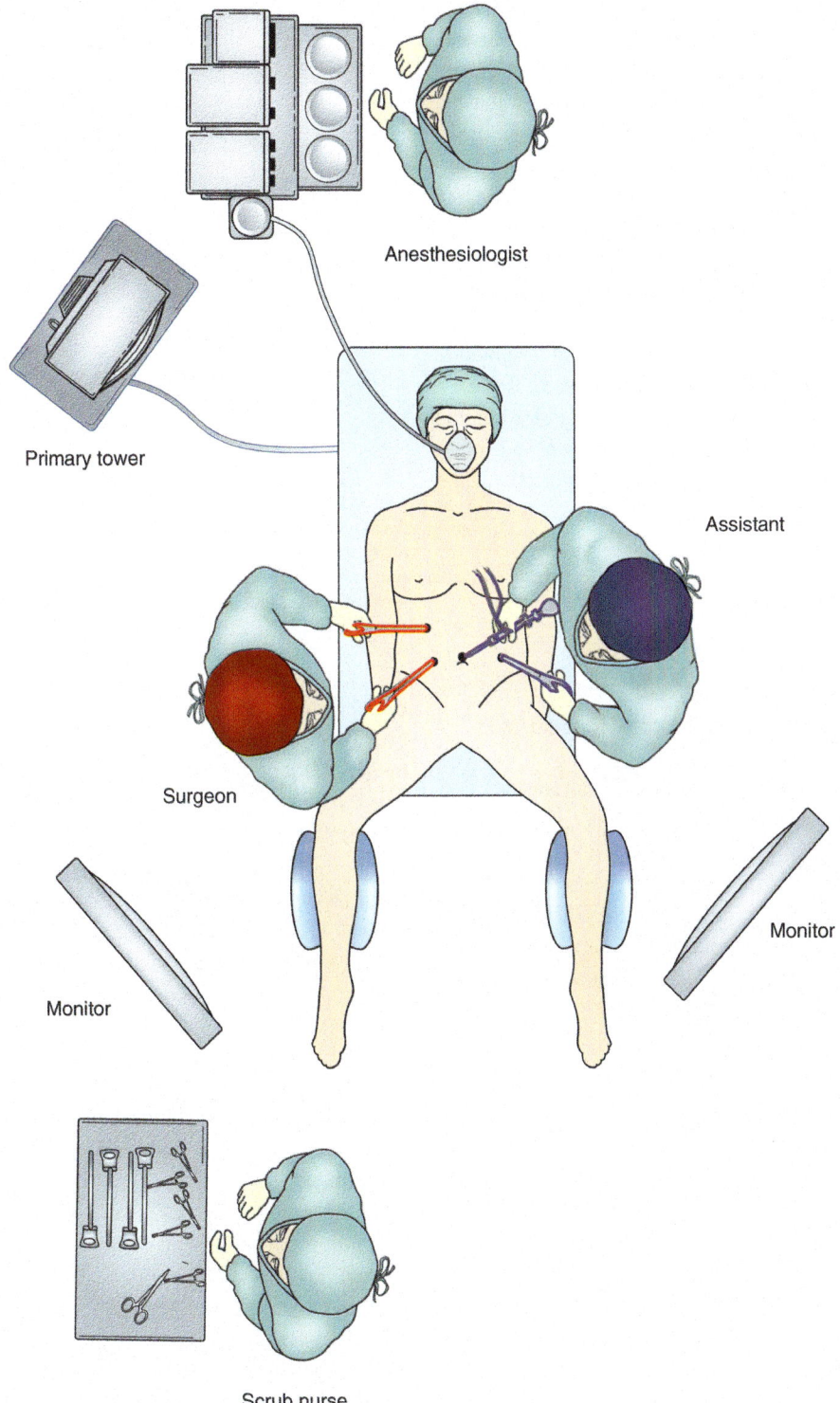

Anesthesiologist

Primary tower

Assistant

Surgeon

Monitor

Monitor

Scrub nurse

Proctectomy room setup. The surgeon will stand on the patient's right with the assistant on the patient's left. The primary monitor will be placed on the patient's left at the level of the thigh. During splenic flexure mobilization, the surgeon may move between the patient's legs

The patient is positioned in modified lithotomy position. Both arms are tucked to allow for surgeon position and manipulation of the instruments. The left arm may be placed on an arm board if necessary, as the dissection will primarily occur on the patient's right side or between the legs. However, leaving the arm out may limit the surgeon's ability to dissect adhesions if encountered in the abdomen. The legs are placed in Yellofin® stirrups (Allen Medical), and the abdomen is prepped and draped in the standard fashion. An orogastric tube and Foley catheter are placed.

The surgeon stands on the patient's right side and the assistant on the left (Insert Tip 6.1). Occasionally, the surgeon will move between the legs for splenic flexure mobilization and adhesiolysis. The primary monitor is placed on the patient's left side at approximately the level of the thigh to allow sufficient visualization for the surgeon while providing adequate room for the assistant to maneuver.

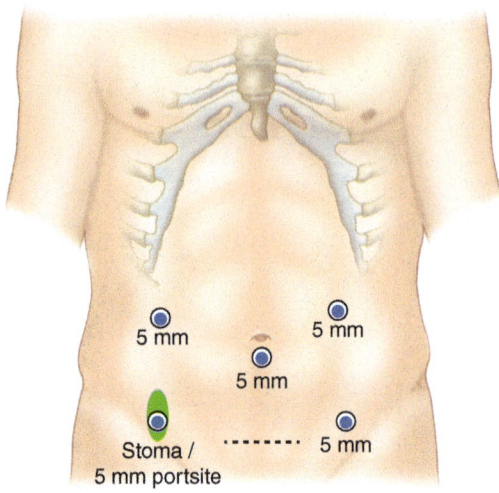

Fig. 6.1 Proctectomy port setup. Entry may be with a 5 mm Versiport through the stoma site or open Hassan technique via infraumbilical incision. Additional 5 mm ports are placed in the right upper and left lower quadrants. If needed, a 5 mm port may also be placed in the left upper quadrant

> 💡 **Tip 6.1 Assistant placement on left colectomy**
> Short assistants may prefer to stand on the patient's right, cephalad to the operating surgeon to facilitate reach to the camera port. For a tall assistant, placement on the surgeon's left may provide better access to assist through the left lower quadrant port. Using a standing stool may help leverage shorter assistants.

Operative Strategy

Step 1: Port Placement (Fig. 6.1)

Abdominal entry can vary depending on surgeon preference. If an ileostomy is indicated, a 5 mm Visiport is placed through the ileostomy site with a 0-degree camera (see Chap. 1). The location of this port is usually determined based on preoperative marking by the enterostomal therapy nurse. If the ileostomy site has not been marked preoperatively, it can be determined operatively based on multiple factors. It should be in a flat location on the abdominal wall, away from skin scar/creases/folds, not at the belt or waistline, easily visible to the patient, within the rectus muscle, and away from bony structures. After pneumoperitoneum is obtained, switch the camera to a 5 mm 30-degree scope. Place additional 5 mm infraumbilical, right upper quadrant, and left iliac fossa ports. Move the camera to the umbilical port.

Alternatively, pneumoperitoneum can be obtained via an infraumbilical 10 mm Hassan. Place additional 5 mm right upper and lower and left lower quadrant ports under laparoscopic guidance.

Occasionally, an additional left upper quadrant 5 mm port is needed for mobilization of the splenic flexure (see Step 9).

The ileostomy site port can be used as the working port for the pelvic dissection and rectal transection. In this case, the surgeon can initially place a 5/12 mm adaptable trocar to accommodate the stapling device. However, if the ileostomy port is not in a location favorable for the pelvic dissection, an additional 12 mm port is placed at least one handbreadth either superior or inferior to the ileostomy port depending on anatomy.

Step 2: Staging Laparoscopy (For Neoplastic Disease If Indicated)

Upon entry, the surgeon should assess the abdomen to rule out inadvertent damage during placement of initial ports. In addition, the surgeon should assess to ensure that it is appropriate to proceed laparoscopically. In cases of significant adhesions or unexpected anatomy, it may be prudent to consider a variation of the planned technique such as possible conversion to hand assist or open.

Laparoscopic staging is performed at the beginning of the surgery in cases of neoplasia to look for metastatic disease or adjacent organ involvement. In cases of Crohn's disease, the small bowel is inspected to look for additional areas of disease.

Step 3: Identification of Pathology

For neoplastic disease, the exact distance and location of the tumor relative to the anal verge should be noted preoperatively to facilitate a distal 2 cm oncologic margin. If the tumor is below the peritoneal reflection on preoperative imaging or in the mid to distal rectum, preoperative marking with endoscopic tattoo or planned intraoperative endoscopy should be considered as the tumor location may not be evident intraoperatively. The bowel is gently occluded with a laparoscopic bowel grasper proximal to the area of suspected pathology when insufflating to prevent propagation of air.

The patient is placed in Trendelenburg position and rotated with the patient's right side down. This allows gravity to move the small bowel out of the operative field and expose the sigmoid colon mesentery (Tip 6.2).

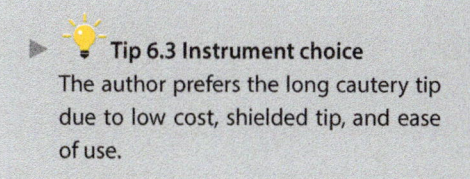

> 💡 **Tip 6.2 Right-sided pelvic adhesions**
> Adhesions from the cecum or terminal ileum may prevent retraction of the right colon and small bowel to the upper abdomen, out of the operative field. Occasionally, dissection of adhesions in this area may be necessary to provide appropriate exposure.

Step 4: Creation of the Retroperitoneal Plane

A bowel grasper is placed through the superior right-sided port in the surgeon's left hand, and the cautery or energy device is placed through the inferior right-sided port. A variety of devices can be used for cautery such as an extra-long cautery tip (Tip 6.3), scissors with attached cautery, or the bipolar device with the cautery tip.

> 💡 **Tip 6.3 Instrument choice**
> The author prefers the long cautery tip due to low cost, shielded tip, and ease of use.

Dissection begins in the right pararectal gutter with the surgeon standing on the patient's right and the assistant on the patient's left. The right ureter is lateral to the dissection plane and is not routinely identified during this portion of the dissection. The rectosigmoid mesentery is grasped at the level of the sacral promontory and retracted upward towards the abdominal wall and cephalad to put the mesentery under moderate tension. This tension should reduce all of the redundancy of the rectum and sigmoid in the pelvis. In order to position the assistant, the surgeon uses two bowel graspers and walks the graspers distally down the colon until traction is sufficient, and the root of the inferior mesenteric artery is placed under adequate tension (Fig. 6.2). Pass the position of tension to the assistant, prior to changing the right hand to an electrocautery.

Fig. 6.2 To expose the IMA, the surgeon will retract the sigmoid out of the pelvis using a hand-over-hand technique. Appropriate retraction is achieved when the IMA is visualized at the sacral promontory

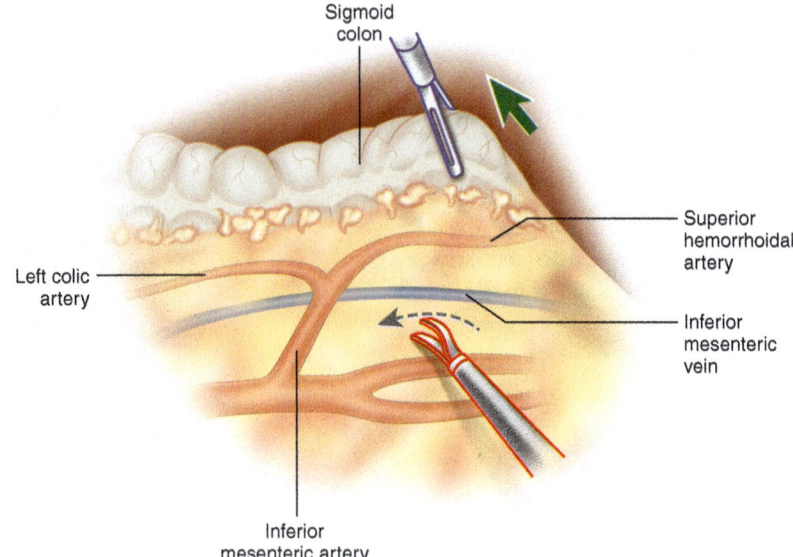

Fig. 6.3 The plane below the inferior mesenteric artery is scored using electrocautery in order to visualize the mesorectal plane. Hypogastric nerves in this plane should be identified and preserved with the retroperitoneal tissues

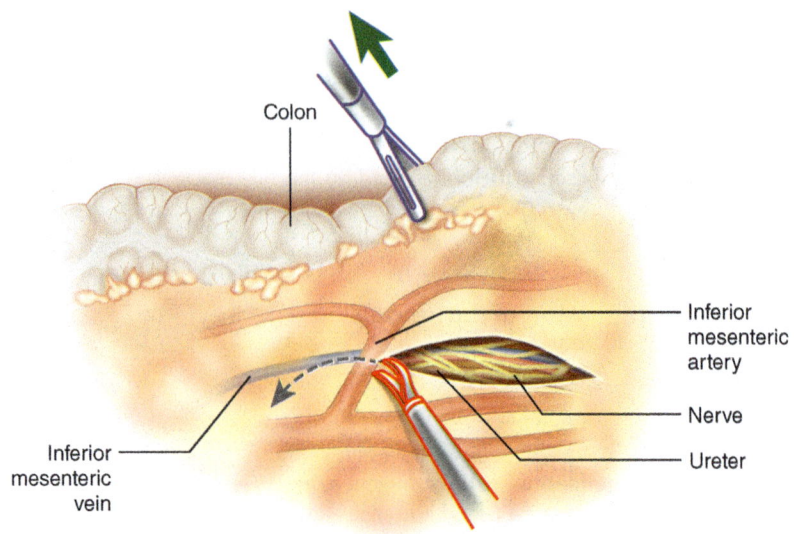

When a hand port is used, the surgeon stands on the patient's right side and places his left hand into the hand port. The index and middle finger are spread apart to create tension on the peritoneum in the right pararectal gutter. Dissection begins between these fingers and proceeds proximally and medially in a similar fashion to straight lap. The areolar tissue planes can be further developed bluntly with finger dissection proximally to the IMA and distally down into the pelvis.

Use electrocautery to score the peritoneum in the groove between the inferior mesenteric artery (IMA) and the retroperitoneum. Air can often be seen tracking in the retroperitoneal avascular planes once the peritoneum is divided. The plane is then developed by dividing the areolar tissue cephalad towards the IMA and caudally over the promontory down into the pelvis. This allows the mesentery to be elevated off of the retroperitoneum and presacral hypogastric nerves (Fig. 6.3). If the nerves are visualized, they should gently be pushed posteriorly towards the sacrum or laterally towards the pelvic sidewall to minimize risk for injury.

Fig. 6.4 Prior to ligation of the IMA, the ureter is identified and preserved with the retroperitoneal structures

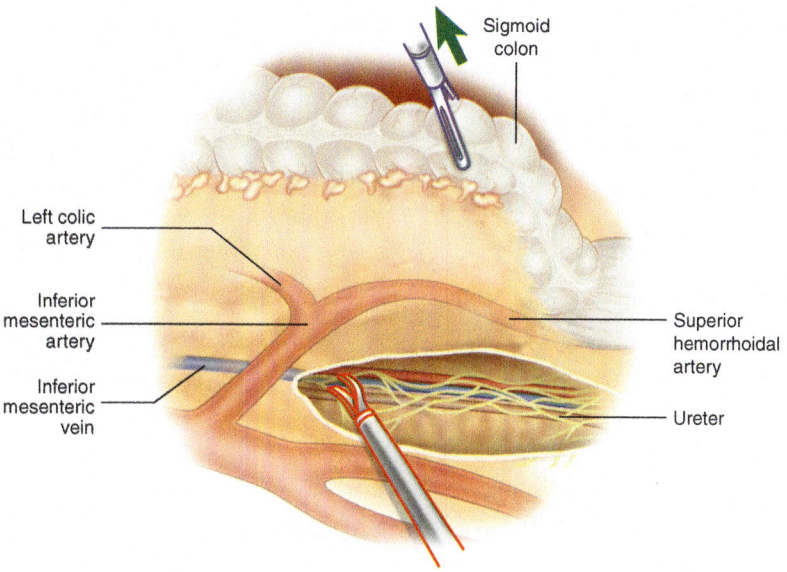

Dissection should then be continued anterior or medial to the nerves.

The dissection plane should be just behind the IMA. If the plane isn't clear, change tension on the rectosigmoid to better visualize the planes. Sweep all of the additional attachments down with the retroperitoneum to widen the plane (Tip 6.4).

> 💡 **Tip 6.4 Tension at rectosigmoid**
> If the mesorectal plane isn't developing well, try changing tension with the left hand. Adhesions from the rectosigmoid to the anterior abdominal wall or left sidewall may prevent adequate retraction. Freeing these adhesions may be necessary to visualize the plane.

Step 5: Identification of Inferior Mesenteric Artery (IMA) and Left Ureter, with High Ligation of IMA

Once the plane has been developed between the IMA and retroperitoneum, continue the dissection cephalad to the origin of the IMA in preparation for high ligation (Tip 6.5). To prevent injury to the left ureter, the ureter must be located and visualized in the retroperitoneal tissues prior to

IMA ligation. The ureter lays medial to the gonadal vessels and dorsolateral to the appropriate mesorectal plane (Fig. 6.4).

> 💡 **Tip 6.5 High ligation of the inferior mesenteric artery**
> A high ligation is a ligation of the IMA at its bifurcation from the aorta. This typically requires ligation of the left colic artery, which branches about 2 cm distal to the aorta. Although high ligation ensures a good lymphatic dissection, it may also compromise the blood supply to the descending colon and may not be required in cases of benign disease.

If the ureter cannot be immediately located, the dissection is likely too deep, and the ureter has been lifted with the IMA pedicle and retroperitoneal fascia. This increases the risk of injury to the hypogastric nerves, as well as the ureter. Readjust the plane with the left hand by isolating the inferior mesenteric artery on its dorsal aspect. Gently push any adherent tissue down with the right hand to bluntly free the ureter and hypogastric nerves.

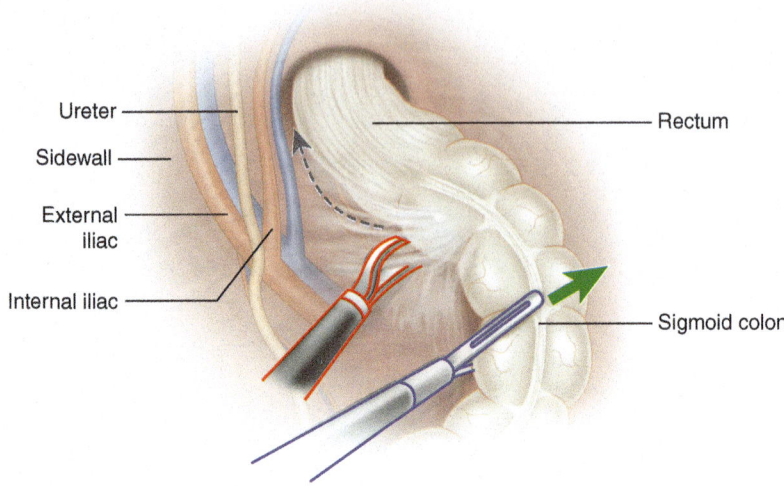

Fig. 6.5 Lateral approach and identification of the ureter. Preserve the white line of Toldt over the retroperitoneal structures. Medial retraction of the colon helps visualization of the correct plane

If the ureter still cannot be located, a lateral-to-medial approach can be used (Fig. 6.5). This requires medial tension on the left colon to free attachments to the pelvic brim and left sidewall. The surgeon's left hand retracts the colon medially, while the right hand carefully divides the thin filmy attachments of the colon and epiploica to the lateral sidewall. As the ureter has not yet been located and may lay just below the dissection field, care must be taken to prevent deep dissection in the area. Continue the lateral dissection proximally towards the splenic flexure and medially until the ureter is identified within the retroperitoneum and separate it from the inferior mesenteric artery and mesocolon by gently pushing it laterally. Alternatively, the ureter can be located near the renal hilum and tracked distally. In redo pelvic surgery, extensive fibrosis, or inflammatory conditions, ureteral stents may be helpful as well (Pitfall 6.1).

Once the ureter has been located and preserved with the retroperitoneum, the IMA is divided with the energy or stapling device. The location of division of the IMA depends on the purpose of the surgery. For neoplastic disease, a high ligation, proximal to the takeoff of the left colic artery, is recommended to ensure appropriate lymphadenectomy. This is generally 2–3 cm inferior to the duodenum at the ligament of Treitz, significantly cephalad to the aortic bifurcation (Fig. 6.6). In benign disease, ligation can occur distal to the left colic artery, preserving retrograde blood flow to the descending colon. When a hand port is used, the IMA can be grasped and occluded with the surgeon's fingers in the unfortunate event of an energy or a stapling device misfire. This will allow the surgeon to reattempt ligation or convert to open if necessary.

The vessel should be isolated from the hypogastric nerves and retroperitoneum prior to ligation. Release tension on the vessel prior to sealing when using an energy device. Excessive tension can impede the energy device from achieving a good seal on the vessel (Tip 6.6).

 Pitfall 6.1 Ureter stents

The presence of stents has not been shown to reduce the risk of ureteral injuries. Placement of stents during the surgery may help the surgeon visually identify the course of the ureter, if movement of the ureter is observed laparoscopically. The tactile feedback that stents provides is not useful unless an open or hand-assisted approach is used.

 Tip 6.6

Prior to sealing, "feel" the vessel with a bowel grasper. Energy devices cannot seal well through excessive calcification, and excessive bleeding may occur. If excessive calcification is noted, change approach to use either an endovascular stapler or endoloop.

Fig. 6.6 IMA ligation. The IMA is transected proximal to the left colic artery takeoff, approximately 1 cm from the aorta. No tension should be placed on the vessel during transection to allow adequate hemostatic control of the vessels

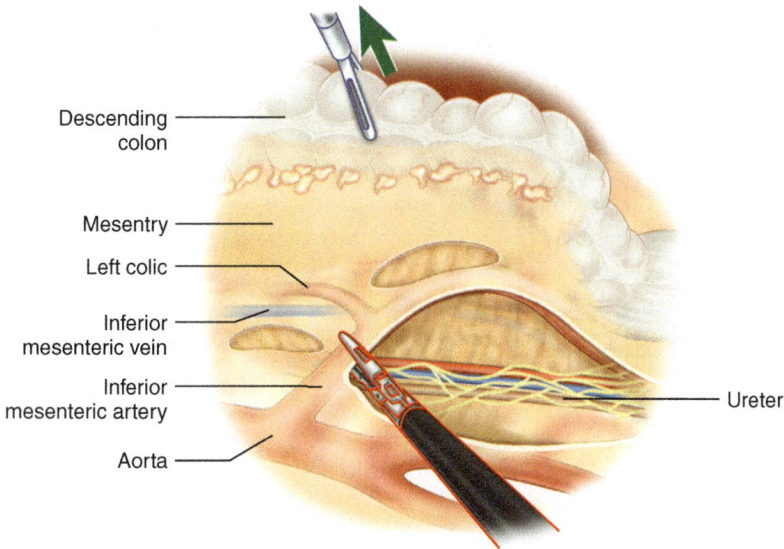

Descending colon
Mesentry
Left colic
Inferior mesenteric vein
Inferior mesenteric artery
Aorta
Ureter

Fig. 6.7 Medial dissection. Optimizing the medial dissection helps to facilitate lateral dissection as well as entry into the lesser sac. The dissection can continue laterally under the colon, superiorly to the border of the pancreas, and inferiorly to the pelvic brim

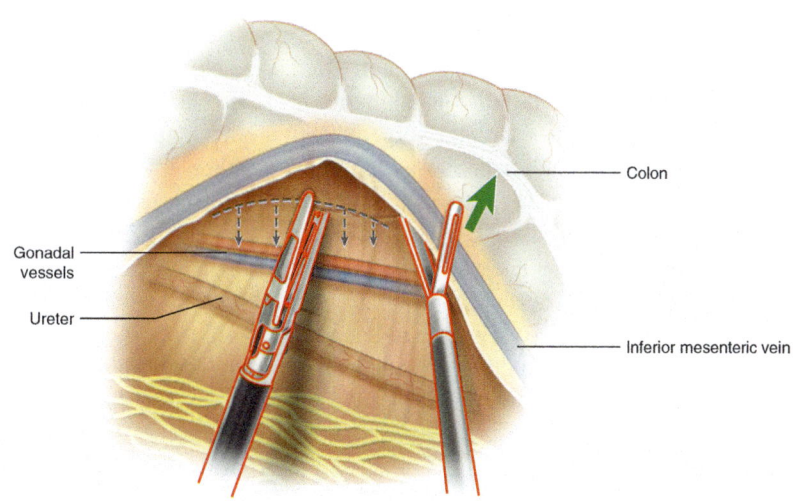

Gonadal vessels
Ureter
Colon
Inferior mesenteric vein

After dividing the vessel, dissect the mesocolon from the retroperitoneum using a medial approach. The left bowel grasper gently lifts the colon and mesocolon towards the abdominal wall, while the right hand divides the areolar tissue under the colon mesentery and above Gerota's fascia. Dissection is carried out laterally to the white line of Toldt, superiorly towards the inferior border of the pancreas, and inferiorly to the pelvic brim, sweeping all retroperitoneal structures and fascia down with the retroperitoneum (Fig. 6.7). Occasionally, this area will not separate easily, and use of cauterization or bipolar will be necessary, but in most cases, blunt tension and counter-tension with a gentle sweeping just anterior to the white line will be avascular and hemostatic.

Step 6: Inferior Mesenteric Vein (IMV) Ligation

The inferior mesenteric vein is visualized during this portion of the dissection and is ligated if additional length is needed for a tension-free anastomosis. Free any adhesions to the duodenum with the electrocautery by gently pulling the duodenum medially away from the adhesions. Isolate the IMV with the left hand by creating a window above and below the vessel. The assistant can create tension by holding the mesentery above the IMV anteriorly and towards the camera to better view the IMV. After isolation, a vessel sealer can be used to transect the IMV (Fig. 6.8). Transecting the IMV close to the inferior border of the pancreas provides optimal lengthening of the left colon and splenic flexure.

Step 7: Mobilization of the Sigmoid and Descending Colon

Once the descending and sigmoid colon are mobilized posteriorly, the only remaining attachment of the descending colon is the peritoneum to the abdominal wall at the white line of Toldt. The colon is grasped and pulled medially to the right side of the abdomen with the surgeon's left hand. If the posterior mobilization was sufficient, a purple hue from bruising is seen through the attachments. Cautery is used to divide the peritoneum. Mobilizing too far laterally can easily lead under the kidney into a retroperitoneal plane. The correct plane is generally very close to the colon wall. If angles are difficult during this dissection, the surgeon can move between the patient's legs

and use the left lower quadrant trocar for retraction and the right lower quadrant port for the cautery. Because this area is thin and avascular, this step should proceed relatively quickly as long as adequate tension is maintained (Fig. 6.9).

Step 8: Splenic Flexure Mobilization

Generally for a proctectomy, splenic flexure mobilization will be required to ensure adequate tension-free length for the anastomosis. The more distal the rectal transection, the more likely splenic flexure mobilization will be required.

The patient is placed in reverse Trendelenburg position, and occasionally the surgeon has to rotate between the patient's legs for easier dissection. An additional 5 mm port to assist with retraction of the greater omentum can be placed in the left upper quadrant. An additional port can assist with gentle retraction of the omentum and colon without placing tension on the splenic capsule. The lateral attachments should be divided to the level of the splenic flexure and posteriorly until the colon is freed completely from Gerota's fascia.

Enter the lesser sac by dividing the greater omentum from the colon. The assistant retracts the greater omentum anteriorly to the abdominal wall from the right upper quadrant port or the left upper quadrant port mentioned in the last paragraph. The surgeon pulls the transverse colon

Fig. 6.8 IMV transection. Transection of the IMV at the inferior border of the pancreas facilitates optimal reach of the splenic flexure into the pelvis for a true coloanal anastomosis

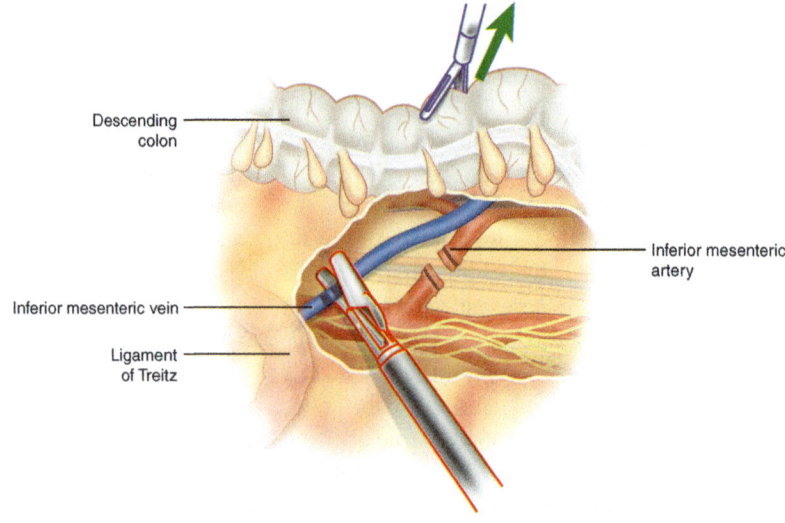

Descending colon

Inferior mesenteric artery

Inferior mesenteric vein

Ligament of Treitz

Fig. 6.9 White line of Toldt dissection. The lateral dissection continues superiorly in an avascular plane to the splenic flexure. Prior medial dissection helps to expedite this dissection

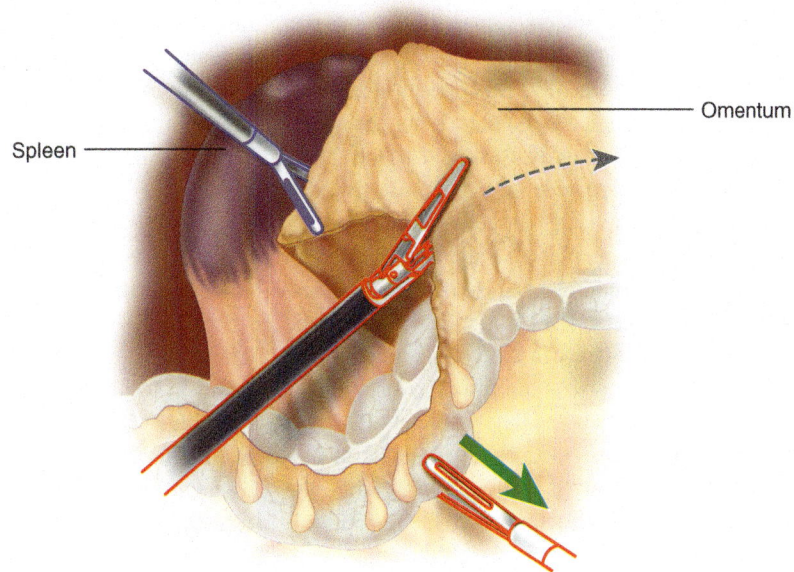

Spleen

Omentum

Fig. 6.10 Splenic flexure. The omentum is separated from the colon to enter the splenic flexure and release attachments for creation of a colon conduit. A subtle change in fat signals the plane between the colon epiploica and omentum

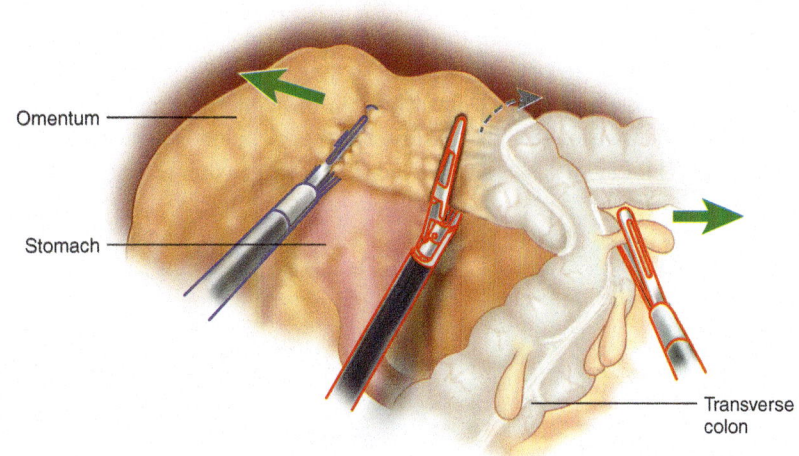

Omentum

Stomach

Transverse colon

inferiorly to aid in visualization of the avascular plane, which is usually within 1 cm from the colon edge. Electrocautery is often sufficient to open the planes. Occasionally, an energy device may be necessary to free the omentum from the colon if the plane has bulky adhesions. If bleeding is encountered, it is usually because the surgeon has deviated into the omentum and transected omental vessels. If this occurs, the surgeon should back up and reevaluate for the correct plane after obtaining hemostasis (Fig. 6.10).

Finding the lesser sac can be difficult, particularly if the patient has a thin omentum. It can occasionally appear that the lesser sac has been entered, only to find out a hole simply has been made through the omentum. The omentum is fused at the midline just left lateral to the falciform ligament, and this is generally the easiest location to separate the colon from the omentum and enter the lesser sac. Reorient by returning to the patient midline and reidentifying the planes. Entry into the lesser sac is confirmed when the posterior wall of the stomach can be visualized.

Once the lesser sac is entered, continue dissecting this plane distally towards the splenic flexure. Care must be taken to prevent injury to the spleen and splenic capsule by minimizing torsion on the attachments to the spleen. Generally, the surgeon should hold the attachments, while the assistant retracts the colon caudally. This prevents excessive torque on the splenic attachments. It may be necessary to switch to an energy instrument as the spleen is approached to provide better hemostasis. Stay close to the colon during dissection to prevent getting out of the proper plane. Straightening the colon distal to the dissection plane also prevents inadvertent injury to the colon. The surgeon should be mindful of redundancy in the colon and carefully separate the transverse colon from the omentum.

Once the attachments to the spleen are freed, the dissection plane meets the prior lateral dissection that occurred while mobilizing the descending colon. Attachments to the retroperitoneum are then freed behind the colon by grasping the flexure and pulling it to the right lower quadrant. Additional tips for splenic flexure mobilization are included in Chap. 4.

If a hand port is being used, the greater omentum can be retracted towards the anterior abdominal wall. The assistant retracts downward on the colon to provide tension such that the lesser sac can be entered. Once in the lesser sac, the index finger

can be placed into this space. Dissection proceeds distally around the splenic flexure by dividing the omental attachments off the colon. The splenic flexure is then pulled inferiorly and medially, and blunt finger dissection is used to gently free the flexure from the retroperitoneal attachments.

Step 9: Rectum Mobilized for Appropriate Resection Margins

The patient is placed in steep Trendelenburg position to allow the small bowel to fall out of the pelvis. The surgeon returns to the patient's right side for this portion of the procedure. The assistant grasps the rectosigmoid colon and retracts it upward and out of the pelvis for exposure. This retraction creates tension on the posterior mesorectum and is critical to be able to locate the avascular plane. If holding the rectum anteriorly and superiorly out of the pelvis doesn't create enough tension, an open bowel grasper can be placed on the inferior aspect of the mesorectum, and the rectum is lifted from below anteriorly and superiorly to create better tension (Fig. 6.11).

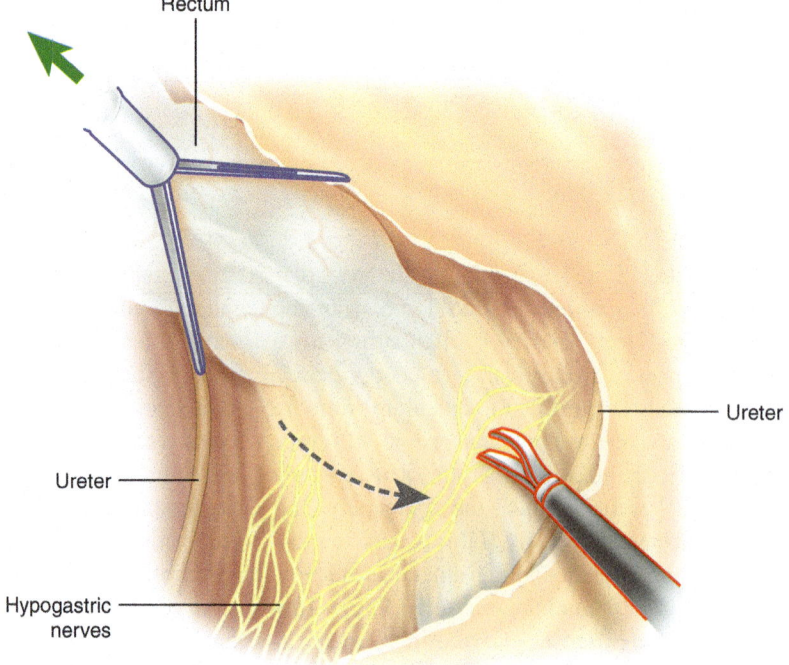

Fig. 6.11 Posterior mesorectal plane. The rectum is lifted and retracted out of the pelvis to create tension on the posterior mesorectum and expose the correct avascular plane

Fig. 6.12 Lateral dissection. The colon is retracted to the contralateral side, creating tension on the mesorectum and fascia. The thin plane is scored using electrocautery

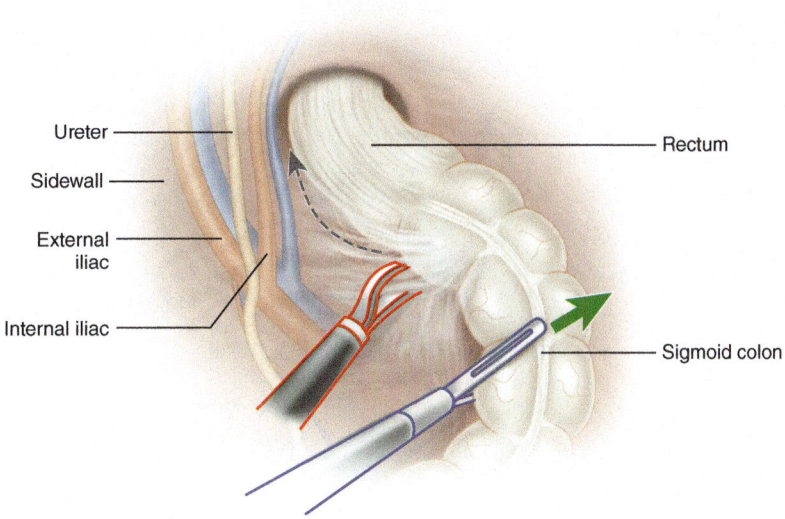

Ureter

Sidewall

External iliac

Internal iliac

Rectum

Sigmoid colon

The surgeon's left hand grasps the mesentery closer to the base of the inferior mesenteric artery for finer dissection. Distal dissection is performed with the electrocautery in the surgeon's right hand through the right lower quadrant port. Dissection begins in the avascular plane between the mesorectal fascial envelope and the presacral fascia. The plane can be seen as a distal continuation of the initial dissection from Step 4. Score the plane gently with an electrocautery. The hypogastric nerves should be preserved deep and lateral to the dissection. Dissection starts posteriorly in a U shape, deepest directly posterior and veering slightly anteriorly on either edge of the mesorectum. The plane is generally a filmy clear plane and does not require any vessel ligation. Occasionally, in radiated patients, thicker tissue may be encountered and require an energy device.

The dissection proceeds inferiorly with the assistant gently pulling the rectosigmoid colon cranially and anteriorly to create counter-tension. As tension is lost, the assistant can replace the left hand distally, recreating tension. Eventually, tension on the lateral aspects will limit posterior dissection. The assistant pulls the rectum to the left, to create tension along the patient's right side of the mesorectum. The surgeon dissects the lateral attachments, staying just lateral to the mesorectal envelope. Again, the plane should be filmy and avascular (Fig. 6.12). Tension is adjusted to pull to the rectosigmoid colon to the patient's right side, and the rectum is freed along the left pararectal gutters in a similar fashion to the right side.

Occasionally, as the surgeon approaches the lateral stalks, the middle rectal vessels are encountered. They can be transected using an energy device. Any other bleeding indicates the surgeon has deviated out of the avascular plane medially into the mesorectum or laterally into the pelvic internal iliac veins. Hemostasis should be obtained and the correct plane reidentified by returning proximally and reevaluating. From the right side, the surgeon can mobilize the rectum on the right and posterior sides all the way to the pelvic floor. A portion of the left side can be mobilized from the right as well by extending the posterior dissection to the left, but to complete the left sided dissection, the rectum is generally pulled inferiorly to the right, and the attachments are divided from an anterior approach.

Remain vigilant to stay in the mesorectal plan and prevent veering laterally to either side of the rectum as the ureter, hypogastric nerves, and internal iliac arteries and veins can be injured. In addition to standard dissection around the mesorectum from the right side, the surgeon must also be aware of the potential for loss of the correct plane when mobilization of the left side of the rectum is done from the patient's right side as it can be difficult to determine how lateral the dissection actually is. Additionally, injury can occur while the assistant is rotating the colon. Lastly, caution is taken to ensure the posterior presacral veins are not injured by veering too far posteriorly away from the mesorectum (Pitfall 6.2).

>  **Pitfall 6.2**
>
> The presacral veins do not respond well to cautery, and large volume blood loss can occur in very short time period. Conversion to open may be necessary to control the bleeding if this occurs.

At the bottom of the sacrum, at the location of the coccyx, the direction of dissection changes from parallel to the mesorectum, to slightly anterior as Waldeyer's fascia is entered. The dissection follows the curve of the sacrum and coccyx down to the anal canal.

The anterior dissection is performed last. The assistant grasps the peritoneum overlying the posterior portion of the dome of the bladder in a male, or vagina in a female, and retracts it firmly anterior. The initial incision is made in the peritoneum approximately 1–2 mm anterior to the pouch of Douglas, and the plane is developed in the area of the loose areolar tissue. Finding the plane between the seminal vessels or vaginal apex and the rectum can be particularly difficult if adequate tension is not applied. At times, a Maryland is necessary to carefully raise that tissue and create tension. If the tumor is located anteriorly, Denonvilliers' fascia should be taken with the specimen (Fig. 6.13).

Step 10: Rectal Transection

The location of the distal resection margin should now be determined. If the tumor involves the anal ring, abdominal perineal resection may be considered (see Chap. 7). If adequate margins can be achieved, a coloanal anastomosis with hand-sewn reconnection may be considered and is covered in special considerations. If an adequate margin can be achieved, a double-stapled technique is preferable to optimize function of the neorectum. Verification of the distal extent of tumor can be obtained by intraoperative proctoscopy or identification of endoscopic tattooing distal to the tumor.

Fig. 6.13 Anterior dissection. Depending on tumor location, the dissection will either remove or retain Denonvilliers' fascia. Anterior upward traction on the bladder or vagina helps to delineate the planes of dissection

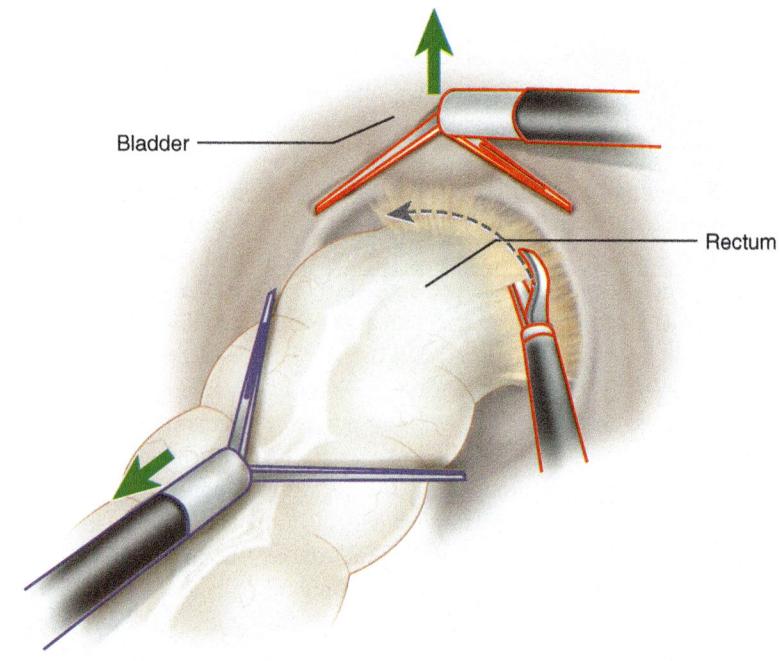

Ideally, mobilization continues 3–4 cm beyond the gross edge of the tumor. There are several reasons for continuing the dissection beyond the tumor, that is, (1) ensures an adequate margin, (2) provides mobility to the rectal stump, (3) decreases tension on the anastomosis, and (4) prevents inadvertent incorporation of the vagina or bladder into the staple line. If 3–4 cm mobilization is not possible, margins as small as 1 cm may be taken.

To transect the rectum, any mesorectum is dissected from the rectal wall. Distally, at the anal ring, the mesorectum dissipates and does not require dissection. For more proximal tumors, the mesorectum is divided circumferentially. Care is taken to prevent injury to the rectum. The assistant retracts the rectum superiorly. Score the peritoneum with electrocautery on the right side of the rectum at the site of planned transection (Tip 6.7). The mesorectum is gently dissected posterior to the rectum by using an energy instrument or bowel grasper to spread the mesorectum parallel to the rectum, displacing the mesorectal tissue. Once the posterior wall of the rectum is visualized, tissue posterior and lateral is taken with the energy device. Branches of the superior hemorrhoidal vessels traverse the mesorectum and require appropriate ligation to prevent bleeding. The tissue is swept away from the rectum with small progressive bites. First, the tissue is displaced, the rectum is then identified, and the tissue is then transected laterally and posteriorly. This continues until the right and posterior aspect of the rectum are cleared of mesentery. The rectum is then retracted to the right side of the patient, and a similar dissection ensues on the left side of the rectum (Fig. 6.14). Failure to completely remove the mesorectum can lead to bleeding at the staple line, or the tissue could be too thick such that the stapler is unable to fire coss.

>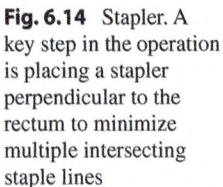
> **Tip 6.7 Pelvic angles**
> Because instrumentation enters the deep pelvis oblique to the rectum, the surgeon's natural tendency is to progress distally as you clean the mesorectum. The surgeon must take care to make mesorectal transection perpendicular to the rectum, to prevent leaving devascularized rectum at the anastomosis, which may increase the risk of anastomotic leak.

When the hand port is used, it is often easier to locate the plane between the rectum and mesorectum. Once this plane is developed, the mesorectum can be easily divided with the energy device. Additionally, tactile sensation can be used to ver-

Fig. 6.14 Stapler. A key step in the operation is placing a stapler perpendicular to the rectum to minimize multiple intersecting staple lines

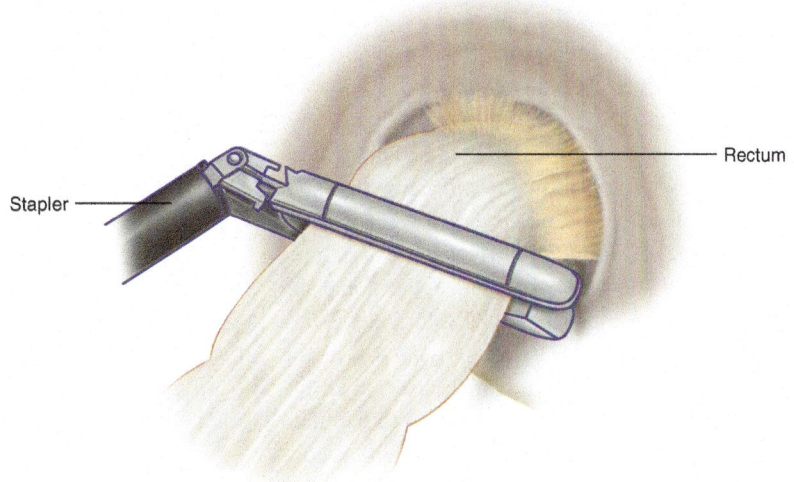

ify an adequate distal margin and site of intended transection of the rectum. Visual confirmation endoluminally, therefore, is usually not required.

Once the mesorectum is divided, the rectum is transected with a laparoscopic stapling device. One trocar is upsized to 12 mm in order to facilitate the stapler, unless one had been previously placed. The right lower quadrant port, left lower quadrant port, or adding a suprapubic port can each be used for stapling. If the angles are not appropriate, making a Pfannenstiel incision and placing an open curved or straight linear stapler through this incision may allow for more distal transection. The Pfannenstiel incision can then be used as an extraction site.

Stapling across the rectum may require multiple stapler fires to completely transect the rectum, but ideally the rectum is transected with a single firing of the stapler. This decreases crossing staple lines or oblique angulation, which may increase the risks of anastomotic leaks. A narrow pelvis may be too wide for a 60 mm stapler, and even a 45 or 30 mm stapler may be tight. The more perpendicular the stapler is to the rectum, the better, as this helps minimize the chance of multiple firings. When multiple firings are necessary, each staple line should be placed in continuity to the prior staple line to prevent angulation.

Once the rectum is divided, a bowel clamp is closed on the proximal staple line to facilitate externalization once the extraction site is created.

Step 11: Colon Exteriorized and Specimen Resected

The colon can be exteriorized in one of three locations. (1) A left lower quadrant incision is made, often as an extension of the left lower quadrant port site. (2) A Pfannenstiel incision can be created. (3) If an ileostomy is planned, the stoma site trephine can be widened and used for exteriorization. The incision can be partially closed at the end of the operation to facilitate creation of the ileostomy. A wound protector is used to facilitate exposure and extraction, as well as prevent contamination. This can be twisted closed to restore pneumoperitoneum after the colon is placed into the abdomen for the anastomosis (see Chap. 1). If

a hand port was placed, the cap is removed and the specimen extracted through the hand port.

The surgeon passes the rectum to the extraction site, where the assistant grasps it using a Babcock. It should be gently brought out through the incision, with care not to pull too hard, or the bowel can be ripped. Once exteriorized, the location of proximal resection margin is chosen. Margins for cancer should be 5 cm proximal from the tumor and always include the full inferior mesenteric artery pedicle to ensure appropriate lymphadenectomy. The left colon will be vascularized by the marginal artery from the middle colic vessels. A balance must be obtained between a proximal transection to maintain adequate blood supply and a distal transection to allow sufficient length for a tension-free anastomosis. Once the appropriate location of transection is determined, the colon mesentery is divided with the energy device or 0 braided absorbable or silk ties (Tip 6.8). Once the colon is divided, brisk oozing should be noted from the mucosa. If sufficient bleeding is not present, a more proximal transection should be performed.

Once the mesentery is divided, a purse-string

> 💡 **Tip 6.8 Checking the blood supply**
> Prior to transection of the left colon marginal artery, the blood supply should be checked to ensure pulsatile flow to the anastomosis. A hemostat is placed to occlude the marginal artery at the site of the anastomosis but is not clamped. The artery is transected with scissors. If flow is adequate, the clamp is closed and the vessel tied off. If the flow is inadequate, a more proximal location is chosen and the flow checked again at that location.

clamp or auto-purse-string device is placed on the colon and the colon divided. Alternatively, a manual purse string can be placed. A 0-polypropelene suture on a small bore needle can be used in a baseball fashion. Take full-thickness bites on the colon, including all layers of the bowel wall, approximately 2 mm from each other until the suture is placed circumferentially. The anvil of a circular stapling device is inserted and the purse string tightened making sure the mucosa is snug against the anvil shaft.

The colon is returned to the abdomen. Gloves are changed and dirty instruments passed off the field.

Step 12: Anastomosis

The wound protector is closed. Pneumo-peritoneum is reestablished. The extraction site port can be closed with fascial sutures or the wound protector closed by twisting it and occluding with a large Kelly clamp. If a Pfannenstiel incision was used, the anastomosis can also be performed under direct visualization.

Length is verified to ensure that the distal colon will reach into the pelvis without tension. If length is not sufficient at this time, various maneuvers can be performed: full splenic flexure mobilization (if not already completed), division of the IMV, or completely mobilizing the descending colon mesentery from the underlying retroperitoneal attachments. Occasionally, the greater omentum will be attached to the descending colon preventing it from adequately straightening out, so this should be freed up as well. Transverse slits can be made in the colon mesentery to help lengthen it as well. If the colon still does not reach (usually due to tethering of the colonic mesentery), small portions of the mesentery can be taken to provide more length. In rare cases, ligation of the mesentery can continue proximally such that the mesentery of the entire transverse colon can be divided, including the middle colic artery. The colon is then rotated 180 degrees, thereby relying on the ileocolic artery for blood supply. Sufficient blood supply at the distal portion of the colon may need to again be verified if division of this much mesentery is required. Once adequate length is obtained, the mesentery should be checked to ensure it is not twisted. This is done by following the free edge of the mesentery through its length from the staple line proximally to the retroperitoneum or tracking a single tenia down into the pelvic making sure it is straight. In addition, the colon should be checked to ensure that the small bowel does not cross under the conduit. Small bowel under the conduit can create postop-erative bowel obstructions or foreshorten the colon making an anastomosis more difficult.

If a stapled anastomosis is being performed, the circular stapler is gently inserted through the anus. The assistant moves between the patient's legs and first dilates the anus using 2–3 well-lubricated fingers to facilitate smooth placement of the stapler into the rectum.

For a coloanal anastomosis, care must be taken so as not to insert the stapler handle too forcefully and disrupt the rectal staple line. The stapler should be inserted carefully and slowly, following the curve of the sacrum. The surgeon watches progression of the stapler laparoscopically and directs the assistant. Have the scrub nurse or second assistant hold the camera during this portion of the operation.

Once the stapler reaches the top of the rectum, it should be situated so that the linear staple line is in the middle of the circular stapler (Fig. 6.15). The stapler should be checked to ensure that the device is flush with the proximal end of the rectum. The surgeon can place gentle traction on the end of the rectum with a bowel grasper, while the assistant withdraws and reinserts the stapler correctly into position. Once the stapler is situated, the spike is advanced posterior to the rectal staple line. During this process, the assistant keeps the stapler stable, preventing withdrawal or redirection. The surgeon takes the distal portion of the conduit and reattaches the anvil to the spike (Tip 6.9). The stapler is closed full and then fired. After opening the stapler according to the manufacturer's instructions, the stapler should be gently withdrawn with a twisting motion. The two anastomotic donuts are inspected to make sure they are complete full-thickness rings of colon and rectum. In cancer cases, they can be sent as an additional margin.

> 💡 **Tip 6.9 Attaching the circular stapler anvil**
> Directing the rectum, and the spike of the anvil, slightly towards the patient's left, away from the camera, facilitates visualization of the end of the stapler. Use two bowel graspers on the anvil to direct the anvil smoothly into the stapler.

Fig. 6.15 Circular
stapler. The circular
stapler may be extruded
through the end of the
rectum anterior or
posterior to the staple
line. Posterior location
may help protect
inadvertent inclusion of
the vagina in low
anastomoses

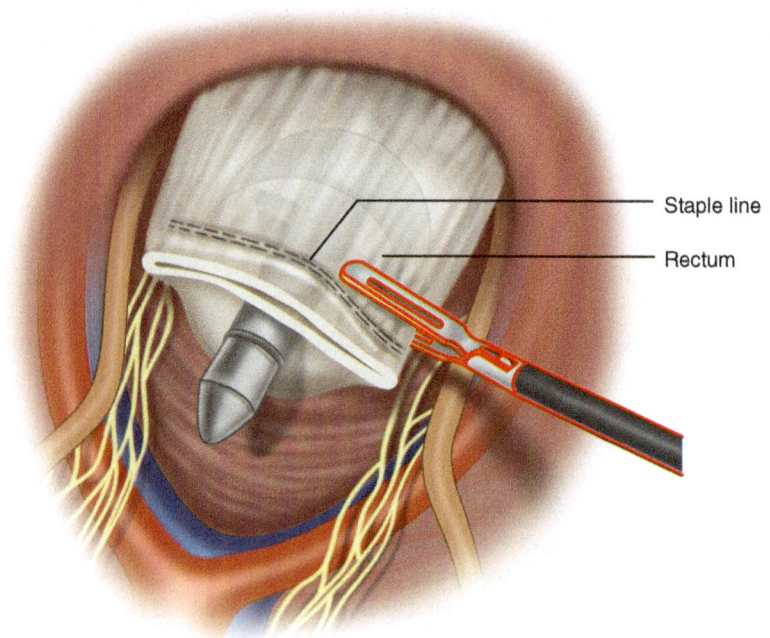

Staple line

Rectum

Once the stapler is removed, test the anastomosis by filling the pelvis with water and inflating the colon using a bulb syringe, proctoscope, or flexible endoscopy. Any leak should be addressed by either placement of sutures, recreation of the anastomosis, and/or diversion based on the surgeon's judgment.

Step 13: Formation of Loop Ileostomy (If Indicated)

If indicated, a loop ileostomy is created. The previously marked stoma location may have been used as an extraction site. If so, this incision is enlarged to create a trephine large enough to admit two fingers. Otherwise, the incision will be made de novo. Use of appendiceal retractors helps to create a small trephine but allows for adequate depth of retraction. The anterior and posterior fascia should be sequentially opened and dilated to the size of two fingers. The rectus muscles should be spared and simply retracted to either side.

The ileum is run proximally from the ileocecal valve until the location for a stoma is deter-

mined and to ensure the small bowel is not twisted. The stoma location is chosen in the ileum to allow for sufficient distal length so as not to compromise nutrition but proximal enough to allow for enough redundancy to complete an ileostomy takedown at a later time. Generally 20–30 cm proximal to the ileocecal valve is sufficient. A laparoscopic grasper is placed on the ileum to mark the spot and prevent twisting. A Babcock is placed through the trephine, and the assistant passes the small bowel to the Babcock after checking orientation of the bowel laparoscopically. The proximal limb is, by convention, placed superiorly and the distal limb placed inferiorly. Once all port sites are closed, the ileostomy is matured in a standard Brooke fashion.

Step 14: Closure

If a drain is placed, it can be brought out through one of the port sites. The fascia of the extraction site and 12mm port site are closed. The skin is then closed on all sites with a subcuticular closure.

Special Considerations

Hand-Assisted Laparoscopic Surgery (HALS)

The approach to proctectomy may need to be varied based on the patient's anatomy, disease process, and surgeon comfort. A common variation is a hand-assisted resection. A gel port is first placed through either a Pfannenstiel or vertical midline incision, with location varying based on surgeon preference. A Pfannenstiel incision is more cosmetic and allows for open dissection and better visualization of the pelvis when the port is removed. A midline incision allows better access to the splenic flexure and can be easily converted to a laparotomy if needed.

There are several benefits to this technique:

- Better mobilization and handling of thick mesenteries in obese patients
- Better identification of tumors when the distal limit is not clear based on external inspection of the rectum
- Shorter operative times

For vertical midline incisions, the gel port is placed first after an incision is made through the fascia large enough for placement of the surgeon's hand. Pneumoperitoneum is obtained, and a 5 mm suprapubic port and 12 mm RLQ port are placed (Fig. 6.16). Typically if a hand port is placed, it essentially replaces two regular ports. As in a pure laparoscopic case, occasionally the 12 mm port can be placed through the intended ileostomy site.

Steps of the operation are then carried out much like a pure laparoscopic proctectomy except the descending colon and sigmoid colon are mobilized in a lateral to medial approach.

See notes throughout the chapter for specific ways the hand is used compared to straight laparoscopy instruments.

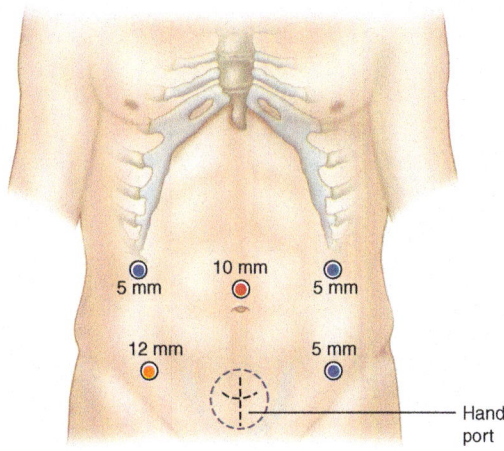

Fig. 6.16 HALS port placement. A HALS port may be placed as a Pfannenstiel or midline port. Other ports must be placed far enough from the hand port to prevent collisions

Types of Colorectal and Coloanal Anastomoses (Fig. 6.17)

Various types of colorectal and coloanal anastomoses exist (straight colorectal, hand-sewn coloanal, Baker, colonic J pouch), and which one to use in each situation can depend on multiple factors: colonic and distal rectal stump length, tumor location, surgeon preference, and patient anatomy. What defines a colorectal versus a coloanal anastomosis is a matter of debate due to the differences in definitions of the surgical anal canal and the anatomic anal canal. For the purposes of this discussion, we will define an anastomosis to the surgical anal canal as an ultralow colorectal anastomosis and a hand-sewn anastomosis to the dentate line as a coloanal anastomosis. For all of these discussions, the mobilization of the abdominal portion of the colon is the same regardless of anastomotic technique employed.

The most commonly performed anastomosis is a straight stapled colorectal anastomosis, the technique of which is described above in Step 9.

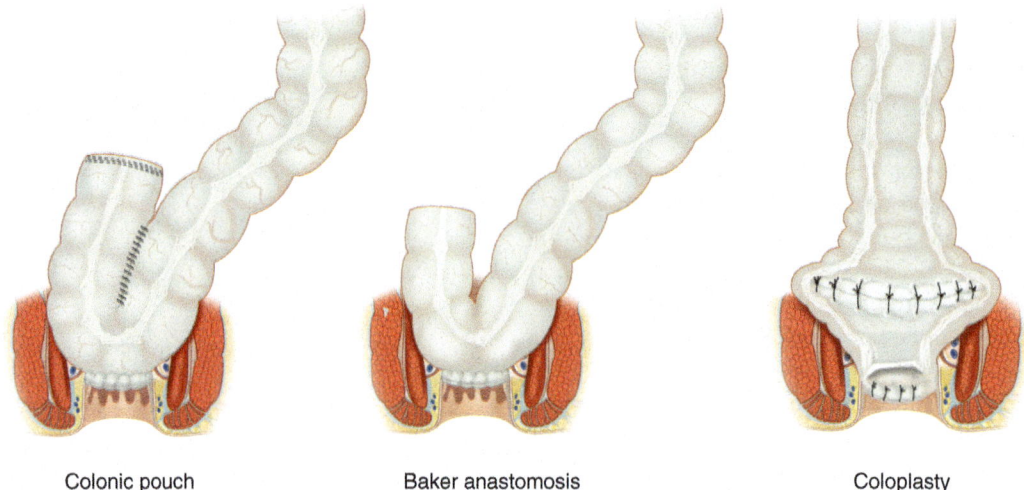

Colonic pouch   Baker anastomosis   Coloplasty

Fig. 6.17 Coloanal anastomosis. Three configurations for coloanal anastomosis are well described: colonic J pouch, Baker anastomosis (side to end), and coloplasty. These may help improve initial capacitance issues after a complete proctectomy

It is used when, after transecting and removing the specimen, enough distal rectum remains to accommodate the handle of the circular stapling device.

In an effort to improve postoperative bowel dysfunction associated with straight colorectal and coloanal anastomoses, a colon J pouch or end-to-side (Baker-type) anastomosis can be performed. Data have demonstrated that function may be improved by creating a larger reservoir in the neorectum. Long-term functional results are similar between a straight anastomosis, J pouch, and Baker anastomosis. Both J pouch and Baker techniques involve additional staple lines compared to a conventional end-to-end anastomosis. Additionally, in patient with a narrow pelvis or insufficient colonic length, these two techniques may not be possible.

To create a colonic J pouch during Step 9 above, while the proximal colon is extracted, the pouch is created. A colonic J pouch is constructed in a similar fashion to an ileal J pouch but is much smaller. The distal colon is folded to create a 6–8 cm pouch. A colotomy is made at the proximal extent of the pouch, and a linear stapler is fired down the common wall of the pouch to enlarge the neo-rectal reservoir. The anvil of the circular stapler is placed at the apex of the pouch and secured into place with a 2-0 absorbable suture. The colotomy is then closed either with a transverse stapler or with a two-layer hand-sewn closure, ensuring that the inlet to the pouch is not narrowed. The colonic pouch is then returned to the abdomen as above.

An end-to-side or Baker anastomosis is easier to perform and offers similar functional results as compared to a colonic J pouch. Rather than creating a colonic pouch, the colon is transected at the proximal resection margin and the colon left open. The anvil is placed through the open colon to the apex of the colon, approximately 4–5 cm from the colotomy. The open end of the colon is then closed with a linear stapler, and the colon is returned to the abdomen (Pitfall 6.3).

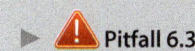

> ⚠️ **Pitfall 6.3**
> When creating a Baker anastomosis, a minimum of 3 cm should be maintained between the circular stapler and the linear stapler. Less than 3 cm may result in an ischemic area between staple lines and increase the risk of anastomotic leak.

Hand-Sewn Coloanal Anastomosis

Occasionally, the rectal tumor is low enough that a sufficient margin cannot be obtained from an abdominal approach. In this situation, the distal transection has to be performed transanally, with the colon brought down and sewn directly to the dentate line. To perform this, the perineal portion of the dissection is begun using a Lone Star retractor, which everts the anal canal allowing for better exposure to the dentate line. After local infiltration of the rectal mucosa with epinephrine, the rectum is transected with electrocautery roughly 1 cm proximal to the dentate line. A circumferential transection through the rectal wall frees the proximal rectum (and tumor) from the anus. The specimen is then extracted, either transanally through the proctotomy or through the abdominal extraction incision, if the rectum and mesorectum are too

bulky to allow for transanal extraction. A Babcock forceps can be used to guide the rectum through the anus.

Once the rectum is extracted, a full-thickness colotomy is made in the colon proximal to the

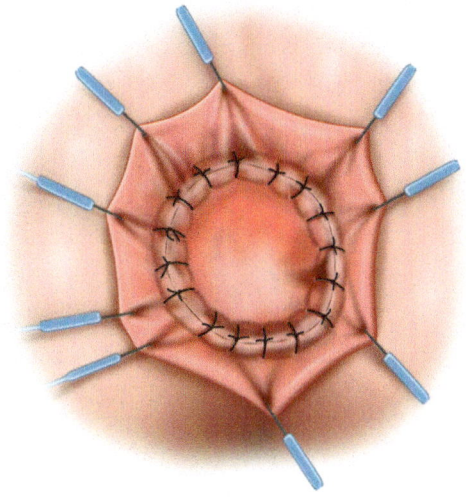

Fig. 6.18 Hand-sewn coloanal anastomosis. A Lone Star Retractor® is placed to facilitate effacement of the anus to allow for placement of multiple sutures. Generally, 3, 6, 9, and 12 o'clock sutures are placed using full-thickness bites, with multiple mucosal/submucosal sutures placed in between

tumor and mesentery. A hand-sewn anastomosis is performed with interrupted 2-0 Vicryl sutures (Tip 6.10). Full-thickness bites of the colon and rectum are used. Enough sutures are placed to approximate the mucosa without gaps (Fig. 6.18). Proximal diversion is performed as described above.

Abdominal Perineal Resection

Bradley J. Champagne and Mark L. Manwaring

Introduction

Laparoscopic abdominal perineal resection involves resection of the sigmoid colon, rectum, and anus with the surrounding pelvic floor musculature. An end colostomy is created. It is commonly performed for low rectal cancer or recurrent anal cancer. Occasionally, it is performed for inflammatory bowel disease or a gynecological malignancy.

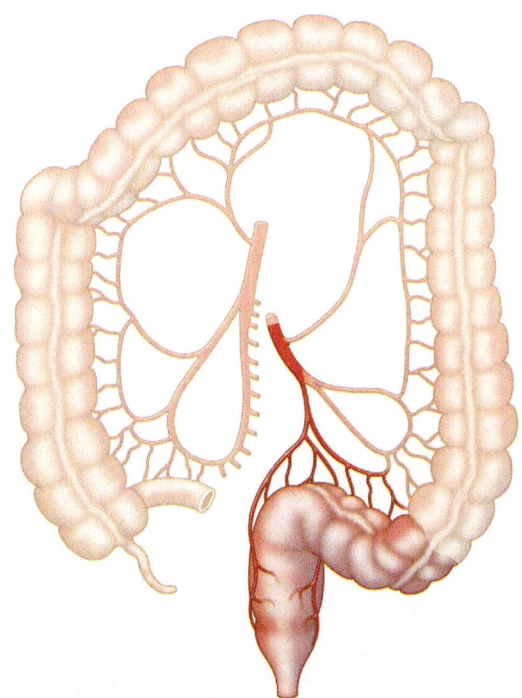

B. J. Champagne (✉)
Department of Surgery, Cleveland Clinic Fairview Hospital, Cleveland, OH, USA
e-mail: Bradley.Champagne@UHhospitals.org

M. L. Manwaring
Saint Thomas Medical Partners in Murfreesboro, Greenville, TN, USA
e-mail: mark.manwaring@me.com

Indications
- Distal rectal cancer
  - In patients with tumor
    - Invading the puborectalis or sphincter muscle
    - Having inadequate distal margin without taking sphincter muscle
  - In patients with preoperative incontinence or poor fecal continence

© Springer Nature Switzerland AG 2020
S. L. Stein, R. R. Lawson (eds.), *Laparoscopic Colectomy*,
https://doi.org/10.1007/978-3-030-39559-9_7

  - In elderly, frail, or ill patients who cannot tolerate the risk of a colo-anal anastomosis and subsequent operation
  - In patients who prefer a colostomy to compromised bowel function
- Recurrent rectal cancer where the location prevents anastomosis
- Anal cancer
  - Recurrence after failed primary radiation chemotherapy
  - Patients unable to undergo chemoradiation
- Failed colo-anal anastomosis
- Perianal Crohn's disease refractory to medical and lesser surgical management

Preoperative Planning
- Preoperative staging for malignancy:
  - Digital rectal exam and flexible sigmoidoscopy or rigid proctoscopy
  - Endorectal ultrasound or pelvic MRI for local staging (T (tumor) and N (nodal))
  - Colonoscopy to exclude synchronous lesions
  - Computed tomography (CT) of the chest, abdomen, and pelvis
  - Carcinoembryologic antigen
- Consider neoadjuvant chemoradiation.
- Preoperative counseling for stoma care, education, and marking (see special considerations).
- Evaluate fecal incontinence preoperatively.
- Mechanical bowel preparation with oral antibiotics.
- Deep venous thrombosis prophylaxis.
- Preoperative antibiotics.
- Urologic, gynecologic, and plastic surgeons as needed:
  - Consider bilateral ureteral stents.

  - Consider hysterectomy and bilateral salpingoopherectomy.
  - Consider musculofascial cutaneous flap for skin and soft tissue coverage.

Steps of the Operation
Patient Setup
1. Step 1: Port placement.
2. Step 2: Assessment for metastatic disease.
3. Step 3: Restore anatomy.
4. Step 4: Retract/expose the inferior mesenteric artery and ureter identification.
5. Step 5: Inferior mesenteric artery and vein division.
6. Step 6: Mobilization of the left colon.
7. Step 7: Total mesorectal excision.
8. Step 8: Division of the mesocolon and sigmoid colon.
9. Step 9: Omental pedicle flap.
10. Step 10: Colostomy creation and closure.
11. Step 11: Perineal dissection.

Tools of the Operation
- 5 mm ports (3–4).
- 12 mm balloon port (1) (umbilicus).
- 10 mm 30-degree camera.
- Laparoscopic bowel graspers.
- Laparoscopic scissors with electrocautery.
- Bipolar energy device for vessel ligation.
- 1 endolumenal stapler with tissue loads.
- Separate bottom table with open instruments for perineal dissection.
- Lonestar or other retractors.
- Second electrocautery unit.

Patient Positioning for Laparoscopic Abdominal Perineal Resection

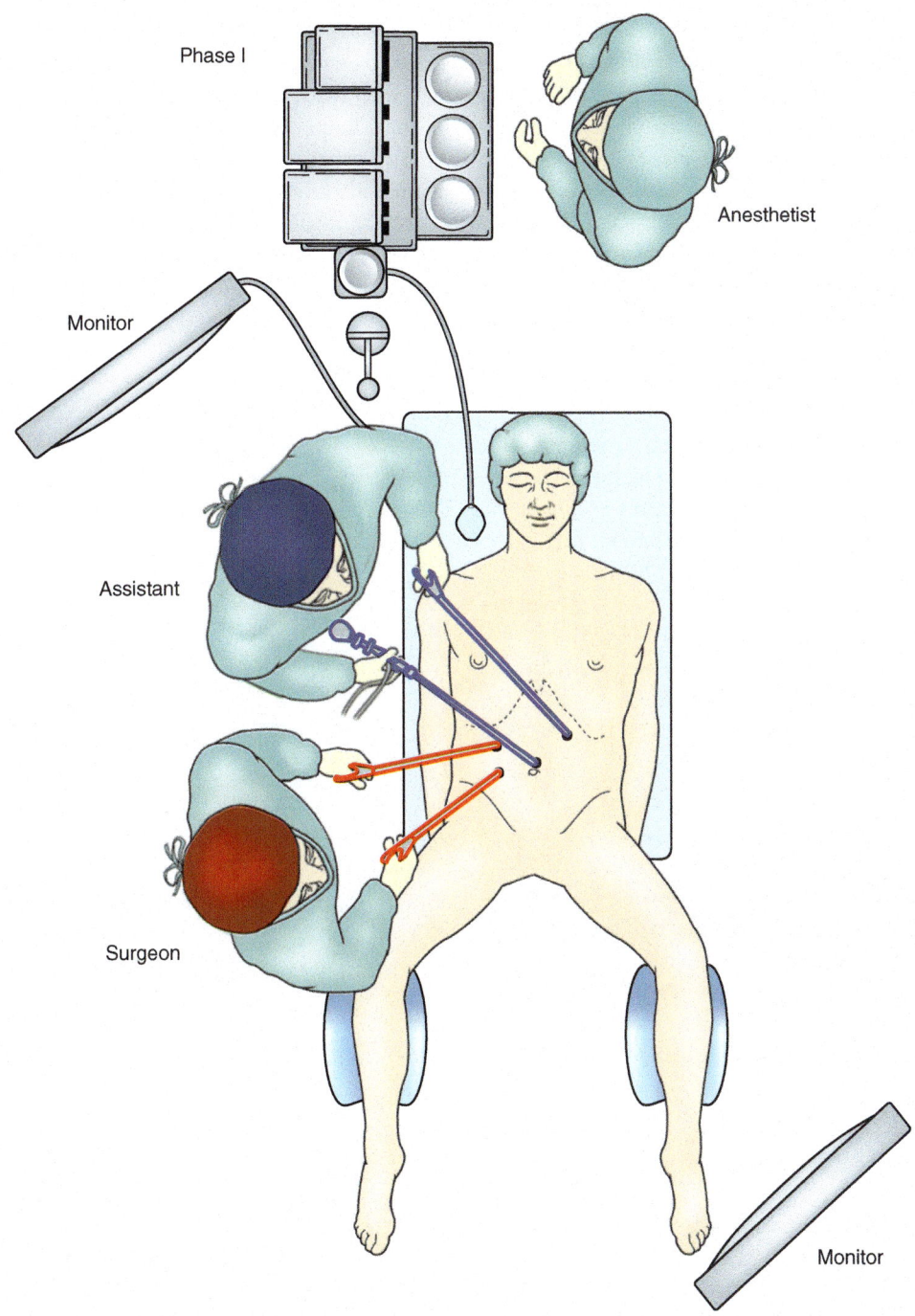

Patient positioning and room setup. The patient is placed in modified lithotomy position with the right arm tucked. The left arm can be tucked or left out if needed by anesthesia. During the laparoscopic portion of the operation, both surgeon and assistant will be on the right side of the patient, with primary monitor off the patient's left foot

In the operating room, the patient is placed in lithotomy position and secured to the bed with a beanbag or gel pad. Padding is placed to protect all vulnerable contact points. The right arm must be carefully tucked in at the patient's side. The left arm can be tucked or left out if needed by anesthesia.

To facilitate the perianal phase of the operation, patient placement on the bed is very important. The fulcrum of the stirrups should be at the level of the hips so the patient can be transitioned to a high lithotomy position for the perineal phase of the operation. The patient should be placed low enough on the caudal extent of the bed so that the bed is halfway between the apex of the gluteal cleft and the anus.

The surgeon will stand primarily on the patient's right during the operation. After port placement the assistant will generally also stand cephalad to the primary surgeon on the right side of the patient. The monitor will ideally be placed near the patient's left hip.

A digital exam is performed to reinforce the location of the tumor prior to prepping. The rectum is irrigated with a dilute betadine solution and drained thoroughly with a mushroom catheter to ensure minimal stool burden. The anus is closed with two 0-monofilament polypropylene sutures to minimize stool contamination (Tip 7.1).

Sterile prep and drape of the perineum follows and a urinary catheter is placed.

roscope using a Hassan technique with a purse-string suture in the fascia. This optimizes seal and is beneficial for closure at the end of the case.

Once the abdomen is insufflated and a laparoscopic view obtained, two right-sided 5 mm trocars are placed. The right lower quadrant trocar is placed 2 fingerbreadths lateral and superior to the anterior superior iliac spine after pneumoperitoneum is established. The right upper quadrant trocar is placed one hand width cephalad and parallel to the right lower quadrant port. Another 5 mm trocar is placed at the preoperatively marked stoma site on the left side (Fig. 7.1 and Tip 7.2).

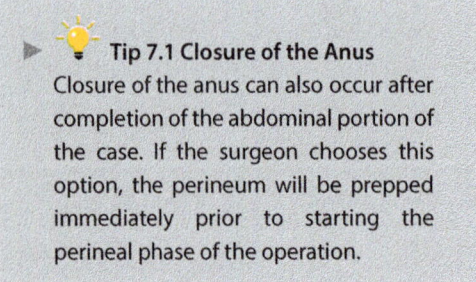

> 💡 **Tip 7.2 Pneumoperitoneum in the Obese**
> In obese patients, an alternative initial trocar placement is Veress needle insufflation followed by optical trocar placement at the same location.

> 💡 **Tip 7.1 Closure of the Anus**
> Closure of the anus can also occur after completion of the abdominal portion of the case. If the surgeon chooses this option, the perineum will be prepped immediately prior to starting the perineal phase of the operation.

Operative Strategy

Step 1: Port Placement

Initial abdominal access for laparoscopic abdominal perineal resection (APR) is similar to other left colon operations and may be performed safely in a number of ways as detailed in Chap. 1. The authors' preference is an infraumbilical 10–12 mm trocar, accommodating a 10 mm lapa-

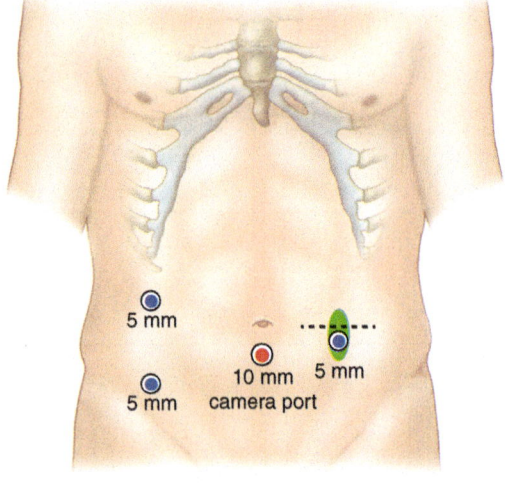

■ Stoma/colostomy site

Fig. 7.1 Port placement. Camera port is an infraumbilical 10–12 mm port to accommodate a Hassan technique with purse string, optimizing seal and closure. Two additional 5 mm ports are placed in the right upper and lower quadrant, and a single left-sided port is placed at the marked stoma location

Occasionally, an additional 5 mm trocar is required in the suprapubic region for additional anterior retraction depending on the patient's lower pelvic anatomy and the position of the tumor (Fig. 7.2 and Tip 7.3).

> 💡 **Tip 7.3 Uterine Retraction**
> Additional retraction of a large or floppy uterus can be performed with an extracorporeal suture. A monofilament suture on a Keith needle is placed through the abdominal wall looped around the body and back through the abdominal wall, leaving laparoscopic instruments free for future retraction (Fig. 7.2).

For the majority of the case, the surgeon operates with both hands through the right-sided ports, while the assistant holds the camera and retracts the colon and rectum out of the pelvis through the left-sided port and holds the camera.

Step 2: Assess for Metastatic Disease

After pneumoperitoneum is established, the peritoneal surface and liver should be evaluated for metastatic disease. CT scan remains very sensitive for stage 4 disease, but occasionally metastatic disease is detected only at the time of surgery. If multiple peritoneal implants are discovered and the patient does not have obstructive symptoms, the surgeon should consider aborting the operation. If the patient has obstructive symptoms and there are peritoneal and/or diffuse liver implants, a loop sigmoid colostomy can be considered. Biopsies should be taken laparoscopically if stage 4 disease has not been determined previously by tissue diagnosis.

Step 3: Restore Anatomy

This brief, but necessary, step is the first step of any laparoscopic colorectal resection. There are three primary reasons that the patient's intra-abdominal anatomy may be distorted. First, prior adhesions from abdominal surgery often will tether the omen-

Fig. 7.2 Retraction of the uterus. Retraction of the uterus using Keith needle: to retract a bulky or floppy uterus, a monofilament suture is placed perpendicularly through the abdominal wall. The needle is then placed through the broad ligament, just lateral to the uterine body, under the uterus, and back through the contralateral broad ligament and abdominal wall. A hemostat can place upward tension on the uterus, leaving laparoscopic instruments free for dissection and fine retraction. The suture is removed at the end of the case

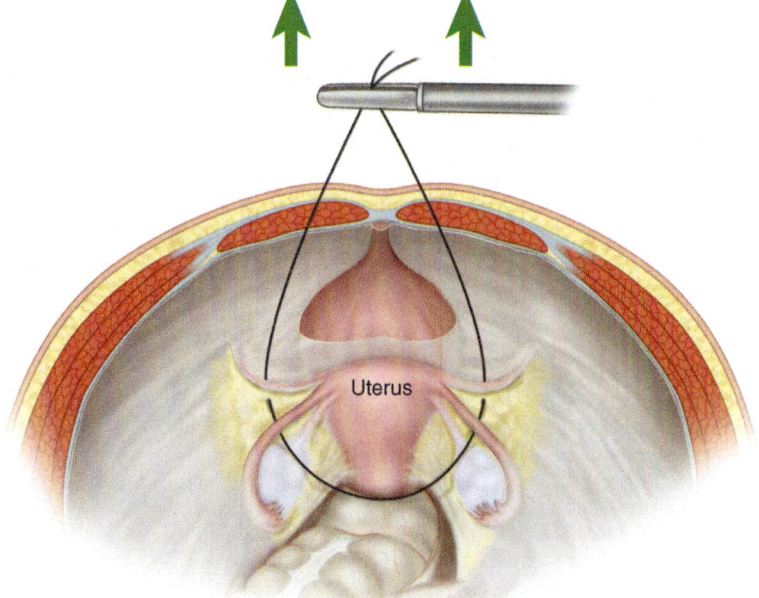

tum, small bowel, or large bowel to the abdominal wall or in the pelvis (prior hysterectomy). These adhesions can prohibit adequate pelvic exposure and must be addressed early. Lysis of adhesions, as described in Chap. 10, may be performed. Second, if the patient has had radiation, the field may have extended to the upper pelvis. The terminal ileum and sigmoid colon should be evaluated for external signs of damage. Occasionally, a small bowel resection is required if the ileum is severely compromised. Lastly, diverticulitis may have fixed the sigmoid colon in an unnatural location. This can be rectified by freeing lateral adhesions from the left abdominal side wall and pelvis, which restores the colon to its normal position as it relates to the location of the inferior mesenteric artery.

Step 4: Expose the Inferior Mesenteric Artery (IMA) and Ureter Identification

Once restoration of anatomy has been accomplished, the patient is rotated slightly, right side down, and into steep Trendelenburg position. Place the omentum over the transverse colon to provide more room for the small bowel. Sweep the small bowel out of the pelvis into the right upper abdomen.

Identify the inferior mesenteric/superior rectal vascular pedicle extending into the pelvis. This is accomplished with anterior traction on the mesentery at the rectosigmoid junction (Tip 7.4). Initially,

the surgeon uses bowel graspers through the left quadrant port to identify the correct location and direction of traction. Traction is in an anterolateral direction. The surgeon achieves appropriate traction with two hands, moving the rectosigmoid until the inferior mesenteric artery is visualized and the peritoneum is under adequate tension. The assistant then assumes this same traction on the mesentery, freeing both hands for dissection.

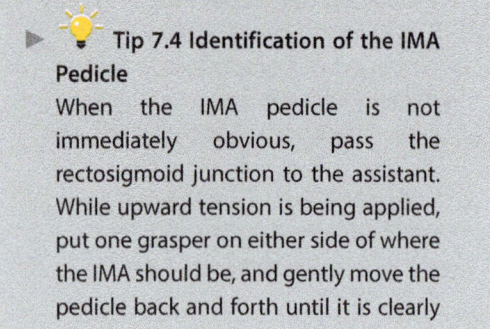

> ▶ 💡 **Tip 7.4 Identification of the IMA Pedicle**
> When the IMA pedicle is not immediately obvious, pass the rectosigmoid junction to the assistant. While upward tension is being applied, put one grasper on either side of where the IMA should be, and gently move the pedicle back and forth until it is clearly identified.

Tension should be created on the tissues behind the IMA pedicle to facilitate opening of the plane. The peritoneum is incised with cautery scissors starting approximately 5 mm anterior to the sacral promontory. The direction of incision is cephalad toward the origin of the IMA. When the correct plane is opened, air will sweep into the plane, further facilitating the direction of dissection (Fig. 7.3).

Fig. 7.3 Entering the mesorectal space. Entry is parallel and deep to the inferior mesenteric artery, facilitated by tension provided by the assistant. Entry occurs with electrocautery anterior to the sacral promontory. When the plane is defined with electrocautery, air will enter this space, further highlighting the correct plane. The plane should be superficial and medial to hypogastric nerves and deep to the mesorectal fascia

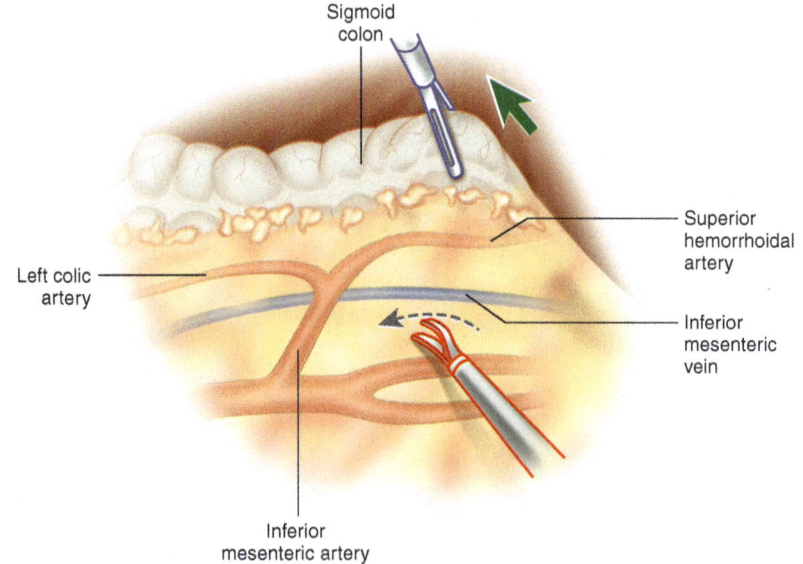

The correct mesorectal plane is just deep to the IMA. Minor adjustment of tension and direction by the assistant on the rectosigmoid demonstrate the hypogastric nerves behind the IMA. The surgeon may add additional traction with the left hand, increasing tension and further exposing the plane. Tissues behind the mesocolon yield a plane connected under the pedicle to a layer over Toldt's fascia. When the window inferior to the IMA has been created, the surgeon's left hand instrument (closed bowel grasper) can be inserted into the plane lifting the distal mesocolon first ventrally and then in a cephalad direction. During dissection, care should be taken not to dissect too deeply, as this increases risk of injury to the iliac vessels or autonomic nerves.

The next key step is to identify the ureter (Pitfall 7.1). It is essential to wait 60 seconds without movement and allow the ureter to vermiculate before continuing dissection after this move (Fig. 7.4). If the ureter is not visualized, the retracting bowel grasper should be pulled back into the port slightly, to ensure the ureter has not been lifted with the mesorectum. If the ureter still cannot be identified, evaluate the anatomy carefully and ensure that the plane is correct. Further dissection distally may help release the rectosigmoid to allow for better identification at the pelvic brim.

If visualization of the ureter remains elusive, grasp the colon with the left hand, and switch to a lateral approach, taking the lateral attachments

> ⚠ **Pitfall 7.1**
> Prior to any use of energy devices or staplers, the ureter must be identified and protected.

with monopolar cautery. This step further allows for elevation of the rectosigmoid and identification of the ureter.

The white line is then divided laterally, opening the plane to identify the ureter from the left side. This separates the ureter laterally from the IMA pedicle. Separation must continue cephalad to allow for safe division of the artery.

Step 5: Inferior Mesenteric Artery and Vein Division

For optimal lymphadenectomy, the inferior mesenteric artery (IMA) is divided near its origin proximal to the left colic. For benign disease or in elderly patients, it may also be divided immediately distal to the left colic artery to preserve improved blood supply to the descending colon and sigmoid.

To safely divide the IMA for malignant disease, a window is created cephalad to the IMA. The 30-degree camera is then rotated coun-

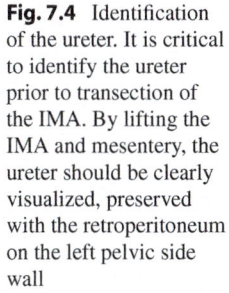

Fig. 7.4 Identification of the ureter. It is critical to identify the ureter prior to transection of the IMA. By lifting the IMA and mesentery, the ureter should be clearly visualized, preserved with the retroperitoneum on the left pelvic side wall

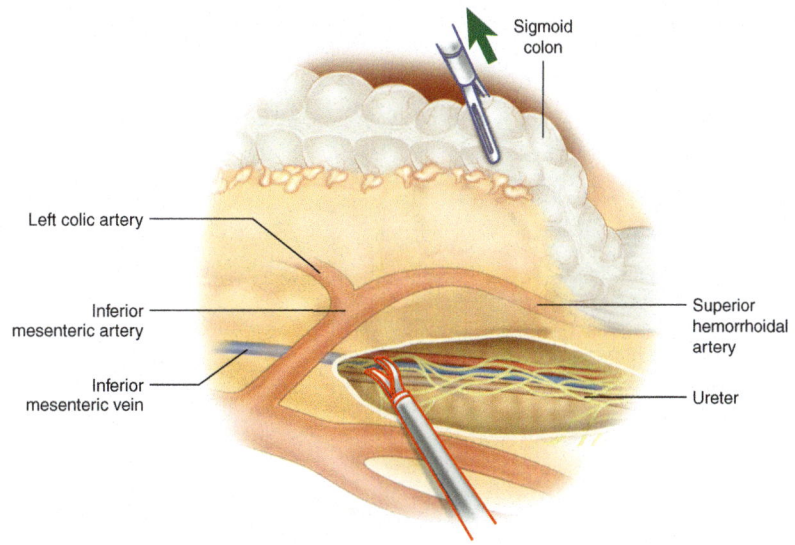

terclockwise. The surgeon holds the IMA in the right hand retracting in a caudad direction. The left hand is used to create the window on the far side of the vessel with monopolar cautery and a Maryland grasper. The assistant retracts the colon more proximally to optimize tension.

The mesentery around the IMA can be taken with bipolar energy prior to ligating the vessel to expose the most proximal extent of the vessel. An endolumenal stapling device with a vascular load is very safe and effective as well (Fig. 7.5). After the high ligation, the IMV can be isolated in a similar fashion and divided, along with the left colic, as they are in close proximity.

After division of the IMA and IMV, medial to lateral dissection can be performed with blunt dissection and gentle sweeping, to facilitate the lateral dissection.

Step 6: Mobilization of the Left Colon

Following division of the inferior mesenteric artery, the left mesocolon is separated from the retroperitoneum in a medial-to-lateral direction using a spreading movement. The patient is taken out of steep Trendelenburg position and airplaned to right side down, as necessary to move the small bowel out of the operating field. Upward traction is maintained on the ligated vessels and mesoco-

lon with the left hand, while the right hand sweeps down additional retroperitoneal attachments. Dissection can continue laterally to the white line of Toldt and left gutter and superiorly toward the pancreas. The more medial the dissection, the easier mobilization of the left colon will be.

The atraumatic bowel grasper is used through the right upper quadrant port to retract the descending and sigmoid colon medially. Scissors are inserted through the right lower quadrant port. Cauterization 1 mm medial to the white line will elevate the left colon and free it from the retroperitoneum. Dissection continues in a cephalad direction just enough to allow adequate reach of the colon to the planned colostomy site to the abdominal wall (Tip 7.5).

> 💡 **Tip 7.5 Stoma Length**
> The end of the colon used for the colostomy should reach without tension to the abdominal wall. Insufflation may falsely overestimate the amount of colon mobilization needed, so desufflating may be helpful when checking length. Additionally, too much length may actually increase the rate of hernia or prolapse.

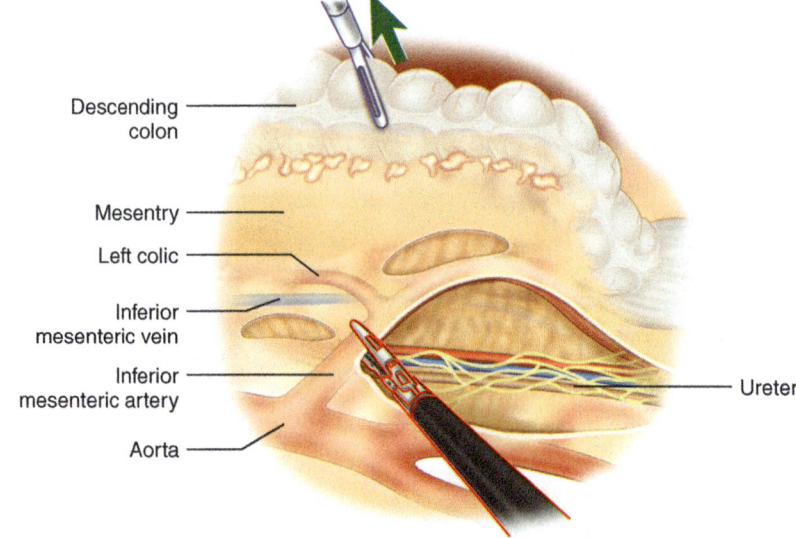

Fig. 7.5 Isolation of the IMA for high ligation. Windows have been created proximal and distal to the vessel, and the mesentery around the IMA has been dissected. The assistant provides proximal tension on the colon, while the surgeon's right hand holds the IMA with caudal retraction. The surgeon's left hand can then create the window on the right side of the vessel

Descending colon

Mesentry

Left colic

Inferior mesenteric vein

Inferior mesenteric artery

Aorta

Ureter

Step 7: Total Mesorectal Excision

The patient is returned to steep Trendelenburg position, and the small bowel reflected cranially. The rectosigmoid junction is elevated away from the sacral promontory, to enable entry into the presacral space. An open atraumatic grasper is used to facilitate traction on the sigmoid and rectum as if mimicking the role of the St. Mark's retractor in an open pelvic dissection (Tip 7.6).

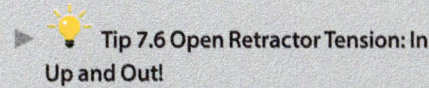

> ▶ 🔆 **Tip 7.6 Open Retractor Tension: In Up and Out!**
> To facilitate retraction in the pelvis, an open long bowel grasper can be placed behind the mesorectum. The direction of traction is gently into the mesorectum, up toward the abdominal wall (anteriorly) and slightly out of the pelvis (cephalad).

A near bloodless plane is expected for the mesorectal dissection except for the caudal lat-

eral stalks, which are amenable to division with bipolar energy or electrocautery. Identify the filmy plane of the posterior mesorectum and dissect with cautery scissors. Take care to preserve the hypogastric nerves laterally as they pass into the pelvis anterior to the sacrum. Continue the dissection in this avascular, loose areolar plane toward the pelvic floor (Fig. 7.6).

When the tension is lost secondary to anterolateral attachments, switch to the peritoneum on the right side of the rectum. Retraction on the rectum should be toward the left side of the pelvis to facilitate traction. Attachments are divided laterally, up to the level of the seminal vesicles or rectovaginal septum. They should be avascular, except at the lateral stalks, where a small amount of adipose tissue and the middle colic vessels cross from the side wall to the mesorectum.

This process is repeated for the peritoneum on the left side of the rectum with the surgeon's left hand retracting the rectum out of the pelvis and to the right, with the assistant providing countertraction on the side wall (Fig. 7.7). This facilitates further posterior dissection along the back of the mesorectum down through Waldeyer's fascia to the anal canal. In many cases, particularly with

Fig. 7.6 Posterior mesorectal dissection. The posterior mesentery makes an inverted "U" providing a visual of the filmy plane for dissection. The assistant facilitates visualization by providing upward tension on the rectum. Caution should be taken to ensure preservation of the hypogastric nerves

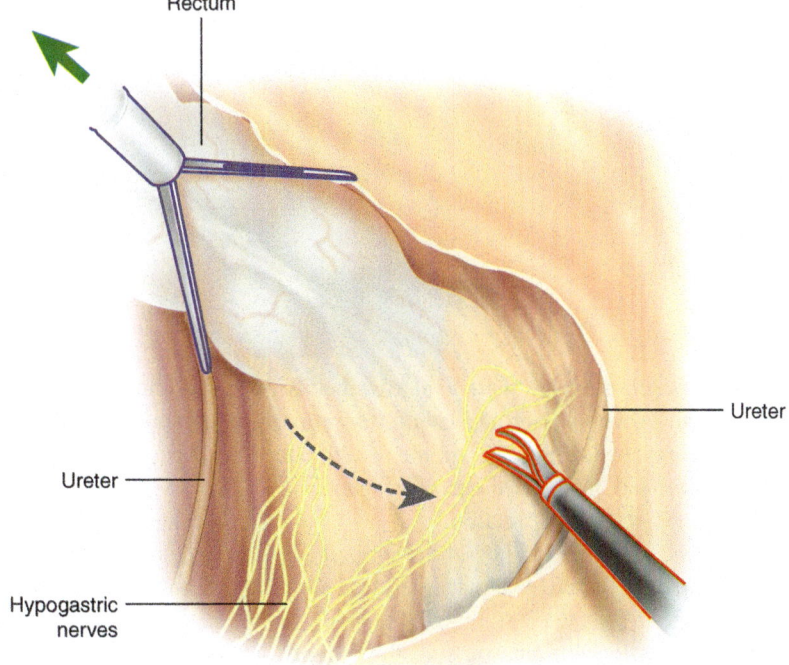

Fig. 7.7 Right lateral dissection. The surgeon's left hand retracts the colon to the left and out of the pelvis, while the assistant tents up the side wall away from the plane of dissection. Dissection proceeds along Denonvilliers' fascia

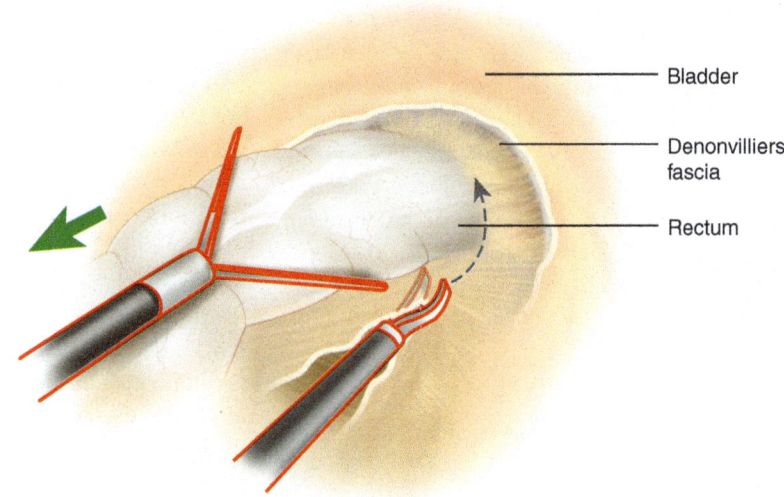

Bladder

Denonvilliers fascia

Rectum

Fig. 7.8 Anterior dissection. Tension is placed anteriorly on the bladder or vagina. The plane is carefully scored with electrocautery, preserving the vagina or seminal vessels unless contraindicated for oncologic margins

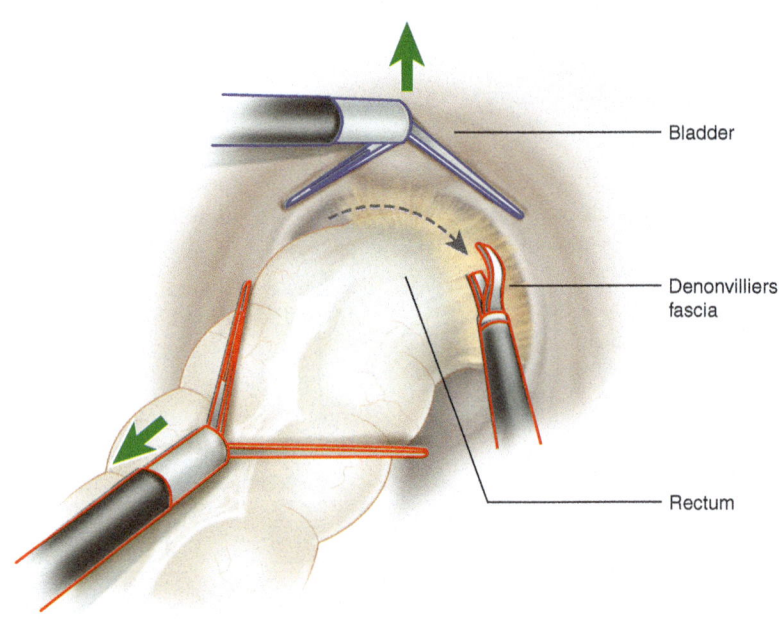

Bladder

Denonvilliers fascia

Rectum

obese patients or males with a narrow pelvis, some or all of the anterior and lateral dissection must be completed to create lift of the rectum out of the pelvis and obtain adequate visualization to complete the posterior dissection.

After the posterior and lateral dissection have been completed, the assistant places an atraumatic bowel grasper, via the left iliac fossa port, to retract the peritoneum anteriorly to the rectum. The rectum is pushed down and pulled out of the pelvis simultaneously. The anterior peritoneal dissection is continued from the free edge of the lateral peritoneal dissection with monopolar cautery (Fig. 7.8). The anterior dissection is an extension of the lateral peritoneal incision from each side of the rectum toward the middle. The plane is developed anterior and parallel to the rectum, leaving Denonvilliers' fascia intact unless contraindicated from an oncologic perspective. The dissection will separate the posterior vaginal wall of the prostate and seminal vessels from the anterior wall of the rectum (Tip 7.7).

> 💡 **Tip 7.7 Vaginal Retraction**
> In females, a sponge stick in the vagina that is elevated in an anterior direction can also help with this dissection.

It is critical not to "waist" the specimen. The mesorectum should be left intact, and attachments/adhesions from the mesorectum to the levator muscles after radiation should be left intact and taken with the specimen (Fig. 7.9).

The difficulty of dissection will vary depending on the body habitus of the patient, the diameter of the pelvis, and the size and level of the tumor. Rectal mobilization can be very difficult to perform laparoscopically under some circumstances. Low bulky anterior rectal tumors, morbidly obese men, or tumors adherent to the

posterior wall of the vagina may need to be completed in an open fashion via a lower midline or a Pfannenstiel incision (Pitfall 7.2).

> ⚠️ **Pitfall 7.2**
> If there is any difficulty determining the difference between tumor and radiation fibrosis in the anterior position, the pelvic dissection should be converted to an open or hybrid approach.

After the anterior dissection is performed, recheck the lateral and posterior planes to determine if more tissue can be divided. The dissection is continued until the levators are visualized laterally and the coccyx is palpated posteriorly. Confirmation with concurrent digital vaginal exam that the extent of dissection has reached tissues accessible from the perineal dissection is helpful (Fig. 7.10).

Step 8: Division of Mesocolon and Sigmoid Colon

The sigmoid mesentery and colon are left in continuity until this point to prevent the sigmoid from falling into the operative field during pelvic dissec-

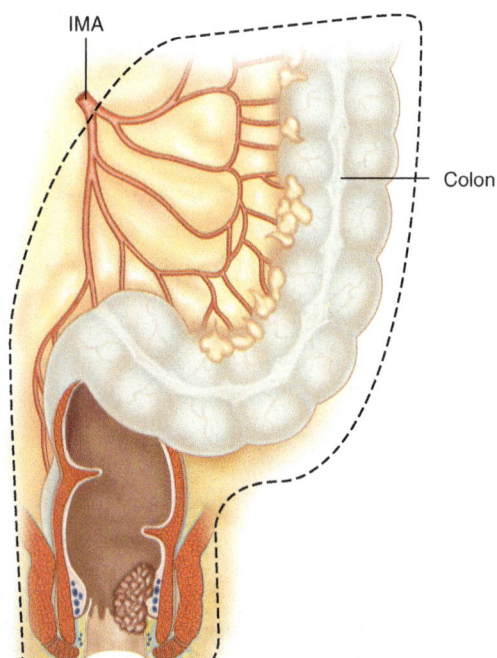

Fig. 7.9 Complete abdominal perineal resection. For a complete abdominal perineal resection, the specimen should contain significant portions of the levator ani without waisting of the specimen. The correct planes for an extra-levator APR are shown above

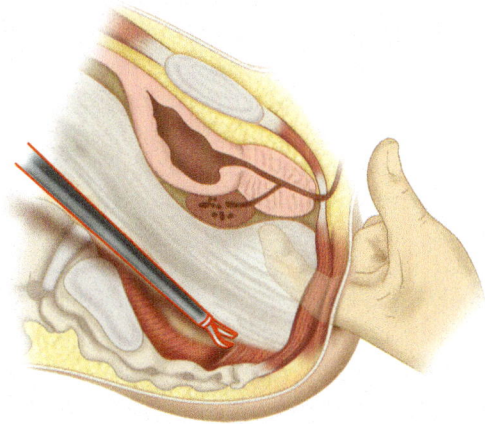

Fig. 7.10 Confirmation of dissection location. When the dissection has reached the levator ani from above, a digital exam can be done to confirm location of the dissection. It is important not to "cone" in on the specimen and to take appropriate oncologic margins including the levator ani for oncologic resection

tion. In some cases, dividing the colon mesentery and sigmoid early in the case may improve exposure and is reasonable if this is the case.

Retract the inferior mesenteric artery pedicle with a bowel grasper through the right lower quadrant port, and insert bipolar energy through the right upper quadrant port. The assistant continues to retract the colon in an anterior fashion. A well-perfused location on the colon with adequate reach to the stoma site should be chosen. The mesentery is divided perpendicular to the colon and proximal to the transected IMA/left colon pedicle. After the residual mesentery is divided completely with an energy device, the colon is divided with a laparoscopic stapler. Introduce the stapler through the 12 mm port at the umbilicus with the assistance of a 5 mm camera from a right port (Fig. 7.11). Care must be taken not to devascularize the terminal of the colon during mesocolic division. Preserving the marginal vessel is typically sufficient to prevent ischemia.

Step 9: Omental Pedicle Flap

Prior to extraction of the descending colon through the abdominal wall, an omental pedicle flap is raised if adequate omentum is available. This helps prevent small bowel loops from entering the deep confines of the pelvis and may reduce the incidence of complicated small bowel obstruction or perineal hernia. The omental pedicle flap is created by releasing attachments of the omentum from the left side of the transverse colon and gastroepiploic arcades.

The gastroepiploic artery is identified and preserved just lateral to the falciform ligament. The energy instrument is used to open the omentum just inferior to the gastroepiploic artery at this point. The energy device is used to continue along the inferior aspect of the gastroepiploic artery to the splenic flexure, freeing all the attachments from the lateral left side wall and spleen.

The omentum is also separated from the colon, starting at the midline. Either electrocautery or bipolar is used to free the omentum from the colon, again continuing to the splenic flexure as described in Splenic Flexure Mobilization, Chap. 4. This should completely free the omentum from the left side, allowing a significant, tension-free extension down into the pelvis.

The omental pedicle can be lengthened to lie down the left paracolic gutter into the pelvis. It can be secured with a 2-0 absorbable braided suture to prevent migration after closure.

Step 10: Colostomy Creation and Closure

The colonic limb is then grasped with an atraumatic clamp through the right lower quadrant port, and attention is turned to making the colostomy site (Tip 7.8).

 Tip 7.8 Timing of Stoma Creation
The creation of the stoma can be delayed until after the perineal phase of the operation. Advantages include ability to continue dissection from the abdomen and ability to irrigate the pelvis fully. Disadvantages are decreased efficiency and return to the abdomen after "dirty" phase of the operation.

The stoma site is created with excision of a nickel-sized piece of skin and vertical incision of the subcutaneous tissues. Appendiceal retractors facilitate visualization and separation (Tip 7.9). Separate the fascia vertically and spread the muscles using a Kelly clamp. The muscles should be spread and not cut. The peritoneum is then scored, which will desufflate the abdomen. If the bowel is close to the incision, the peritoneum can be lifted using Kelly clamps and then incised. The tissues are opened just enough to admit the colonic conduit without vascular compromise; excessive dilation should be avoided as this will predispose the patient to hernia.

 Tip 7.9 Pneumoperitoneum During Trephine Creation
Maintain pneumoperitoneum during creation of the stoma incision. This will help prevent inadvertent injury to the bowel as the peritoneum is opened.

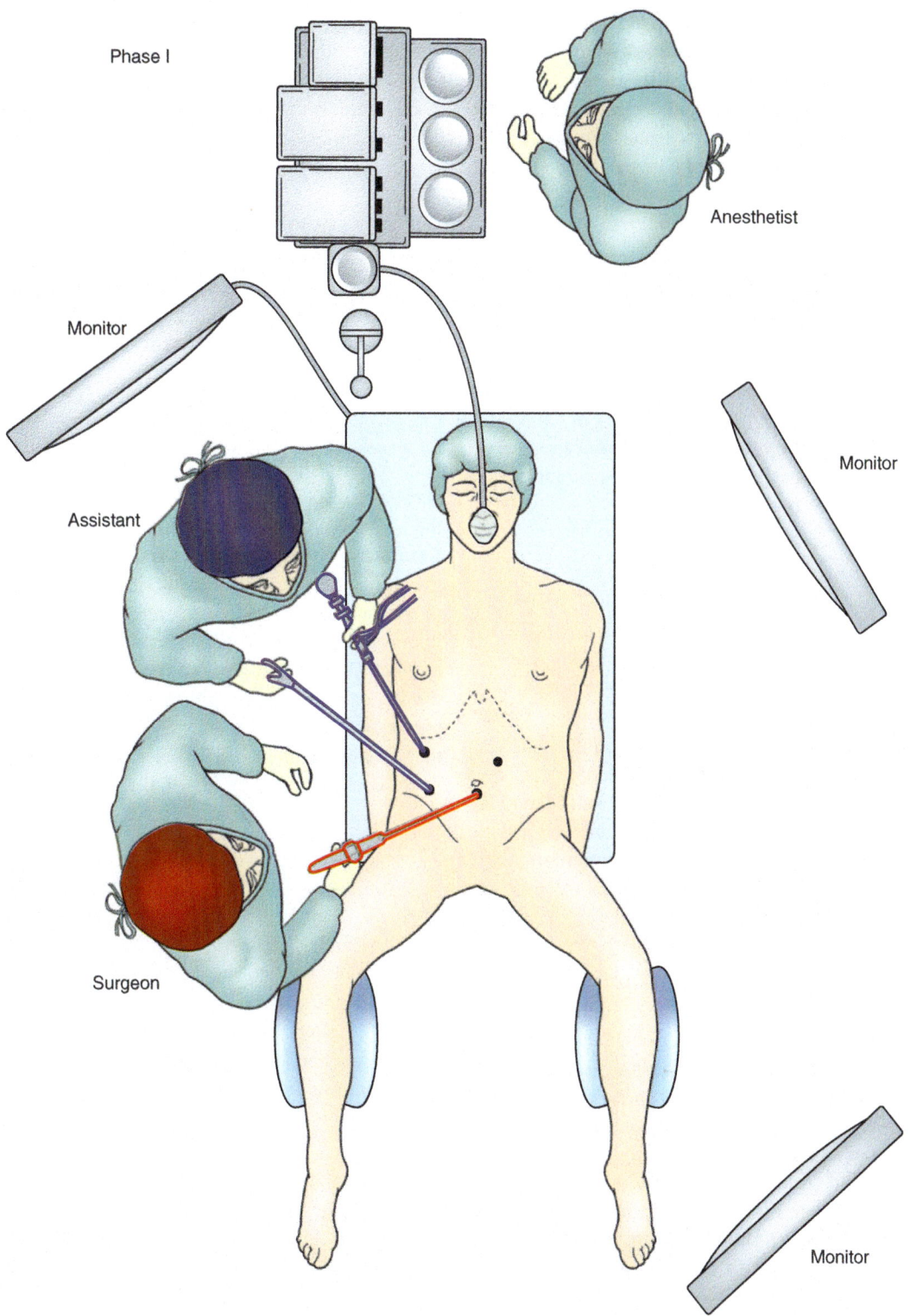

Fig. 7.11 Port relocation for colon transection. To facilitate colon transection, a 5 mm camera is moved to the right upper quadrant port, and the infraumbilical port is used for insertion of the stapler

A Babcock clamp is placed through the stoma incision, and the colon is passed from the laparoscopic grasper to the Babcock (Tip 7.10). The end of the colon is grasped, extracted, and maintained with a Babcock clamp. After reinsufflation, evaluate mesentery to ensure the colon and vascular supply have not been twisted. Follow the free edge of the mesentery to verify absence of mesocolic torsion.

> **Tip 7.10 Recreating Pneumoperitoneum with an Incision**
> If the colon is dropped or there is cause for concern for twisting of the mesentery, the stoma incision can be temporarily closed with penetrating towel clamps.

A JP drain is placed in the pelvis through the right lower quadrant port site. The uterine retraction suture is released, if present, and hemostasis at all sites is assured. Trocars are removed, closing ports larger than 5 mm with a Carter-Thompson suture passer or 5/8 circular needle. The skin is closed at the laparoscopic port sites and the wounds covered with a towel. Mature the stoma by amputating the staple line and sewing the bowel wall to the dermis circumferentially using an absorbable suture.

Step 11: Perineal Dissection

The patient is transitioned to a high lithotomy position, with the table raised, to allow the surgeon and assistant to sit. A small Mayo stand cover or sterile sheet is secured to the surgeon's gown and the drapes to protect instruments from dropping off of the field. A headlight assures adequate lighting. Morbidly obese patients sometimes benefit from a single retraction suture on each buttock to expose the dissection site. A Lone Star Retractor can also be used to facilitate exposure in a complete extralevator dissection (Fig. 7.11 and Tip 7.11). Palpate both ischium and the coccyx and mark the skin for a cylindrical resection. The location and extent of

the dissection is based on pathology and preoperative imaging. Inadequate resection can result in close or positive margins. If primary closure is not possible, secondary to radiation changes or laxity of tissue, consider use of a myocutaneous muscle flap.

There are few external landmarks for use in this

> **Tip 7.11 Perineal Retraction**
> An alternative to a commercial available perineal retractor is 2-0 polysorbable braided sutures. These should be placed wide to the dissection field and placed under tension in a circumferential manner.

portion of the surgery. Using a marking pen, trace the planned borders of the skin incision. Electrocautery is used to score the dissection markings (Tip 7.12). After the dermis has been incised, move the Lonestar (R) retractor into the dermis for improved retraction. As the dissection continues in a cylindrical shape, larger deep retractors including Deaver's may be necessary. Intermittently relax the retraction, and pay close attention to the shape of the developing specimen to avoid coning-in or waisting of the specimen (Fig. 7.12).

> **Tip 7.12 Begin with Posterior Dissection**
> Working posteriorly first can prevent bleeding into the dissection plane and also generally provides the most consistent landmark, the coccyx, for borders of dissection.

Initially when dissecting through the ischiorectal spaces, working circumferentially can maintain the surgeon's sense of the specimen shape and allow for necessary adjustments. Concentrating on the posterior dissection toward the coccyx provides a landmark as the dissection deepens. Make an incision through the ligamentous attachments to the coccyx to open the supra-

Fig. 7.12 Perineal setup and Lone Star Retractor placement. The perineum should be redraped as soilage may have occurred during manipulation of the rectum. Place a suture on the anus to prevent further soilage. Lonestar is placed outside the margins of resection. Starting posteriorly prevents rundown of bleeding and is the most uniform location to enter the peritoneum, secondary to the location of the coccyx

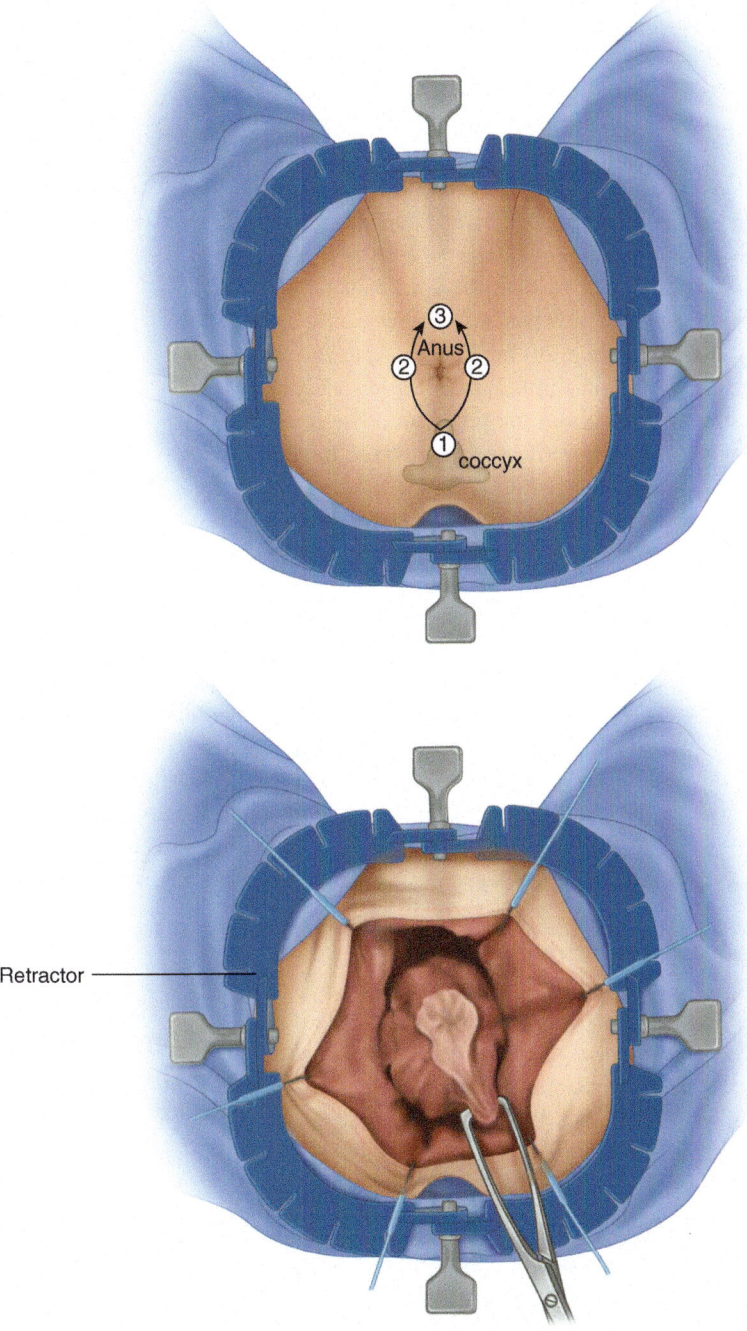

levator space. This should promptly expose the abdominal dissection planes. From this location, extend the incision anterolateral by hooking the levator musculature with a cocked finger or right-angle clamp, and divide the muscle and soft tissue with electrocautery.

The anterior dissection is taken through the rectovaginal septum in women or through the perineal muscles and to the retro-prostatic plane in men. Frequent digital vaginal exams can help avoid inadvertent injury during the dissection. In men, the urinary catheter can be palpated as the urethra passes posterior to the symphysis pubis and is an important structure to avoid during the dissection. Avoid blunt dissection of the levators to decrease the risk of entering the tumor. The dissection is carried anteriorly on both sides staying wide to maintain a cylindrical specimen, leaving only anterior attachments. At this point, the specimen can be folded posteriorly and pulled through the aperture, leaving the anterior prostatic or vaginal attachments. Amputate the specimen in the proper plane from this final attachment.

After assurance of hemostasis, close the incision with interrupted braided absorbable sutures in layers from the perineum. The levators cannot be approximated given fixed lateral attachments to the pelvis. Perform closure of the fatty layers, and position a Penrose drain from the pelvis to the inferior portion of the wound. Prior to skin closure, the wound is irrigated with a Pulsavac (R) (Zimmer) lavage of triple antibiotic solution (1 liter). The perineal skin is closed with 0 nonabsorbable monofilament in a vertical mattress technique. Dry gauze dressing is applied and the legs returned to a low lithotomy position.

Special Considerations

Preoperative Stoma Marking

Preoperative preparation for a laparoscopic abdominal perineal resection must include left-sided preoperative stoma site marking, preferably by a stoma therapist. Placement of the stoma is critical, as this will be a permanent colostomy.

Although every patient is different, a stoma triangle is a well-known concept that facilitates placement of a stoma. A triangle is drawn between the umbilicus, the pubis, and the anterior superior iliac spine. This locates the stoma within the supporting rectus sheath. A location within this stoma triangle is ideal for many patients (Fig. 7.13).

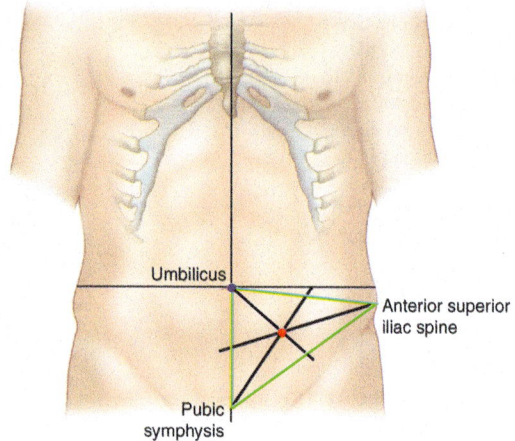

Fig. 7.13 The stoma triangle. The stoma triangle, bounded by the umbilicus, pubis symphysis, and anterior superior iliac spine, is the ideal location for a stoma for many patients

Additional considerations include skin creases as possible and prior abdominal incisions. With supine, sitting, and standing positions, the site should have a flat surface amenable to pouching. It should be visible to the patient, and not interfere with pant lines, belts of daily activities.

Ideally, a site is selected at a preoperative visit designed to educate the patient about postoperative colostomy care.

Varying the Approach

Prone Dissection

In the setting of morbid obesity, limited hip mobility, or tumors requiring an extra-levator dissection based on preoperative MR imaging, a prone perineal-first approach has distinct advantages. Though it adds to positioning time, visualization is superior, and an assistant can be more effective in assisting with exposure. When performed, this approach begins with the patient in the prone jackknife position with the buttocks taped apart to optimize exposure. The perineal dissection, as outlined above, is performed first and taken above the levators into the mesorectal plane. The perineum is then sealed with an occlusive dressing and the patient rotated to the lithotomy position. The trans-abdominal dissection is then performed as outlined.

T4b Tumors

T4b tumors can also be challenging laparoscopically, but may be possible. In a woman who has had a prior hysterectomy, the vagina can be removed en bloc laparoscopically. The vagina can be entered from above with the assistance of a sponge stick in the introitus held by a second assistant standing between the legs. With the sponge stick in place, the vaginal apex can be opened with monopolar cautery. The vaginal walls can then be divided with bipolar energy down each side. This part of the dissection needs to be reserved until after the posterior and lateral dissection is complete to prevent a loss of pneumoperitoneum. In a thin female, this is easily

accomplished from the perineum, but in a morbidly obese patient, it helps to do this from the abdomen. T4b tumors into the prostatic capsule or seminal vesicle should not be approached laparoscopically.

Intra-levator Dissection

Recently, advocates of the complete extra-levator approach have espoused this technique be used in all cases to obtain superior oncologic outcomes. The data has not substantiated this claim and each case should be looked at individually. In elderly patients with several comorbidities and a tumor limited to one location, the radial margin should be wide on the side of the tumor, but it is not necessary on the contralateral side. A massive defect may warrant a complex closure with a flap, adding time and complexity to the operation. The importance of a solid radial margin and complete TME cannot be overstated, but each patient must be evaluated independently.

Subtotal Colectomy

8

Joshua I. S. Bleier and Skandan Shanmugan

Introduction

Laparoscopic subtotal colectomy is the resection of the entire abdominal colon with an end ileostomy or creation of an ileorectal anastomosis. Extent of distal colon resection varies from the sigmoid colon to rectum, depending on the indication and plan for anastomosis. It is performed for both benign and malignant diseases processes.

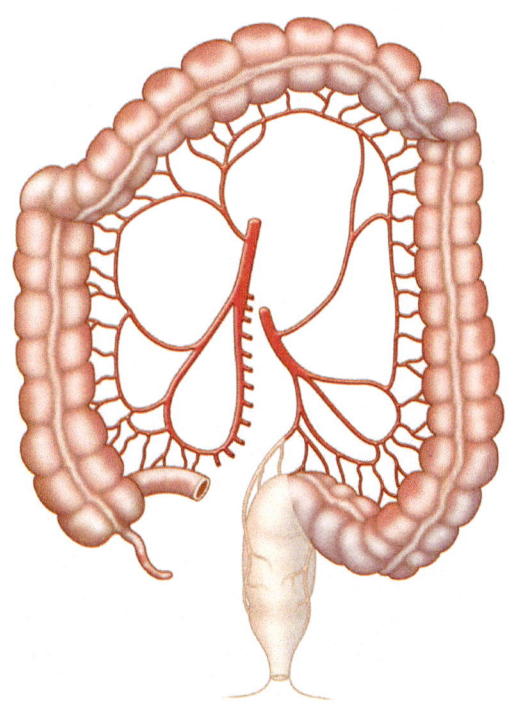

J. I. S. Bleier (✉)
Department of Surgery, Division of Colon & Rectal Surgery, Perelman School of Medicine, Pennsylvania Hospital, Philadelphia, PA, USA
e-mail: Joshua.Bleier@uphs.upenn.edu

S. Shanmugan
Department of Surgery, Division of Colon & Rectal Surgery, Penn Presbyterian Medical Center, Philadelphia, PA, USA
e-mail: Skandan.Shanmugan@uphs.upenn.edu

Indications
- Medically refractory colitis (distal sigmoid division)
- Ulcerative colitis, Crohn's colitis, indeterminate colitis
- Neoplasia requiring total abdominal colectomy (upper rectal division)

© Springer Nature Switzerland AG 2020
S. L. Stein, R. R. Lawson (eds.), *Laparoscopic Colectomy*,
https://doi.org/10.1007/978-3-030-39559-9_8

- Polyposis syndromes (upper rectal division)
- Prophylactic
- Attenuated FAP
- Infectious colitis (mid- or distal sigmoid division)
- Colonic inertia (upper rectal division)

Preoperative Planning
- Colonoscopy to establish diagnosis and confirm distal extent of disease or lesion
- CT scan to rule additional intra-abdominal pathology
- Sitz marker studies to evaluate colonic dysmotility
- DVT prophylaxis
- Mechanical bowel preparation
- Preoperative antibiotics
- Stoma marking (when appropriate)

Steps of the Operation
Patient Positioning
1. Step 1: Port placement
2. Step 2: Staging laparoscopy (for neoplastic disease)
3. Step 3: Right colon medial to lateral dissection
4. Step 4: Division of the ileocolic pedicle
5. Step 5: Mobilization of the terminal ileum
6. Step 6: Mobilization of the hepatic flexure
7. Step 7: Entry into the lesser sac
8. Step 8: Identification and division of middle colic pedicle
9. Step 9: Inferior mesenteric artery
10. Step 10: Left colon mobilization
11. Step 11: Distal transection of the rectosigmoid
12. Step 12: Extraction of the specimen
13. Step 13: Ileorectal anastomosis
14. Step 14: Creation of an end ileostomy (if necessary)

Tools of the Operation
- 12 mm Hasson port (1)
- 5 mm port (3)
- 12 mm port (1)
- 10 mm 30-degree camera (1)
- Laparoscopic bowel graspers (locking capability) (2)
- Laparoscopic shears with cautery (1)
- Bipolar energy instrument for vessel ligation/mesenteric division
- Laparoscopic stapler (either for bowel or vascular pedicles)
- Small wound protector
- Anastomosis
- 25 or 28 circular endolumenal stapler
- Proctoscope/flexible endoscope for anastomotic assessment/air-leak test

Patient Positioning for Laparoscopic Subtotal Colectomy

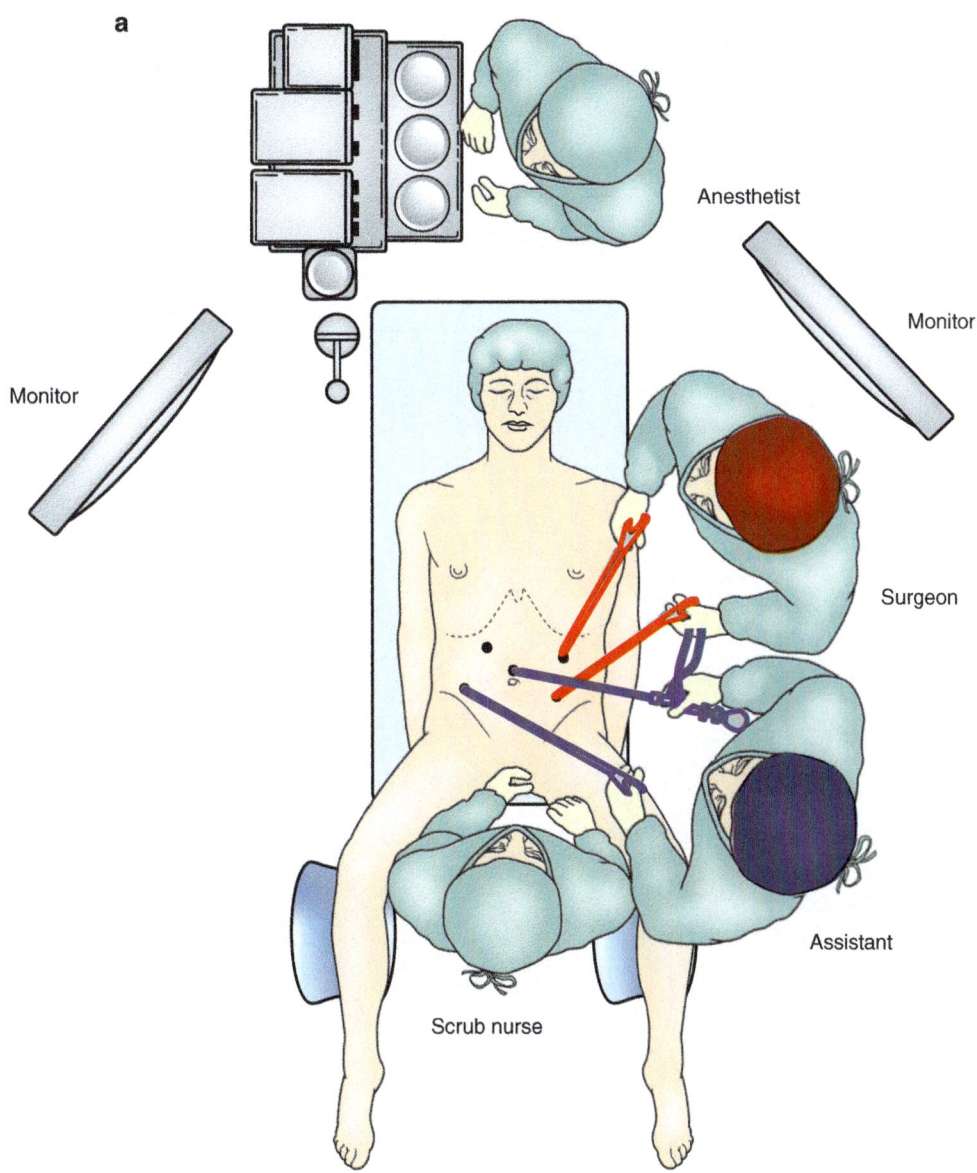

Room setup for subtotal colectomy: the surgeon and assistant will move during various phases of the operation. For the right colon, the surgeon will stand on the patient's left, with the assistant caudal (**a**). For the left colon, the surgeon and assistant will both move to the patient's right side (**b**)

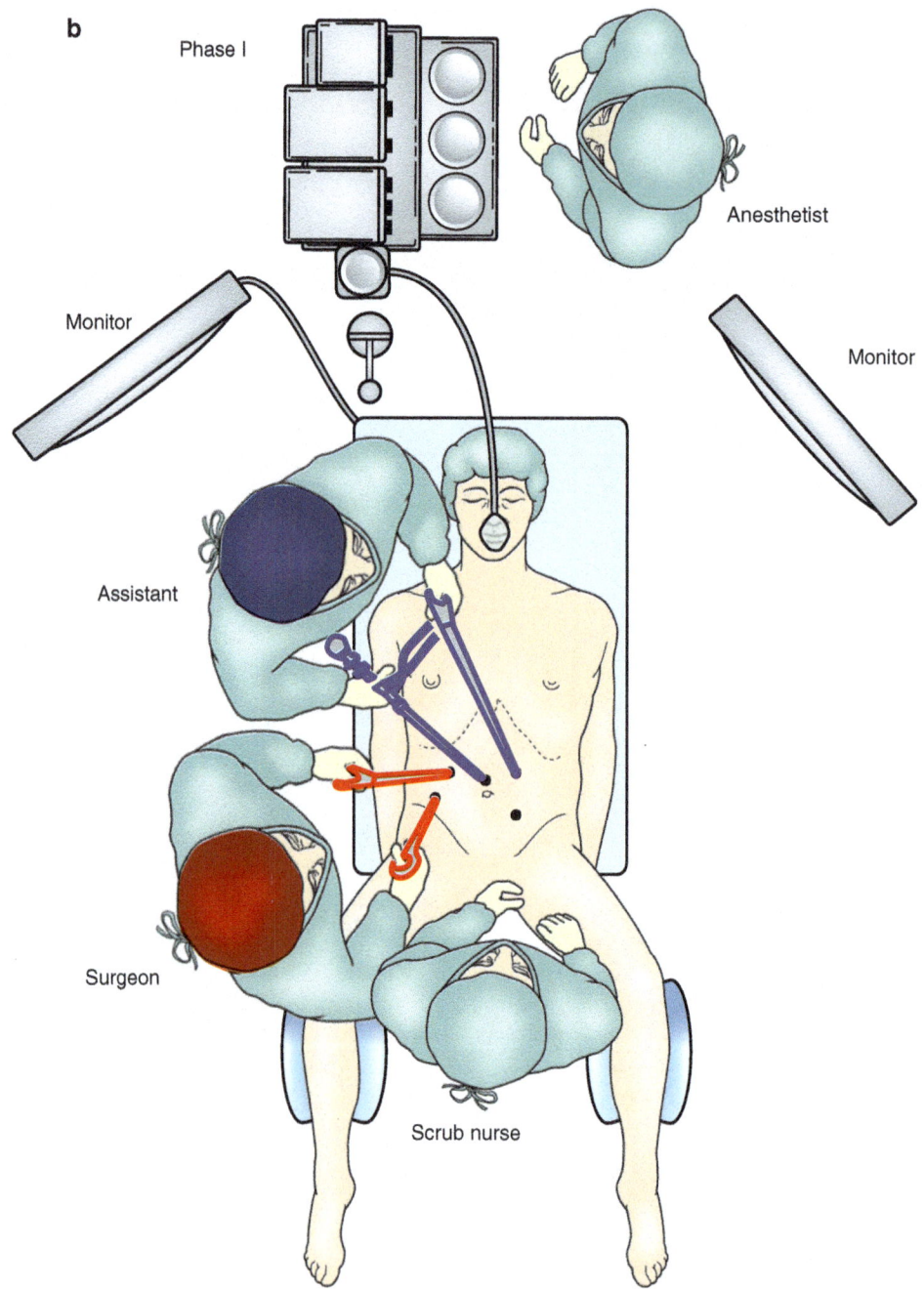

The patient is placed in lithotomy position on the operating table. Both arms are tucked at the patient's side. Take care to pad all pressure points along the course of the superficial peroneal nerve at the knee and the ulnar nerve at the level of the elbows. The abdomen is prepped from the xiphoid down to the pubic symphysis and laterally to each anterior superior iliac spine (Tip 8.1).

The primary monitor is positioned on the right side of the patient toward the patient's head. The secondary monitor is placed on the left side of the patient at the same level. The scrub instrument table is placed between the patient's legs. There should be sufficient space for the surgeon to move to either side of the table and between the patient's legs when necessary.

During mobilization of the right colon, the surgeon and assistant will stand on the patient's left. Mobilization of the transverse colon and splenic flexure may be facilitated with the assistant between the patient's legs to hold retraction. The left colon is mobilized with both the surgeon and assistant on the patient's right side.

Step 1: Port Placement

Abdominal entry is through a 1.5 cm supra- or infraumbilical incision via an open Hasson technique. A 5 mm port is placed in the left lower quadrant two finger breadths medial and superior to the anterior iliac spine and lateral to the inferior epigastric vessels. A second 5 mm port is placed in the left upper quadrant one hand breadth away. Additional two 5 mm ports are placed on the right side, mirroring the left-sided ports (Tip 8.2).

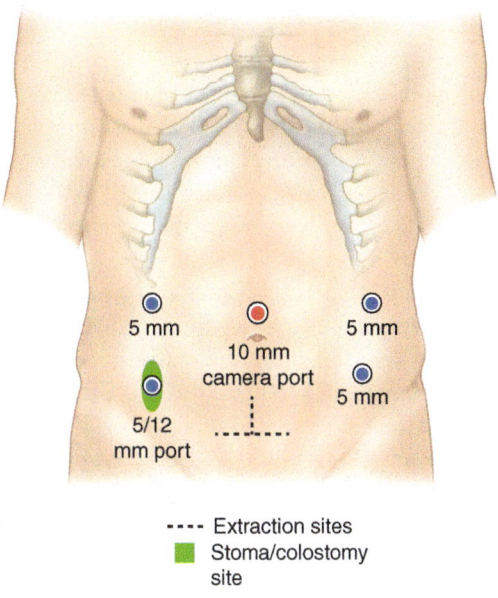

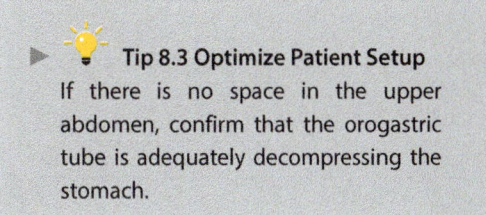

Fig. 8.1 Port placement for subtotal colectomy: a 10 mm port is placed supraumbilically, with 4–5 mm ports placed in each quadrant of the abdomen. If appropriate for dissection, the stoma site may be used for the right lower quadrant port site

All ports are placed under laparoscopic guidance taking care to avoid injury to the epigastric vessels. The right lower quadrant port can be upsized to a 12 mm port to facilitate entry of the endoscopic stapler (see Fig. 8.1).

Step 2: Laparoscopy, If Applicable

The abdomen should be evaluated for signs of injury on entry, metastatic disease, or contraindications to continuing the surgery laparoscopically (Tip 8.3).

Step 3: Right Colon Medial to Lateral Dissection

The mobilization of the right colon is preferably performed as a medial to lateral dissection. The surgeon and assistant stand on the patient's left side with the assistant standing caudal to the surgeon. The patient is rotated with the right side up, to approximately 15–20° tilt. The patient is placed into steep Trendelenburg position.

The surgeon inserts atraumatic bowel clamps through the left-sided abdominal ports. The greater omentum is reflected over the transverse colon so that it lies on the stomach.

The small bowel is moved out of the operative field, allowing visualization of the ileocolic pedicle. The assistant uses an atraumatic bowel clamp through the right lower quadrant port to tent the ileal mesentery medially and cephalad. Occasionally, a third right upper quadrant port may be needed to help hold the small bowel away from the operative field (Tip 8.4).

The ileocecal junction is grasped and stretched anteriorly toward the right lower quadrant port, putting the vessel on stretch and lifting it away from the retroperitoneum. In almost all patients, this demonstrates a sulcus between the

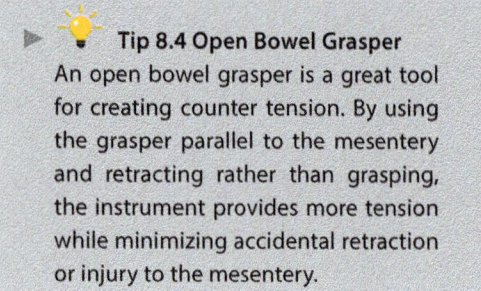

> 💡 **Tip 8.4 Open Bowel Grasper**
> An open bowel grasper is a great tool for creating counter tension. By using the grasper parallel to the mesentery and retracting rather than grasping, the instrument provides more tension while minimizing accidental retraction or injury to the mesentery.

medial side of the ileocolic pedicle and the retroperitoneum as shown in Fig. 8.2. Laparoscopic shears with cautery are then used to incise the peritoneum below the ileocolic vessel along this sulcus line.

Blunt dissection is then used to lift the vessel away from the retroperitoneum. This lifts the descending and transverse mesocolon away from the duodenum medially and the white line of Toldt laterally. The surgeon uses a bowel grasper held open and parallel to the mesentery from the left upper quadrant port to facilitate tenting of the mesentery upward. A second bowel grasper is inserted from the left lower

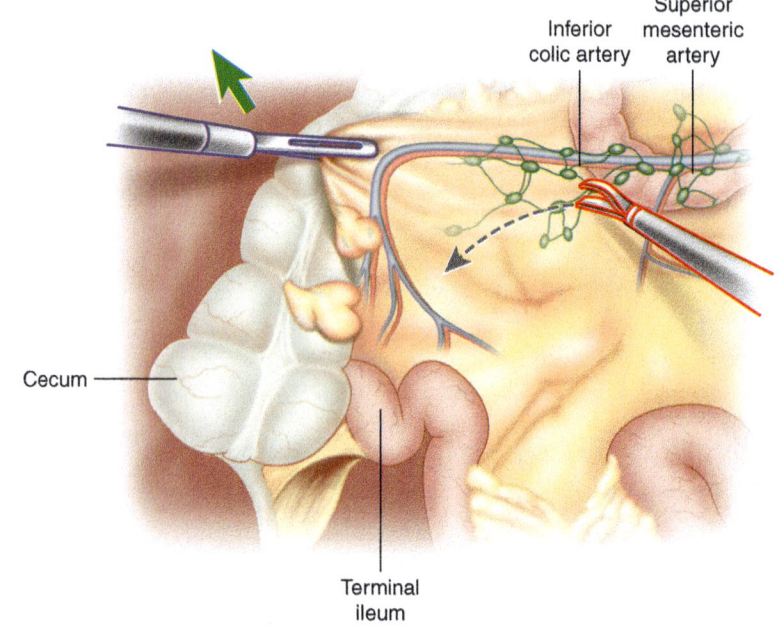

Fig. 8.2 Ileocolic pedicle is placed under tension by lifting the assistant's grasper anteriorly and laterally to demonstrate the sulcus between the mesocolon and retroperitoneum. Entry into the peritoneum is just below the ileocolic pedicle

Fig. 8.3 After entry into the peritoneum, the mesocolon is gently retracted anteriorly, while the retroperitoneum and duodenum are swept downward

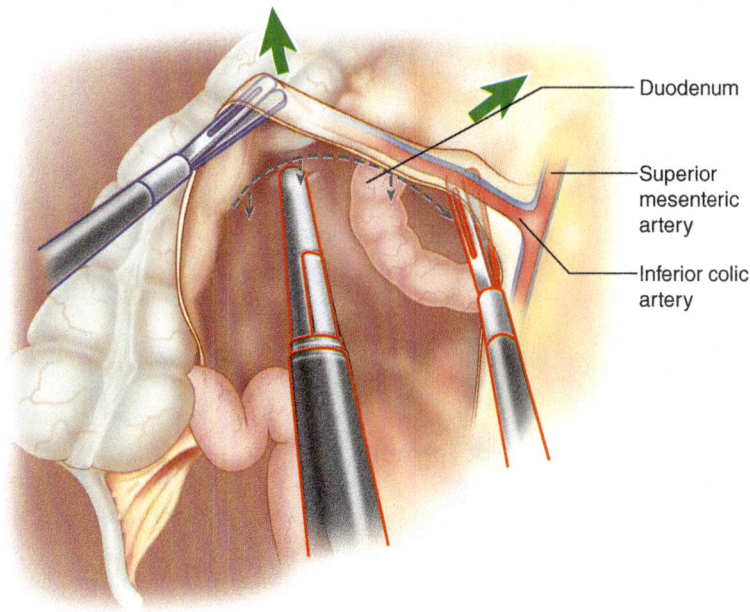

Duodenum

Superior mesenteric artery

Inferior colic artery

Fig. 8.4 Division of the ileocolic pedicle. The ileocolic pedicle is divided with the bipolar, clips or stapler within 1 cm of the takeoff from the SMA if the surgery is being performed for oncologic indications

Ileocolic artery

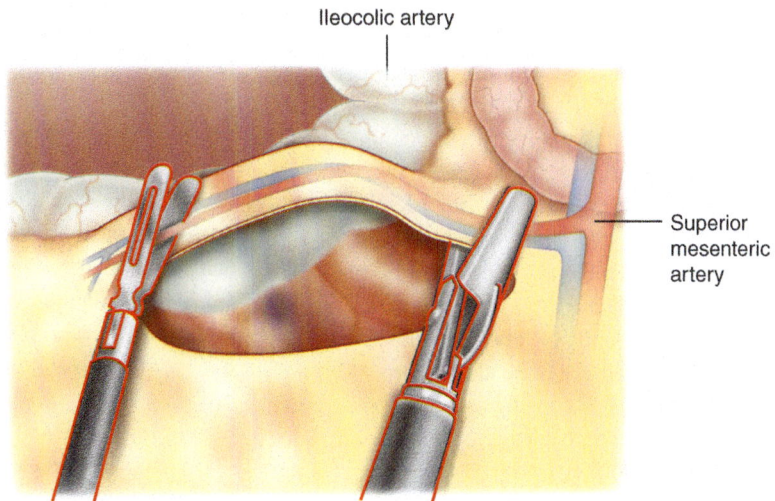

Superior mesenteric artery

quadrant port to dissect attachments to the mesentery with gentle sweeps toward the retroperitoneum.

The duodenum is carefully swept downward and medially creating a plane beneath the middle colic pedicle and the transverse mesocolon (see Fig. 8.3). The dissection should be carried laterally to the line of Toldt and superiorly under the transverse colon toward the hepatic flexure.

Step 4: Division of the Ileocolic Pedicle

Cautery is used to open a window in the peritoneum on either side of the ileocolic pedicle. Once the ileocolic pedicle is visualized and adequately mobilized away from the duodenum, it is ligated with a bipolar energy device or an endoscopic stapler with a vascular load (Fig. 8.4 and Tip 8.5).

Tip 8.5 Bulky Mesentery

A vascular pedicle can be skeletonized using precise dissection with the laparoscopic shears or the bipolar energy device in situations where the mesentery of the ileocolic pedicle appears bulky. This provides optimal visualization of the vessel and ensures that the vessel lumen is safely transected.

Step 5: Mobilization of Terminal Ileum

The terminal ileum and cecum are reflected superiorly with the surgeon's left hand exposing the junction of the visceral peritoneum and the retroperitoneum at the right pelvic brim. Tension on the appendix facilitates this dissection. The surgeon uses laparoscopic shears with cautery to dissect the terminal ileum off the retroperitoneal structures. The assistant may also assist with tension on the cecum, freeing the surgeon's left hand for finer dissection.

Usually there is only a thin layer of peritoneum requiring division, which is easily visualized with good tension on the cecum. This line of dissection extends from the ileocecal junction toward the origin of the superior mesenteric artery at the base of the duodenum. Although cautery can be used during this initial dissection, the more proximal aspect of the mobilization should be performed with scissors alone to avoid injury to the third part of the duodenum.

A plane between the retroperitoneum and the terminal ileum is developed, and the terminal ileum can be reflected medially and cephalad. The iliac vessels, right ureter, and gonadal vessels all remain safely beneath the parietal peritoneum. It is important to ensure that the terminal ileum has been freed to the level of the duodenum to facilitate delivery of the complete specimen at the end

of the case through a small extraction site without tension or tearing of the mesentery (Pitfall 8.1).

Pitfall 8.1

Residual bleeding may occur with any vessel ligation. It is critical to have tools such as Endoloop or laparoscopic clips available in the operating room prior to ligation to facilitate rapid use if needed.

Step 6: Mobilization of the Hepatic Flexure

The patient is placed in slight reverse Trendelenburg position. An atraumatic bowel grasper through the left lower quadrant port is used to deliver the omentum inferiorly, exposing the hepatic flexure. The surgeon grasps the hepatic flexure with the left hand, reflecting it medially and inferiorly. The surgeon's right hand holds laparoscopic monopolar shears with cautery. The assistant uses a bowel grasper through the right lower quadrant port to maintain upward retraction on the greater curvature of the stomach. This puts the hepatic flexure under tension facilitating division of the gastrocolic ligament. Alternatively, a bipolar energy device can also be used for this dissection. The surgeon continues to progress along this plane drawing the hepatic flexure inferiorly and medially.

As this dissection continues, the purple hue from the previous medial to lateral mobilization becomes apparent (Fig. 8.5). The purple filmy tissue is the only remaining attachment of the ascending colon along the lateral line of Toldt. This white line of Toldt is divided inferiorly to the base of the cecum (Pitfall 8.2).

The right colon is now completely dissected free from the underlying duodenum and retroperitoneum and reflected entirely to the

Fig. 8.5 Hepatic flexure mobilization from above. The remaining attachments from the colon to liver are transected

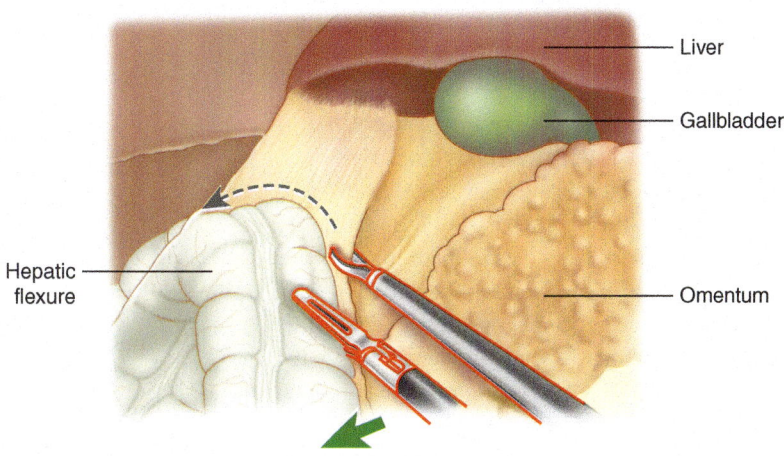

Liver

Gallbladder

Hepatic flexure

Omentum

⚠ Pitfall 8.2
Care must be taken to avoid injury to the gallbladder and second part of the duodenum that are encountered below as the hepatic flexure is mobilized.

tmidline completing the hepatic flexure mobilization.

Step 7: Entry into the Lesser Sac

Full mobilization of the lesser sac facilitates access to the middle colic vessels to ensure a safe ligation. This superior mobilization provides critical exposure to both sides of the mesentery for safe dissection of the middle colic vessels (Tip 8.6).

If the surgeon desires to resect the entire omentum with the specimen, the lesser sac can be entered by creating a hole through the omentum below the gastro-epiploic vessels. The plane can be dissected using a bipolar energy device to transect omental branches and continued to the splenic flexure.

If the omentum is to be left in situ, the assistant retracts the omentum through the right upper quadrant port, and the surgeon will retract the transverse colon, tenting it inferiorly. An energy device is used to divide the attachments along the antimesenteric wall of the colon, entering into the lesser sac. Position is confirmed by visualization of the back wall of the stomach. If this technique is used, the greater omentum will be divided at the proximal transverse colon, leaving a portion attached to the hepatic flexure (Tip 8.7).

 Tip 8.7 Omentum
Leaving the omentum in situ may be helpful for creating omental flaps, or for further infectious processes, such as in Crohn's disease. However, there appears to be an increased risk of small bowel obstruction associated with keeping the omentum after subtotal colectomy.

Tip 8.6 Entry into the Lesser Sac
Because of the variability in adherence of the lesser sac at the proximal colon, the easiest point of entry into the lesser sac is below the greater curvature of the stomach, proximal to the pylorus.

Step 8: Identification and Division of Middle Colic Pedicle

If the subtotal colectomy is being conducted for benign disease, a mid-mesenteric dissection may be performed whereby the transverse colon mesentery is divided close to the bowel wall. This dissection can be continued from the previously ligated mesentery from the right colon mobilization. The surgeon can stand at the patient's right side, and the assistant positions themselves between the patient's legs. The surgeon uses the right upper quadrant port to retract the proximal transverse colon, while the assistant uses the left lower quadrant port to retract the distal colon at splenic flexure. A bipolar energy device is used from the right lower quadrant port to find the cut edge of the right colon mesentery. The surgeon uses the energy device to divide the branches in the transverse colonic mesentery just below the colon. This dissection can be continued to the splenic flexure.

If malignancy is suspected, then a high ligation of the middle colic pedicle at its bifurcation should be undertaken (Pitfall 8.3). For malig-

> ⚠ **Pitfall 8.3**
> During a superior transection of the middle colic vessels, it is easy to be more posterior than expected. Lifting the transverse colon away from the pancreas and duodenum while retracting inferiorly helps to ensure the proper plane.

nant disease, the omentum is often preserved with the specimen to ensure negative margins. The assistant stands between the patient's legs and uses the left upper quadrant port to elevate the splenic flexure. The surgeon stands to the patient's right and uses the right upper quadrant port to elevate the hepatic flexure whereby the transverse colon is tented and exposes the middle colic pedicle (Fig. 8.6). The surgeon uses the right lower quadrant port to score the mesentery on each side of the middle colic vessels. The transverse colon can also be tented inferiorly to visualize the middle colic pedicle from above, through the lesser sac.

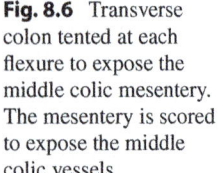
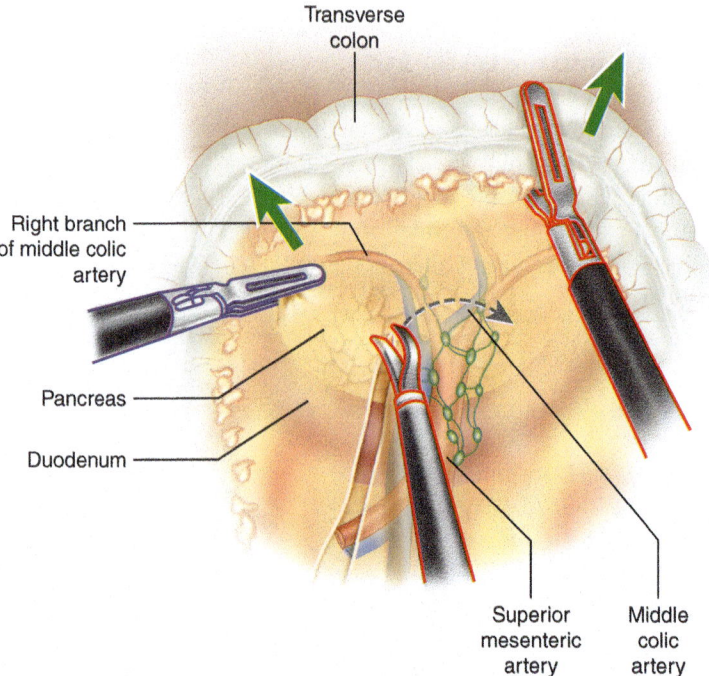

Fig. 8.6 Transverse colon tented at each flexure to expose the middle colic mesentery. The mesentery is scored to expose the middle colic vessels

The correct vascular pedicle is confirmed prior to division. The superior mesenteric artery and vein lie deep to the dissection line. The pancreas is fully exposed as dissection progresses. Once the avascular windows have been created on either side of the pedicle, the middle colic vessels can be ligated from either side of the patient depending on the ease and angle (Fig. 8.7). Each branch is transected with either a bipolar energy device or as a group with a laparoscopic stapler. A bowel grasper is maintained at the base of the pedicle to maintain proximal control in case of back bleeding.

The remaining colonic mesentery leading up to the splenic flexure can then be divided with the surgeon working from the patient's right side while the assistant retracts the splenic flexure inferiorly.

Step 9: Inferior Mesenteric Artery (IMA)

Once the transverse colon has been mobilized to the splenic flexure, attention is turned to the left colon, starting with a medial to lateral dissection of the sigmoid colon at the level of the sacral promontory. Both the surgeon and assistant move to the patient's right side with the patient positioned in steep Trendelenburg and tilted to the right side. This moves the small bowel away from the operative field.

An atraumatic grasper is used to reflect the greater omentum over the transverse colon. The assistant uses a bowel grasper through the left upper quadrant port to retract the descending colon anterior and cephalad out of the pelvis.

The surgeon places an atraumatic bowel grasper on the rectosigmoid mesentery at the level of the sacral promontory, approximately halfway between the bowel wall and the promontory itself, drawing it anteriorly. In most cases, this tension will help to demonstrate a groove between the right or medial side of the inferior mesenteric pedicle and the retroperitoneum (Fig. 8.8 and Tip 8.8).

Laparoscopic shears with electrocautery are introduced through the right lower quadrant port and used to score the peritoneum along this groove. This plane is opened proximally to the origin of the inferior mesenteric artery and distally past the sacral promontory. The surgeon

Fig. 8.7 The middle colic vessels are ligated after creating windows on either side of the middle colic artery

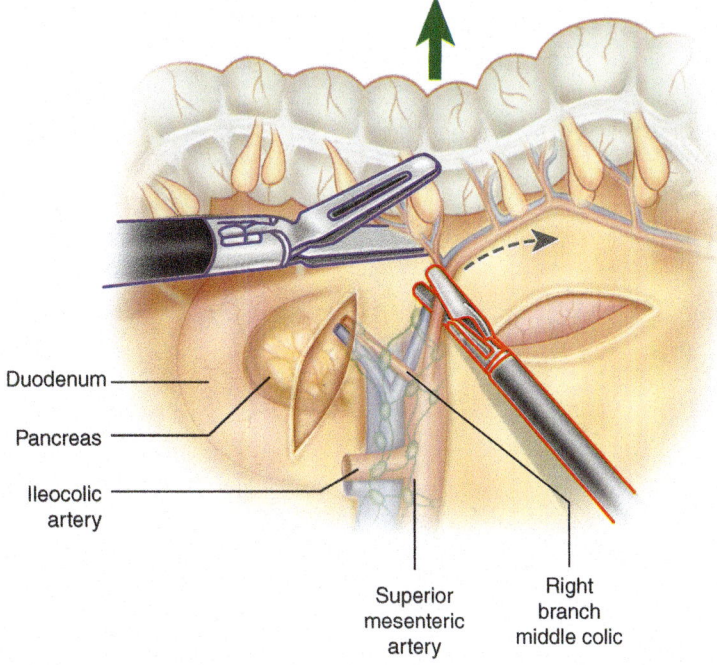

Duodenum

Pancreas

Ileocolic artery

Superior mesenteric artery

Right branch middle colic

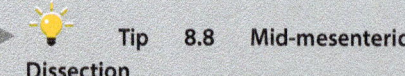

Tip 8.8 Mid-mesenteric Dissection

In the setting of benign disease, high ligation of the IMA pedicle may be unnecessary. The mesentery of the left colon may be divided close to the bowel wall. Although more vessel branches will be encountered, this prevents injury to the hypogastric nerves and ureters.

releases the mesentery and uses blunt dissection to lift the inferior mesenteric artery pedicle anterior, away from the retroperitoneum and the presacral sympathetic autonomic nerves.

The left ureter is demonstrated anterior and lateral to the left common iliac artery through this medial window (Fig. 8.9 and Pitfall 8.4).

The dissection is continued proximally to the origin of the inferior mesenteric artery. The IMA is carefully defined and divided using a high ligation with either a bipolar energy device or laparo-

Fig. 8.8 Sigmoid tented anteriorly and cephalad to demonstrate the loose areolar plane of dissection underneath the IMA pedicle

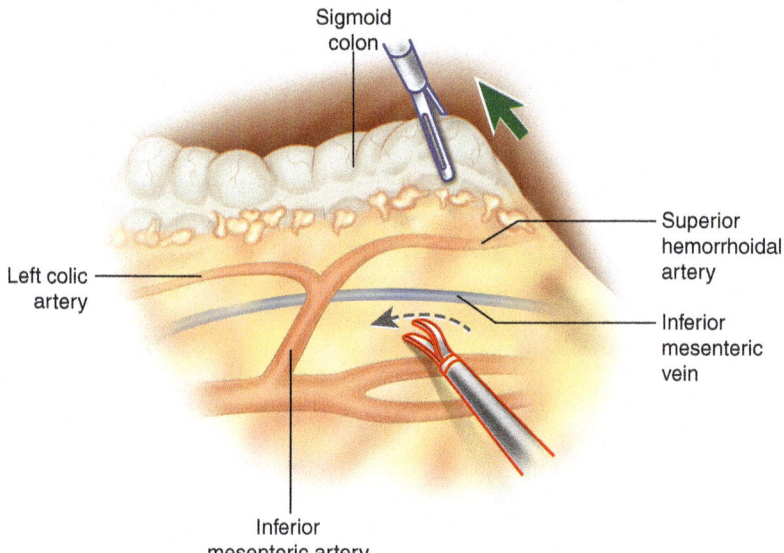

Fig. 8.9 The left ureter is identified from the medial aspect to ensure it is preserved prior to transection of the IMA pedicle

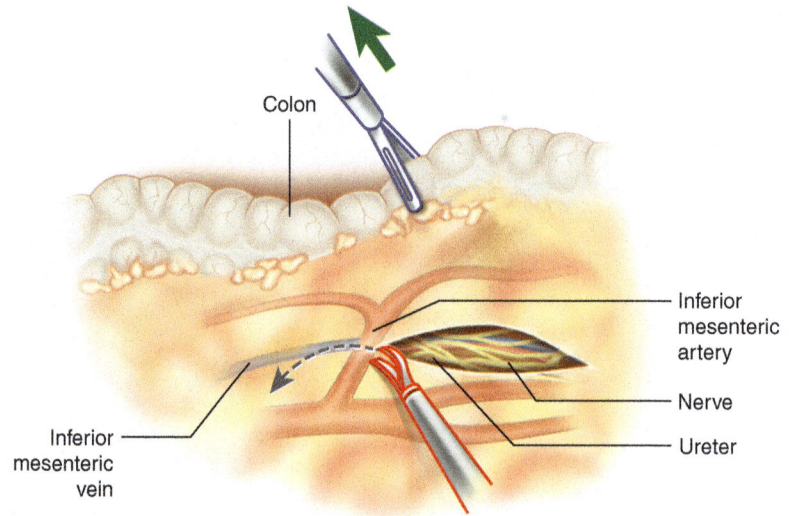

Pitfall 8.4 Left Ureter
If the left ureter cannot be seen from the right side, the plane should be verified. The ureter should be just deep to the parietal peritoneum and just medial to the gonadal vessels. If it is still not visualized, vary the approach to a lateral dissection to ensure that the ureter is not injured.

scopic stapler. If a high ligation of the IMA pedicle is not warranted, then the colon can be divided at the rectosigmoid junction, and the mesentery may be ligated with a bipolar device close to the bowel wall. This dissection can be carried upward to the splenic flexure to meet the dissection above from the transverse colon mobilization.

Step 10: Left Colon Mobilization

After dividing the inferior mesenteric vessels at the origin of the artery, the plane between the descending colon mesentery and the retroperitoneum is developed laterally, using the left hand to elevate the mesentery and right hand to sweep the retroperitoneum posteriorly. This continues laterally to the line of Toldt and superiorly over the

anterior surface of Gerota's fascia toward the splenic flexure. This clearly exposes the inferior mesenteric vein lateral to the ligament of Treitz, where it can be divided (Tip 8.9).

 Tip 8.9 Using the Colon as a Retractor
Elevating the descending colon and drawing it anterior and medially is useful to keep small bowel loops out of the operating field.

The surgeon grasps the rectosigmoid junction with a bowel grasper in the left hand and retracts it to the patient's right side. This exposes the white line of Toldt for division, freeing the left colon from the remaining lateral attachments (Fig. 8.10). Bruising can be seen in this area from the previous retroperitoneal mobilization of the colon from the medial to lateral dissection. Dissection now continues 1 mm medial to the white line of Toldt, toward the splenic flexure (Tip 8.10).

As the dissection continues, the surgeon's left-hand instrument gradually moves proximally along the descending colon to keep the lateral attachments under tension. In this way, the lateral

Fig. 8.10 The left colon is mobilized toward the splenic flexure at the white line of Toldt with retraction of the left colon medially

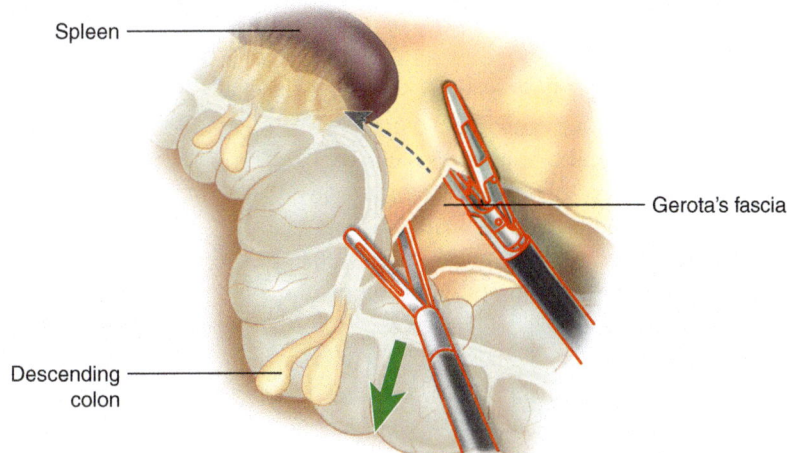

Spleen

Gerota's fascia

Descending colon

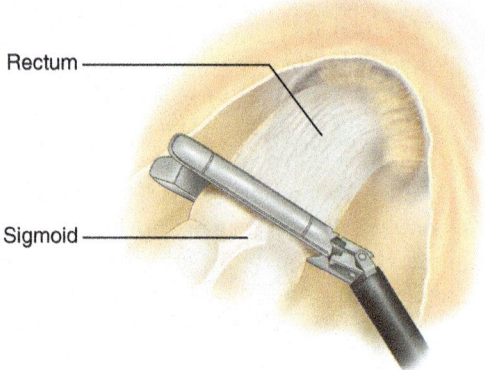

Rectum —

Sigmoid —

Fig. 8.11 Laparoscopic stapling of distal colon at the rectosigmoid junction. The rectum is identified by decussation of the tenia coli

and any remaining posterior attachments are freed, medializing the left colon and sigmoid.

The surgeon may move between the patient's leg, and the surgeon's right hand instrument is moved to the left lower quadrant port site. This will provide for greater reach along the descending colon and up to the splenic flexure. If the small bowel is an impediment to dissection, the operating table can be repositioned into the reverse Trendelenburg position. This will allow gravity to keep the small bowel away from the site of dissection.

At this point, splenic flexure mobilization from below is met with the previous plane of dissection from above. The left colon is retracted medially and the dissection plane now enters into the lesser sac. The colon at the flexure is retracted caudally and medially and any residual restraining attachments divided, bringing the entire left colon to the midline.

the mesentery perpendicular from the rectosigmoid junction to the bowel wall. The entire colon is now completely mobilized and free of any attachments and/or mesentery.

A laparoscopic stapler is introduced by upsizing the right lower quadrant port and then used to divide the rectum (Fig. 8.11). Once the entire colon is completely mobilized, the abdomen should be inspected for hemostasis (Tip 8.11). Care should be taken not extend the retromesorectal dissection too deeply, and preserve the area around the superior hemorrhoidal pedicle. This will facilitate rectal dissection by maintaining a virgin plane, should future operations require proctectomy.

Step 11: Distal Transection of the Rectosigmoid

A point of transection is determined by the pathologic process. In some cases, the proximal or distal sigmoid may be the point of division.

Identification of the rectosigmoid can be determined by anatomical landmarks such as the sacral promontory or anterior peritoneal reflection. The surgical definition of the rectum is the location where the taenia coli coalesce.

The mesentery at the level of the inferior mesenteric artery pedicle is grasped, and the peritoneum of the mesentery is scored perpendicular to the colon with laparoscopic cautery shears. A bipolar energy device is used to divide

Step 12: Extraction of the Specimen

There are several incisional options for extraction sites, but the two most common options include a lower midline or a Pfannenstiel incision. The size of incision depends on the pathology and size of the specimen, as well as patient body habitus. The specimen can be delivered through the incision with the assistance of a laparoscopic bowel grasper and then grasped with the Babcock through the incision. The entire colon and terminal ileum should be delivered onto the abdominal field (Tip 8.12).

> 💡 **Tip 8.12 Use of a Hand Port**
> As with all laparoscopic procedures, if encountering difficulty a hand port may be placed to perform a hand-assisted approach prior to considering an open procedure. A hand-assisted approach may facilitate surgery when encountering many adhesions or phlegmon, and dealing with vascular control of bulky mesentery. It may also be an invaluable tool when assessing for residual inflammatory disease elsewhere in the small intestine and to manually break up fistulous communications.

Step 13: Ileorectal Anastomosis (Side to End (Baker Type) or End to End)

An area free of disease on the small bowel should be identified. The terminal ileum is carefully evaluated for tension-free reach into the pelvis. It is inspected to ensure that it has excellent blood supply. The remaining mesentery is scored and transected with the bipolar energy device or between Kelly clamps and suture ligatures. A linear stapler is used to divide the small bowel and the specimen is passed off the field (Pitfall 8.5).

> ⚠️ **Pitfall 8.5 Contamination**
> Any instruments used for the creation of anastomosis should be passed off the sterile field after handling open bowel. The surgeon and assistant change gloves to decrease the rate of infections.

Side-to-End (Baker) Anastomosis (Tip 8.13)

To perform a side-to-end (Baker) anastomosis, the staple line is resected using electrocautery, and the small bowel lumen is then dilated to accommodate either a 28 or 25 mm circular stapler. The anvil with spike is then introduced into the lumen and extruded through the antimesenteric border of the small bowel approximately 7–10 cm from the staple line. The lumen is once again closed with the firing of linear stapler.

> 💡 **Tip 8.13 Baker Anastomosis**
> In cases of size mismatch between proximal and distal bowel, a side-to-end or side-to-side anastomosis can be made. This can facilitate placement of a circular stapler in the small bowel.

A 3-0 prolene suture is used to place a purse string around the anvil at the antimesenteric exit site (Fig. 8.12). The anastomosis can be performed through the open incision or laparoscopically depending on incision location.

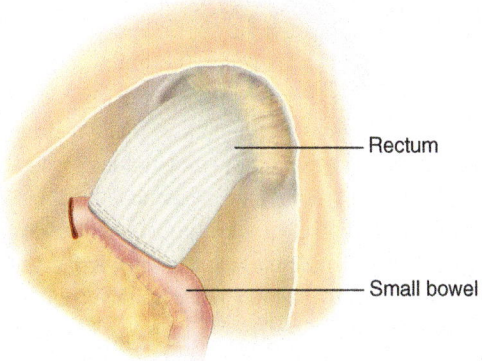

Rectum

Small bowel

Fig. 8.12 Baker anastomosis: side-to-end ileorectal anastomosis is performed using a circular stapler. A hydropneumatic leak test is performed to ensure anastomotic integrity

End-to-End Anastomosis

An alternative approach is an end-to-end anastomosis. After the ileum is divided, a hand-sewn purse-string closure may be created using a 2-0 prolene suture, run as a baseball stitch around the end of the ileum. Alternatively, an auto-purse-string device may be used. The anvil is placed into the end of the ileal lumen and the purse string is tied down. This may require the use of a smaller circular stapler to accommodate the size of the small bowel.

After completion of the ileal portion, all instruments and gloves are changed. A circular stapler is introduced into the anus and rectum with the spike piercing through the midportion of the rectal staple line. The spike is removed from the small bowel anvil, and the terminal ileum with anvil is engaged with the circular stapler and stapler is then fired (Pitfall 8.6).

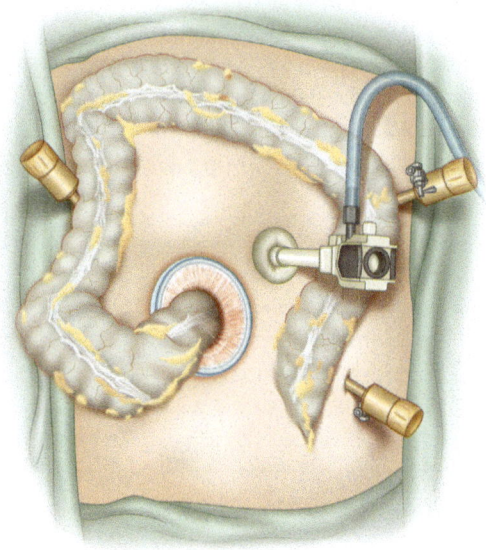

Fig. 8.13 Stoma site used as extraction site. The entire abdominal colon is resected

---

> ⚠ **Pitfall 8.6 Anastomosis**
> Prior to attaching the small bowel to the stapler, the mesentery of the small bowel is orientated to ensure that there are no twists. Loops of small bowel should be placed over the anastomosis to prevent postoperative herniation and obstruction.

The anastomosis is tested for leaks with irrigation solution through the abdomen and visualization via a rigid proctoscope through the rectum.

To perform the anastomosis laparoscopically, the terminal ileum with anvil in place is dropped into the abdomen, and the incision is closed with a running suture. The abdomen is then re-insufflated, and the anastomosis is performed under laparoscopic guidance using a laparoscopic Babcock to engage the anvil with the circular stapler (Fig. 8.12).

Step 14: Creation of an End Ileostomy (If Necessary)

If an end ileostomy is planned over an ileorectal anastomosis, the stoma site can be used as an extraction site (Fig. 8.13). The distal margin of the resection is grasped on the staple line and brought to the stoma site in the right lower quadrant.

The stoma incision is made.

The colon staple line is transferred via the laparoscopic grasper to a Babcock placed through the incision. If the specimen is too bulky for the stoma incision, the posterior fascial incision can be enlarged for specimen delivery. Once the terminal ileum is divided and the specimen is passed off the field, the rectus sheath is closed to the normal size using interrupted nonabsorbable suture. The stoma can then be created in a Brooked fashion as described previously, after all port sites have been fully closed.

Laparoscopic Proctocolectomy with the Construction of an Ileal Pouch-Anal Anastomosis

9

David B. Stewart

Introduction

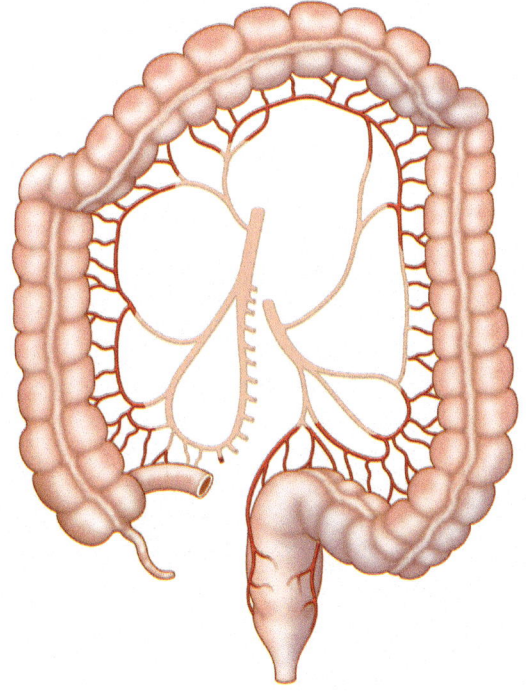

Laparoscopic proctocolectomy with ileal pouch-anal anastomosis is the removal of the entire colon and rectum with creation of an ileal neo-reservoir. It is performed for patients with inflammatory or neoplastic processes isolated to the colon and rectum with good sphincter control and without involvement of the small bowel or anus.

Indications
- Ulcerative colitis
- Indeterminant colitis without contraindications
- Familial adenomatous polyposis
- Nonhereditary synchronous colon and rectal cancers

Preoperative Planning
- Preoperative colonoscopy to confirm the diagnosis and extent of disease
- Preoperative staging for malignancies:
  - Computed tomography scan of the chest, abdomen, and pelvis
  - Carcinoembryonic antigen level

D. B. Stewart (✉)
Colorectal Surgery, University of Arizona – Banner University Medical Center, Tucson, AZ, USA
e-mail: dbstewart@surgery.arizona.edu

© Springer Nature Switzerland AG 2020
S. L. Stein, R. R. Lawson (eds.), *Laparoscopic Colectomy*,
https://doi.org/10.1007/978-3-030-39559-9_9

- Preoperative optimization of inflammatory bowel disease (IBD):
  - Consideration of limiting or discontinuing steroids and immunosuppressants
  - Optimization of nutritional status (serum albumin and/or prealbumin)
  - Medical optimization
- Preoperative stoma-site marking and counseling session by an enterostomal therapist
- Preoperative evaluation of sphincter function
- Mechanical bowel preparation
- Venous thromboembolic chemoprophylaxis – preferably beginning on the day prior to surgery
- Preoperative antibiotics

Tools of the Operation
- Port options
  - Single site port
  - 2–3 bladeless 5-mm trocars
  - 1 bladeless 12-mm trocar
- Laparoscope
  - Preferably a 5-mm, flexible tip laparoscope.
  - A 5-mm, 30-degree laparoscope is an acceptable alternative.
- Two 5-mm laparoscopic Babcock graspers

- Advanced bipolar device
  - Use of monopolar cautery or "hot" laparoscopic scissors for the proctectomy is an alternative.
- Laparoscopic reticular linear-cutting stapler
- 100-mm open linear-cutting stapler for pouch construction
- Wound protector

Steps of the Operation
Patient Positioning
1. Step 1: Port placement
2. Step 2: Initial inspection of the peritoneal cavity
3. Step 3: Right colectomy – posterior approach
4. Step 4: Hepatic flexure
5. Step 5: Left colectomy
6. Step 6: Transverse colectomy/splenic flexure mobilization
7. Step 7: Externalization of the colon (optional)
8. Step 8: Proctectomy
9. Step 9: Transection of the rectum
10. Step 10: Externalize the specimen
11. Step 11: Construction of the pouch
12. Step 12: Construction of the pouch-anal anastomosis
13. Step 13: Creation of diverting loop ileostomy

Patient Positioning for Laparoscopic Laparoscopic Proctocolectomy with the Construction of an Ileal Pouch-Anal Anastomosis

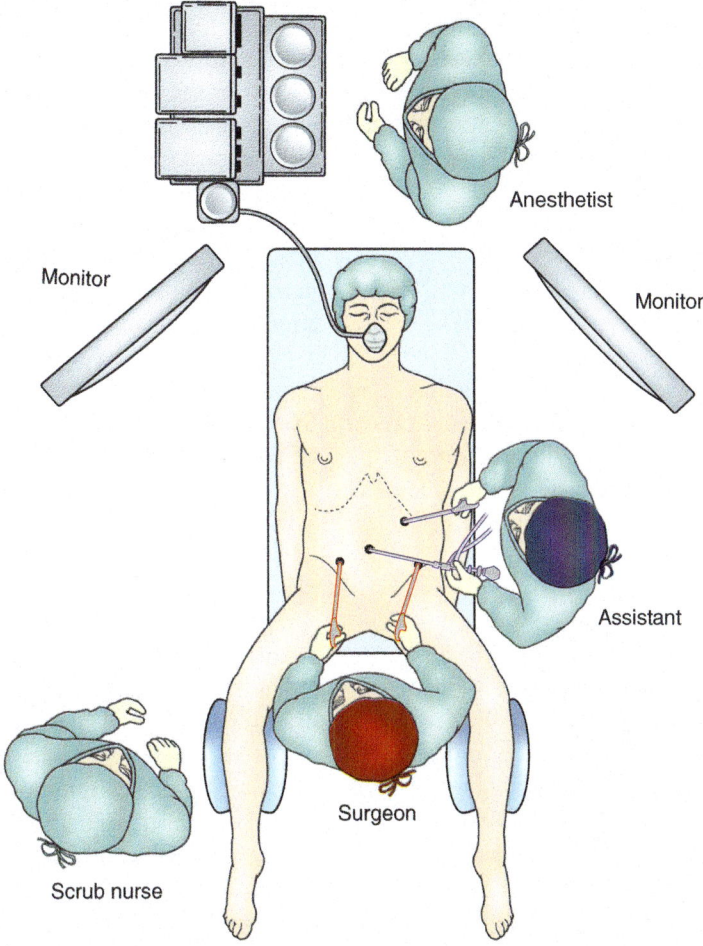

Patient positioning: The patient is placed in modified lithotomy positioning to have access to the perineum for possible mucosectomy or stapling.

The patient is secured to the operating table by stirrups and a beanbag. The anesthesiologist should reassess peripheral venous catheters and blood pressure monitoring devices to ensure they are functioning properly after beanbag inflation. A towel and 2-inch silk tape placed over the patient's chest are then applied to further secure the patient. The patient is placed in steep Trendelenburg to ensure the patient is secure on the table (Tip 9.1).

> **Tip 9.1 Checking Positioning**
> Prior to starting the surgery, the anesthetist should check ventilatory mechanics in steep Trendelenburg. Some patients, particularly obese patients, may have difficulty ventilating. If ventilatory difficulties occur at this juncture, the surgeon should consider performing the surgery via laparotomy.

The surgeon stands on the patient's left side for the portions of the surgery dealing with the right and proximal transverse colon. For the left colon and pouch-anal anastomosis, the surgeon will stand on the right side. The assistant position is typically adjacent to the operating surgeon, though location can vary throughout the operation.

Operative Strategy

Step 1: Port Placement (Fig. 9.1)

Multiple entry techniques are possible and detailed in Chap. 1. A laparoscopic-guided port placement uses the 5-mm laparoscope in the obturator of the camera port. Lift the abdominal wall as the port is advanced into the peritoneal cavity under laparoscopic visualization (Tip 9.2).

> ▶ 💡 **Tip 9.2 Laparoscopically Guided Initial Abdominal Entry**
> Focus on a straight line of entry. Scything will cause an ergonomically unfriendly trocar angle and will fall short of entering the peritoneal cavity.

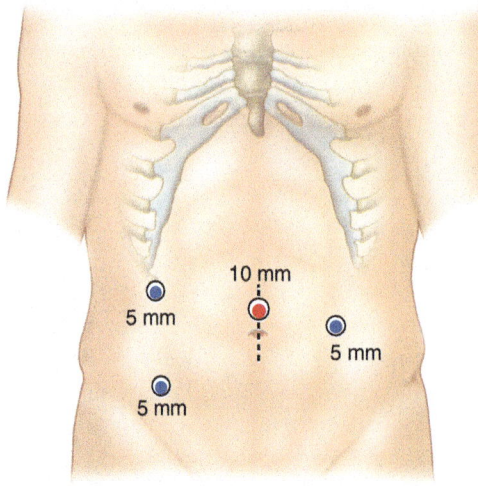

Fig. 9.1 Port placement

Place two 5-mm trocars in the bilateral lower quadrants of the abdomen. An optional third trocar can be placed in either the right or the left upper abdominal quadrant depending on where reach is difficult. A right upper abdomen trocar allows for use during dissection of the left colon and splenic flexure, which is typically the most difficult portion of the case. A 12-mm trocar is placed at a potential stoma site or in a suprapubic position. A suprapubic placement provides a direct path for the endostapler to the anorectal junction and can be used for extraction and creation of the ileal pouch.

Step 2: Initial Inspection of the Peritoneal Cavity

Initial inspection evaluates for any vascular or intestinal injuries, which can occur with port placement.

For patients with ulcerative or indeterminate colitis, the small intestine is run to ensure the absence of enteritis that would indicate a Crohn's disease phenotype. If signs of Crohn's disease are discovered, an IPAA should not be constructed, and a total proctocolectomy with end ileostomy should be considered.

For patients with cancer, it is important to ensure that the primary cancer is resectable, and there is no metastatic disease that would mandate a change to the surgical plan.

Step 3: Right Colectomy – Posterior Approach

A posterior approach immediately places the duodenum and right ureter in view and allows for minimal use of electrical energy until the ureter and duodenum are isolated.

Place the patient in maximal Trendelenburg position with left side down. A Babcock is placed using either of the lower abdominal trocars for retraction. An energy device is placed through the right upper quadrant trocar.

The ileocolic junction is retracted toward the anterior abdominal wall, exposing the confluence between the ascending colon mesentery and the retroperitoneum in the region of the right pelvic inlet (Fig. 9.2). The confluence of the mesentery and the retroperitoneum are scored using the bipolar device, elevating the ascending mesocolon away from the retroperitoneum. This places the confluence on traction and often exposes both the duodenum and right ureter. This dissection continues laterally to the right lateral wall, medial to the duodenum and pancreatic head, and cephalad to the transverse colon. The terminal ileum is pulled medially allowing for transection of the lateral pericolic attachments from the cecum to the hepatic flexure (Pitfall 9.1).

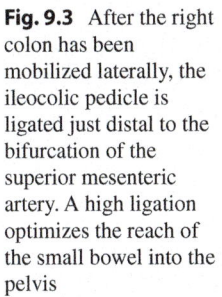

> ▲ **Pitfall 9.1**
> The interface between the right colon mesentery and retroperitoneum is a faint white line. This line should be preserved with the retroperitoneum to prevent violation of the right colon mesentery, poor oncologic margins, and bleeding.

Retraction of the right colon laterally exposes the ileocolic artery. Even in obese patients, there is virtually always an avascular region of the mesentery on either side of the ileocolic artery (Tip 9.3). The avascular planes are opened with an energy device, parallel to the ileocolic artery (Fig. 9.3).

Fig. 9.2 Right colon dissection: A lateral-to-medial dissection expedites the surgery. The cecum is elevated medially and cephalad with a Babcock, and dissection begins at the pelvic brim

Fig. 9.3 After the right colon has been mobilized laterally, the ileocolic pedicle is ligated just distal to the bifurcation of the superior mesenteric artery. A high ligation optimizes the reach of the small bowel into the pelvis

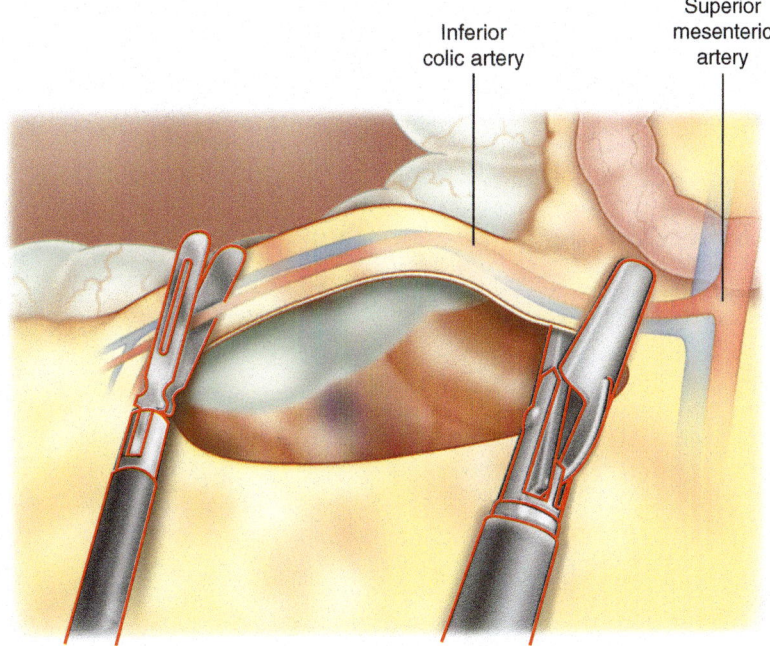

Inferior colic artery

Superior mesenteric artery

Identification of the duodenum prior to transection can assist in preventing iatrogenic duodenal injury. The ileocolic artery is then ligated just distal to the bifurcation from the superior mesenteric artery using bipolar energy, clips, or stapler.

> 💡 **Tip 9.3 Mesenteric Windows**
> Windows through the mesentery represent the peritoneum without underlying adipose tissues or vessels. These windows appear darker than surrounding mesentery. In thin patients they may also appear slightly shiny and translucent.

The energy device is used to free the attachments of the terminal ileal mesentery all the way to the duodenum, maximizing mobility of the terminal ileum for the ileal pouch (Tip 9.4).

> 💡 **Tip 9.4 Ileocolic Artery in Pouch Patients**
> While some surgeons prefer to preserve the ileocolic artery, considering that the pouch apex will be approximately 16 cm from the end of the terminal ileum, a balance between length/tension involving the pouch and blood supply to the pouch must be met.

An energy device is used to transect the terminal ileal mesentery perpendicular to the bowel wall. A stapler is inserted through the 12-mm port at the ileostomy site (Tip 9.5), and the terminal ileum is transected just proximal to the ileal cecal valve. This allows the right colon to be tucked over the liver, out of the way for the remaining portions of the surgery.

> 💡 **Tip 9.5 Bring Tissue to Stapler**
> The endostapler is bulky, and the surgeon should bring the tissue to the stapler, as opposed to moving the stapler in the surgical field.

Step 4: Hepatic Flexure

The hepatic flexure and transverse colon are mobilized to the midline, toward the middle colic vessels. Position the patient in maximal reverse Trendelenburg positioning, and retract the proximal transverse colon caudally and toward the anterior abdominal wall with the Babcock (Fig. 9.4). Separate the transverse colon from the omentum superiorly, and resect any remaining retroperitoneal attachments above Gerota's fascia and the duodenum.

Create avascular mesenteric windows on either side of the right branch of the middle colic vessel to safely isolate the vessels prior to transec-

Fig. 9.4 Hepatic flexure mobilization is expedited by moving the colon anteriorly and caudally, exposing the liver and Gerota's fascia

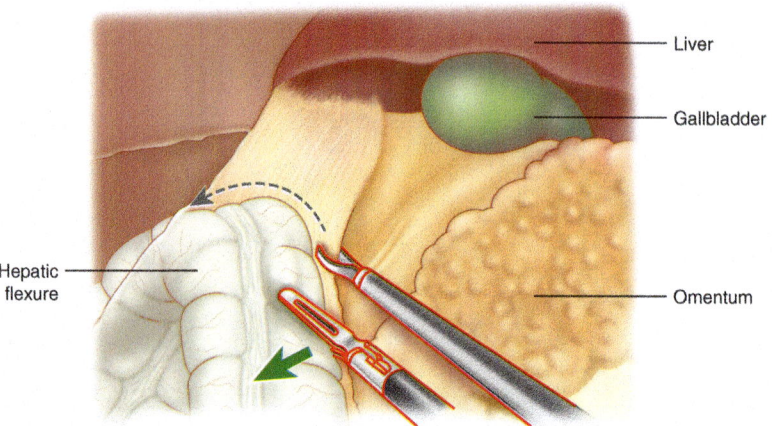

Fig. 9.5 The transverse colon is retracted anteriorly to expose the middle colic vessels which are sequentially transected

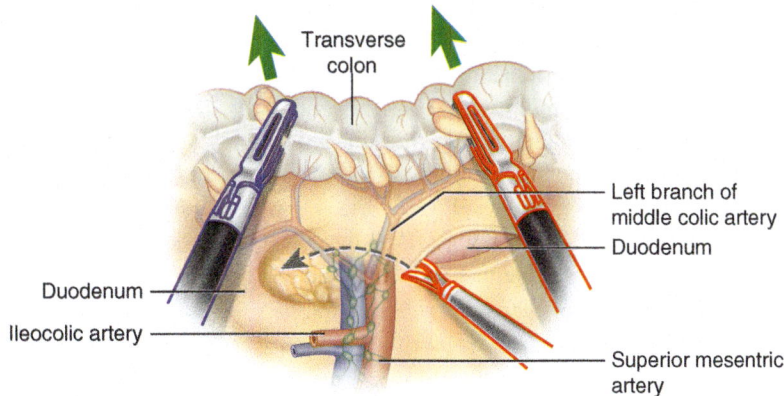

Transverse colon

Left branch of middle colic artery

Duodenum

Superior mesentric artery

Duodenum

Ileocolic artery

tion. The transverse colon is retracted anteriorly to expose the vessels (Fig. 9.5). With the energy device adjacent and parallel to each branch of the middle colic vessels, a window is opened and each vessel transected after isolation (Pitfall 9.2). This process brings the duodenum into view once again, allowing for a medial-to-lateral transection of the proximal transverse mesocolon which will mobilize the hepatic flexure.

> ⚠ **Pitfall 9.2**
> The middle colic vessels are an additional danger point. Proximal ligation can leave a short stump from the MCA that can retract behind the pancreas. Ensure that you have room for ligation and good hemostasis while transecting the MCA.

Step 5: Left Colectomy

Attention is next turned to the left colon. The surgeon moves to the patient's right using a Babcock for retraction in the left hand and an energy device for dissection and ligation of vessels in the right. The assistant stands cephalad to the surgeon, retracting the colon as needed (via which port). The patient is placed in maximal Trendelenburg and right lateral decubitus positioning for this portion of the surgery.

The choice of approach laterally to medial approach depends on the redundancy and natural position of the sigmoid colon (Pitfall 9.3):

> ⚠ **Pitfall 9.3**
> Whether a medial-to-lateral or lateral-to-medial approach is taken, isolation of the ureter away from the IMA is a prerequisite to prevent inadvertent injury to the ureter before the IMA is safely ligated.

(a) For a *lateral-to-medial approach*: The sigmoid colon is retracted medially with the left hand. The energy device is used to elevate the sigmoid colon from the retroperitoneum. Incision of the white line of Toldt reveals a second, deeper "white line" representing the coalescence of the mesentery and retroperitoneum. This white line is preserved and is the correct, bloodless plane of dissection. The sigmoid mesocolon is freed laterally until it is medialized in order to isolate the left ureter from the inferior mesenteric artery (IMA) (Fig. 9.6).

(b) For a *medial-to-lateral approach*: The sigmoid mesocolon is retracted toward the anterior abdominal wall with the left hand. Identification of the IMA at the pelvic brim is beneficial in developing the avascular windows on either side of the IMA, which can then be scored with the cautery. The Babcock is used to grasp the mesocolon and retract medially lifting the colon mesentery away from the retroperitoneum (Tip 9.6). The energy device bluntly sweeps the retroperitoneal tissues and ureters away from the IMA in a lateral and dorsal direction.

Skeletonize the IMA and retract the colon toward the anterior abdominal wall in the midline position. The left ureter should be identified from this medial perspective prior to transection (Fig. 9.7). Ligation of the IMA with an energy device can be performed either proximal to the bifurcation of the left colic artery for malignant disease or distal to the bifurcation in the setting of benign disease.

The remaining sigmoid colon and the descending colon are mobilized (Tip 9.7).

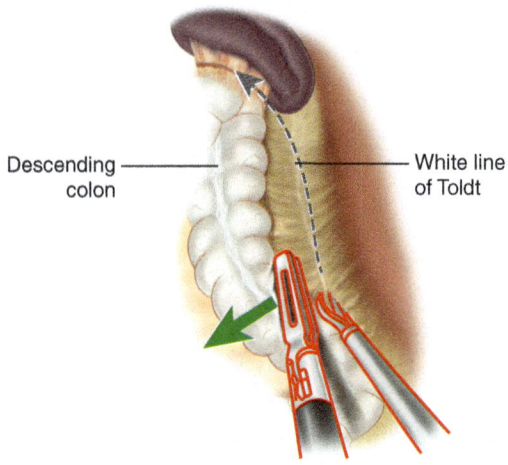

Fig. 9.6 A lateral-to-medial dissection of the sigmoid colon allows for visualization of the left and preservation of the ureter and left pelvic side wall

> 💡 **Tip 9.6 Countertension for Obese Patients**
> Especially for patients with visceral obesity, placing the retracting instrument closer to the junction of the mesocolon and retroperitoneum will provide better countertraction for identification of the IMA and for safe, time-efficient dissection.

> 💡 **Tip 9.7 Retracting in Two Planes**
> Optimized retraction often requires retracting in two different planes. For example, lateral mobilization of the left colon at the white line of Toldt requires retracting the colon medially and anteriorly to provide the best exposure.

Fig. 9.7 The inferior mesenteric artery is transected after the left ureter is identified

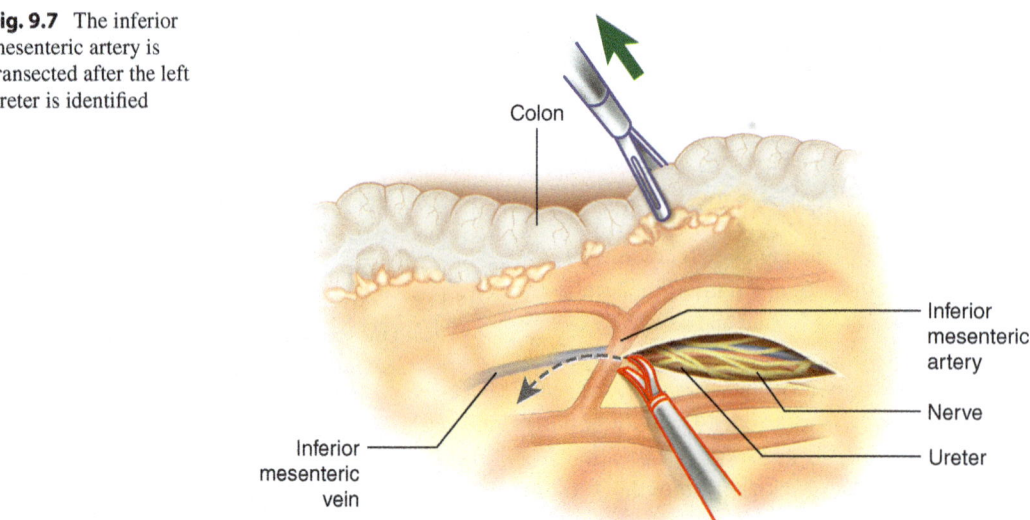

The colon is retracted toward the midline and the anterior abdominal wall, while the energy device is again used to sweep the retroperitoneal tissue laterally, away from the left colon mesentery. This process is continued to the level of the splenic flexure. Any remaining lateral pericolic attachments are transected. Mesenteric resection will include a ligation of the inferior mesenteric vein (IMV) (Pitfall 9.4).

> **Pitfall 9.4**
> The duodenojejunal junction is deep to the transverse colon mesentery at the splenic flexure. Once the avascular window is developed, identifying this segment of the intestine avoids collateral thermal injuries, including those caused by lateral spread from the energy device.

Step 6: Transverse Colectomy/Splenic Flexure Mobilization

This portion of the surgery represents the most potentially dangerous aspect of a proctocolectomy. The splenic flexure is the convergence of the spleen, the stomach, the duodenojejunal flexure, the pancreas, and the transverse mesocolon presenting many organs at risk for injury (Pitfall 9.5).

> **Pitfall 9.5**
> Be certain to reflect the stomach cephalad, avoiding injury to the posterior gastric wall and differentiating the transverse mesocolon from epiploic fat to avoid bleeding.

The patient is placed in maximal reverse Trendelenburg positioning right side down. The surgeon and the assistant move to the patient's right side, with the operating surgeon using a Babcock for retraction and an energy device for dissection and vessel ligation.

Transection of the gastrocolic ligament at its midpoint provides access into the lesser sac. Transection then proceeds toward the inferior pole of the spleen (Fig. 9.8). This provides full exposure of the lesser sac with visualization of the posterior gastric wall, the pancreas, the spleen, and the transverse mesocolon.

Attention is now returned to the middle colic vessels for ligation. Windows are developed mechanically on either side of the remaining

Fig. 9.8 After entering the lesser sac, dissection proceeds toward the inferior pole of the spleen, with full visualization of the posterior gastric wall

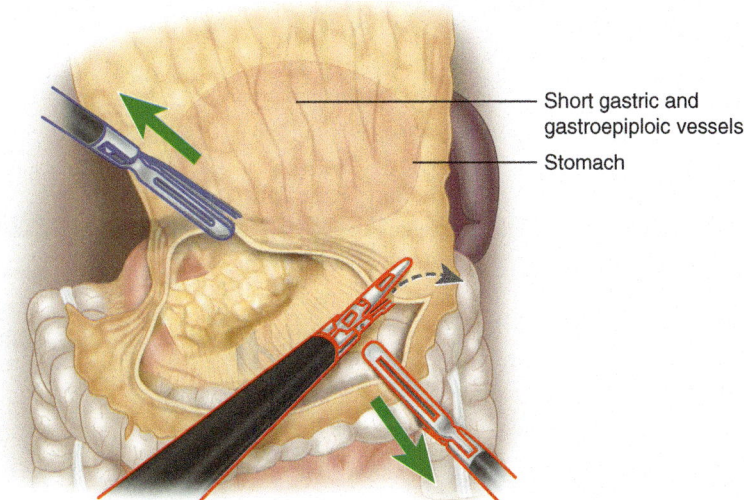

Short gastric and gastroepiploic vessels

Stomach

middle colic vessels. Each vessel is isolated and then transected with an energy device. This approach allows for the non-dominant hand to retract the mesentery anteriorly, away from the retroperitoneum, using the mesenteric windows to isolate each major arterial vessel and using the energy device to ligate these structures. This vantage point allows for a circumferential viewing of each vessel to ensure safety during the ligation process (Pitfall 9.6).

> **Pitfall 9.6**
> The posterior gastric wall can be injured easily and will sometimes extend more caudally than the anterior gastric wall which is readily in view. Opening the lesser sac completely helps to prevent gastric injury.

The remaining transverse mesocolon is freed from the retroperitoneum. Using the right hand, the transverse colon is retracted toward the right abdomen. Additional retroperitoneal attachments are transected using the energy device, freeing the splenic flexure completely. At this point the entire abdominal colon, from the right colon to sigmoid, is freed from its attachments.

Step 7: Externalize the Colectomy Specimen (Optional)

Externalizing the colectomy specimen prior to performing the proctectomy prevents a floppy colon from obscuring visualization during pelvic dissection. This is particularly true with large colon and small peritoneal cavities and in cases of obese patients, where visualization may be difficult. In a single-site approach, the presence of a trocar with removable top facilitates this step by allowing for easy reestablishment of pneumoperitoneum. In a standard laparoscopic approach, an extraction incision is created for removal. This can either be sealed

with commercial device or closed in order to continue laparoscopically. The expense of an additional stapler/resealing device should be balanced against ease of dissection (Tip 9.8).

> 💡 **Tip   9.8   Reestablishing Pneumoperitoneum**
> In multiport surgery, a wound protector with removable top, similar to a hand port, can be used to reestablish pneumoperitoneum after colon extraction and continue with a laparoscopic approach. If a removable top is not available, a small glove can be used to occlude the port.

Step 8: Proctectomy

The assistant moves to the patient's left side. The assistant retracts the rectosigmoid colon with forceps under the mesorectum and putting the mesorectum on stretch in, up, and out (Fig. 9.9). The left ureter is identified, and the energy device is used to transect any remaining attachments of the rectosigmoid mesentery on the left. Transection of the superior rectal artery, after confirming location of the ureter on the left, provides access into the presacral space (Tip 9.9).

Dissection begins in the posterolateral plane, in a "U" shape around the mesorectum. The assistant retracts the rectum anteriorly and cephalad, providing tension and space for dissection in the posterior

> 💡 **Tip 9.9 Mesorectal Dissection for Benign Disease**
> The mesorectum can be preserved in benign disease to decrease the likelihood of pelvic nerve injuries and to provide a cushion of adipose tissue to support the ileopouch. This technique is nonanatomic, it is not a bloodless plane, and it is more time-consuming.

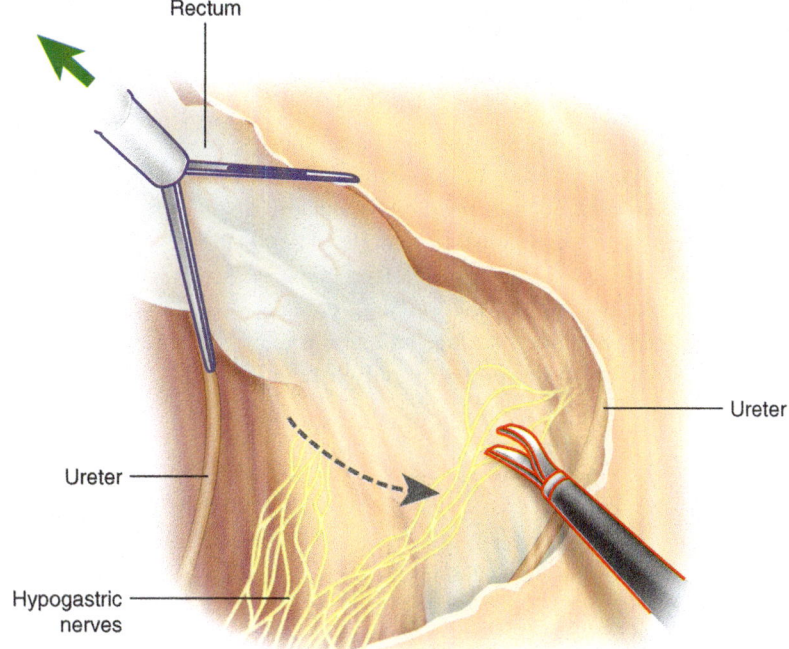

Fig. 9.9 The rectosigmoid is elevated anteriorly to the abdominal wall, exposing the posterior mesorectal plane down into the pelvis

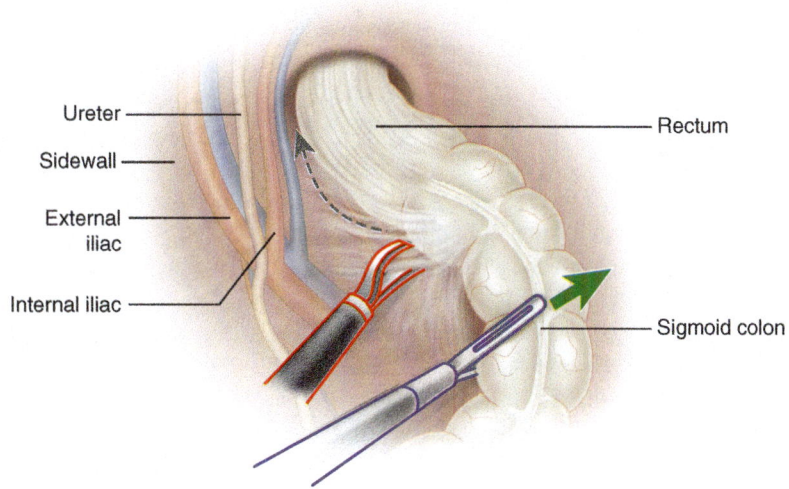

Fig. 9.10 Dissection continues until the pelvic floor is reached. Transection should be just proximal to the top of the levator muscles, minimizing remnant rectal tissue

midline. A thin filmy plane is visualized. With the left hand, the surgeon provides additional upward traction on the mesorectum, while the right hand uses the cautery on the scissors to dissect in the mesorectal plane. The correct plane should leave a filmy surface on the mesorectum anteriorly, while preserving the hypogastric nerves and presacral fascia laterally and deep to the dissection.

As the posterior plane loses tension, the assistant retracts the rectum anterolaterally, to the right or to the left, allowing for lateral mesorectal

mobilization. The surgeon's left hand provides more traction, freeing the right hand to dissect in the filmy, avascular plane on either side of the mesorectum. Posterior dissection continues until tension is lost, and then dissection begins laterally on each side in sequence. As the lateral tissue is freed, greater traction can be obtained posteriorly by replacing the assistant's retractor distally. This is continued in a posterior, lateral fashion until the levator floor is reached (Fig. 9.10).

The most difficult plane of dissection is anterior to the rectum (Tip 9.10). Once the anterior peritoneal reflection is incised, the assistant uses a bowel grasper to push upward on the vagina putting tension between the vagina and rectum or bladder and rectum. The surgeon retracts the rectum proximally out of the pelvis with a slight posterior angle. The dissection is performed with a cauterized scissors or hook, parallel to the rectum, being mindful of the prostate, vagina, and urethra, which lie anterior to the plane by only a few millimeters.

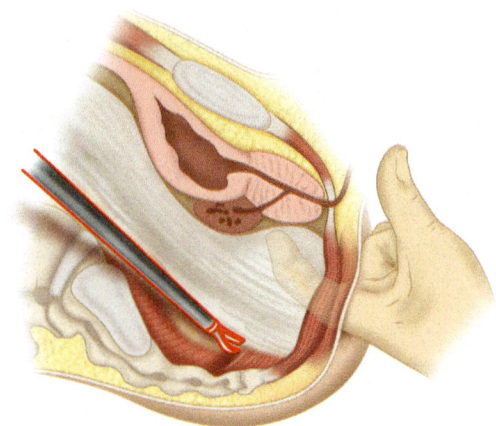

Fig. 9.11 A rectal exam helps to confirm the distal extent of dissection prior to transection of the rectum

💡 **Tip 9.10 Retraction of the Uterus**
A bulky uterus can be secured with a silk suture on a straight needle. A suture is introduced through the suprapubic anterior abdominal wall and is passed through the uterine fundus and back through the anterior abdominal wall. In males, the anterior peritoneal reflection can also be retracted in a similar fashion.

- Appropriate stapler location with respect to disease state (Tip 9.11).
- Straight staple line to prevent ischemia.
- Minimize multiple stapler loads.

💡 **Tip 9.11 Confirming Margins for Rectal Cancers**
For patients with rectal cancers, a rigid proctoscopy after the application of the endostapler but before stapling can confirm adequate margins. The specimen should be opened on a back table to ensure that the cancer has been removed with a proper gross distal margin.

The rectal mobilization is continued circumferentially to the anorectal junction. The goal of this portion of the surgery is to remove the entire rectum. Leaving a cuff of rectum can lead to poor functional outcomes in pouch patients with ulcerative colitis and increased neoplastic risks in patients with cancer or polyposis. A digital anorectal exam confirms the distal extent of dissection (Fig. 9.11).

Step 9: Transection of the Rectum

Laparoscopic stapling at the anorectal junction can be challenging secondary to limited room and the lack of right angle staplers. There is no one right way to approach this portion of the surgery. Keys to proper transection include:

The rectum is retracted proximally and posteriorly to expose the distal rectum at the anal ring. The mesorectum will generally taper off at the anorectal ring, but any remaining adipose tissue near the anorectal junction is transected. This minimizes the volume of tissue introduced into the stapler and prevents bleeding from the staple line.

Although the stapler can be applied in a number of directions, applying the stapler in an anterior to posterior direction is helpful in a narrow pelvis or obese patients. In a female or patient with a wider pelvis, the stapler can be placed from the right lower quadrant port, horizontally across the rectum from right to left. It is crucial that the rectum be manipulated to provide a staple line that is perpendicular to the rectum (Tip 9.12). For this reason, the assistant is often provided the stapler, while the surgeon manipulates the rectum in the stapler jaws.

> 💡 **Tip 9.12 Creating a Perpendicular Stapler Line in the Pelvis**
> With the stapler in place, use the right hand to push the rectum distal to the stapler on the right side of the rectum. Pull the stapler with the left hand proximal to the stapler, in effect moving the rectum within the stapler, rather than moving the stapler around the rectum.

The surgeon performs a close visual inspection of the stapler placement laparoscopically and a digital anal examination to confirm that the stapler is applied in a distal perpendicular position (Fig. 9.12). Every effort is made to transect the intestinal wall with a single stapler application.

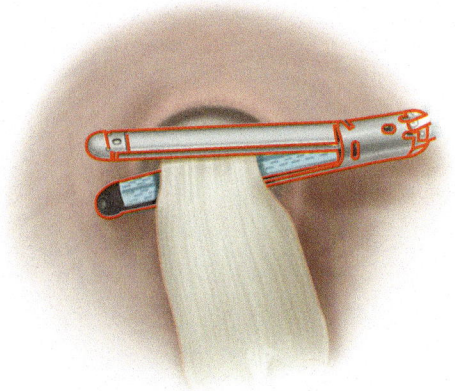

Fig. 9.12 Ensuring that the stapler is applied perpendicularly to the rectum minimizes excess staple loads and may reduce risk of staple line leaks

This single staple line decreases risk of ischemia, leak, or abnormal configuration of the anastomosis. The number of stapler applications applied to surrounding fatty tissue is less important.

Step 10: Externalize the Specimen

The specimen is removed through the single-port device during a single-site approach or through a small extraction incision in the case of a standard laparoscopic approach. It is important to balance the concern of making too many additional surgical sites, with being strategic about sacrificing trocar sites that will be needed later in the operation.

For thinner patients, expanding the site of a 12-mm suprapubic trocar to a Pfannenstiel incision can allow for removal of the specimen, pouch construction, and construction of the pouch-anal anastomosis. Pouch construction may require a larger incision given the distal location of the anastomosis.

Specimen extraction and pouch construction can also be made through the future stoma site. The fascia of the site can be partially closed after pouch construction and then reopened at the conclusion of the surgery to construct the diverting ileostomy.

Step 11: Construction of the Pouch

Initially after externalizing the specimen, the surgeon should verify that there is adequate length for pouch creation. A good rule of thumb for adequate length is if the apex of the pouch reaches to the pubis. Internally, laparoscopic instruments can be used to determine the anticipated apex of the pouch internally and reach it toward the anus as a surrogate evaluation. If the ileum reaches to the anus easily, there should be adequate length for pouch creation (Fig. 9.13).

If the length is inadequate, the surgeon can perform additional maneuvers in order to achieve adequate mesenteric length. First, check to ensure that the mesentery of the small bowel has been fully mobilized to the duodenum. This can provide several centimeters of additional pouch reach. If reach is still inadequate, careful elective ligation of mesenteric vessels may be performed.

If the ileocolic artery is intact, branches of the ileal arcade may be transected, providing additional reach to the apex of the pouch. Prior to transection of any branches, the branch should be occluded transiently, with observation, to ensure that the future pouch does not become ischemic. If further reach is needed, scoring the mesentery in a stair stepping mechanism can provide additional reach (Fig. 9.14 and Tip 9.13).

The pouch is constructed using open surgical staplers through the extraction incision (Tip 9.14). The terminal ileum is externalized, and a sterile ruler is used to measure a 15-cm length for a J-pouch. The choice of the extraction/pouch construction site on the abdominal wall is generally

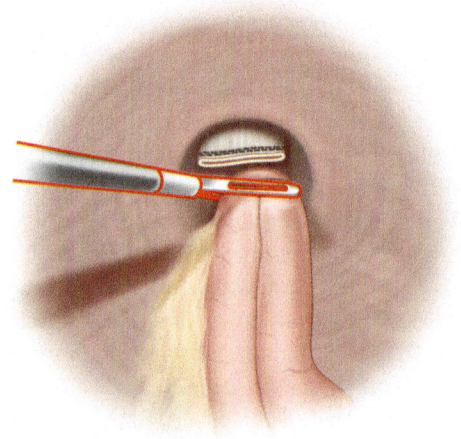

Fig. 9.13 Internally, the reach of the pouch can be confirmed by pulling the pouch deep into the pelvis to the rectal stump. The pouch should reach easily, without tension

> 💡 **Tip 9.13 Failure to Reach**
> If the pouch does not reach to the anus, the pouch can be hitched to anterior sacrum with an absorbable braided suture under a moderate amount of stretch. This allows the pouch to stretch and can be attached during an interval surgery.

> 💡 **Tip 9.14 Pouch Conformation**
> J pouches are most commonly created, with a 15–18-cm pouch. Other conformations such as "S" pouch" and "W pouch" can be created, as each provides a slightly varied apex, which may make reach to the anus easier.

Fig. 9.14 Stair stepping is performed, scoring the peritoneum covering the mesenteric vessels. This is done sequentially to increase reach. Care must be taken to prevent injury to the underlying blood supply to the pouch

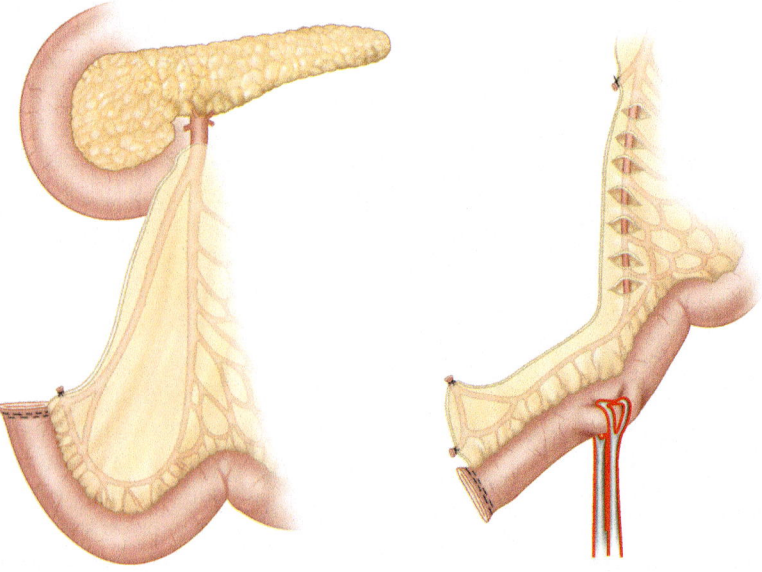

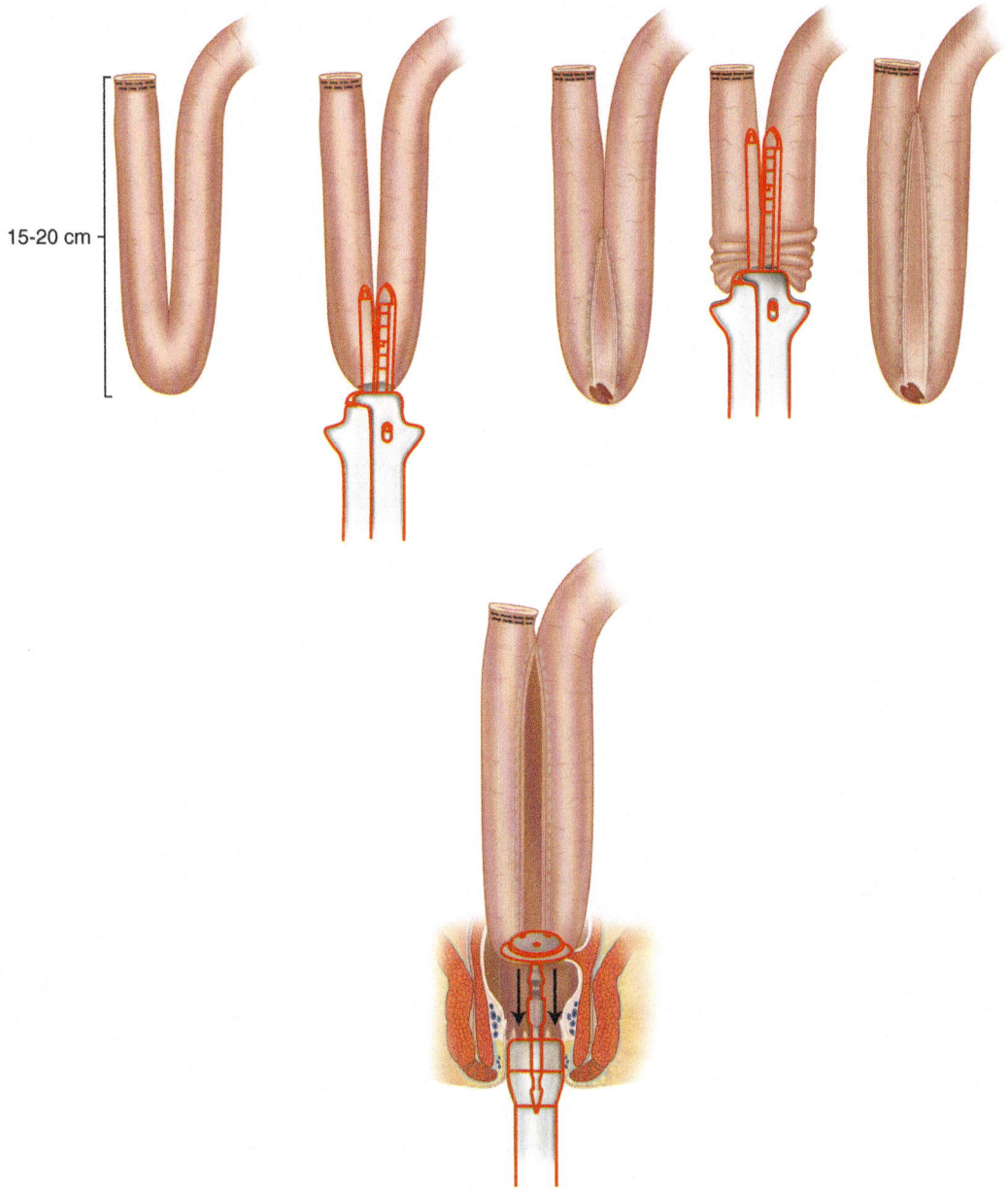

15-20 cm

Fig. 9.15 The pouch is created with the distal ileum by folding the ileum and using two to three firings of a linear stapler to open the entire length of the pouch

dictated by the length of the bowel and ability to expose at least 30 cm of the distal ileum through the incision. For these reasons, either a right or left lower quadrant port, ideally the ultimate stoma port, or a Pfannenstiel incision is generally used for extraction. The ileum is grasped with a bowel grasper approximately 15 cm proximal to the ileal staple line or the distal most portion of the pouch. The two limbs of the pouch are secured with several interrupted seromuscular 2–0 Vicryl pop-off sutures to maintain proper orientation of each intestinal limb (Fig. 9.15).

Cautery is used to create a full-thickness enterotomy at the apex of the pouch, allowing for three applications of a 100-mm linear-cutting stapler to construct the common channel of the pouch. The first stapler is placed through the enterotomy and carefully advanced into each limb of the pouch. Subsequent firings are placed through the enterotomy, deeper into the pouch, until the entire length of the pouch has been opened. The seromuscular sutures allow for proximal retraction on the pouch while the stapler is being advanced. If the patient will not be diverted, the pouch is distended with a red rubber catheter and sterile saline, to ensure that the staple lines comprising the pouch are watertight (Fig. 9.16).

The anvil for a circular, endolumenal end-to-end stapling device is secured in the apex of the pouch using a full-thickness purse-string suture. The pouch is returned to the peritoneal cavity, and pneumoperitoneum is reestablished, either by closing the SSL port or closing the fascia of the incision used for pouch construction.

Step 12: Construction of the Pouch-Anal Anastomosis

The base of the end-to-end stapling device is carefully introduced by the assistant through the sphincters, into the anal stump (Pitfall 9.7). Once the entire outline of the stapler is visualized at the end of the anal stump, the pin of the stapler is advanced through the center of the stump. The surgeon uses laparoscopic graspers to grasp the stapler anvil within the pouch, to the pin of the

> ⚠️ **Pitfall 9.7**
> Care must be taken when inserting the endolumenal stapler through the anus for pouch creation. The anal stump is very short, and inexperienced assistants can accidentally rupture the staple line.

Fig. 9.16 The distal enterotomy is occluded and the pouch is distended with saline. This demonstrates the size of the pouch as well as pouch integrity

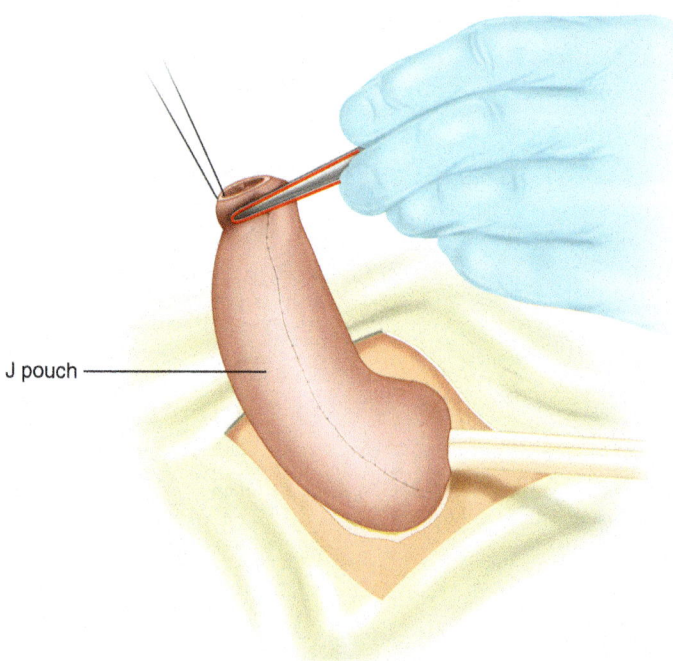

J pouch

stapler base. Having the assistant turn the EEA device away from the surgeon by moving hands to the left facilitates alignment and attachment of the stapler anvil (Tip 9.15).

> ### 💡 Tip 9.15 Protection Against Pouch-Vaginal Fistulas
> Some surgeons prefer to extrude the pin posterior to the staple line to orient the anastomosis in a more posterior position in females. This is an added measure against a pouch-vaginal fistula.

During this process, the surgeon checks to ensure the pouch is not twisted on its own mesentery. The most reliable approach is to visualize the transected edge of the small bowel mesentery from the pouch to the level of the duodenum; a straight line transected edge of the ileal and right colon mesentery can be easily identified. If this line is not straight, it must be corrected prior to stapling (Fig. 9.17). The assistant closes the stapler until the closure feels "tight" and then allows a 15-second delay for tissue

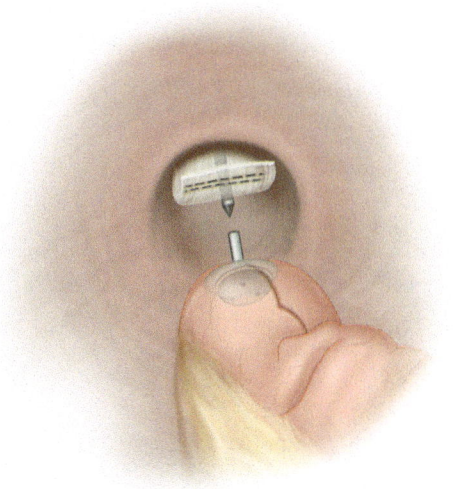

Fig. 9.17 The pouch is brought into the pelvis and a circular stapler is used to create the pouch-anal anastomosis

compression and hemostasis. The stapler is then deployed, with the firing mechanism held closed for an additional 15 seconds prior to relaxation, in order to ensure proper staple apposition and hemostasis.

If the patient is to be diverted, some surgeons will not perform a leak test on the IPAA because this will not alter immediate treatment. If diversion is not planned for in a perfunctory fashion, then an adult rigid proctoscope is used to distend the anastomosis to assess for an air leak. Pelvic drains are placed only if the IPAA is undiverted, in which case drains placed anterior and posterior to the anastomosis are utilized.

Step 13: Creation of Diverting Loop Ileostomy

Prior to closing, a loop ileostomy is created proximal to the pouch. Using the left-sided ports, run the bowel 15–20 cm proximal to the pouch inlet so that the pouch is no longer under tension. To check tension, the surgeon lifts the ileum to the stoma site. It is vital to ensure that the ostomy is not causing tension to the mesentery or to the ileopouch, as this may compromise blood supply. If the stoma is under too much tension, run the bowel more proximally to find a more appropriate ileostomy site. The appropriate positioning of the stoma is a compromise between using a distal stoma which allows for better nutritional and fluid absorption and the mechanical difficulties of preserving blood supply and reach.

Once the appropriate segment of the bowel is identified, a stoma trephine is created. A circular opening is made in the skin, dissecting and opening all layers of the abdominal wall to create a hole large enough for the stoma. Generally, the fascia is divided and the rectus muscle is pushed laterally using appendiceal retractors. As soon as the peritoneum is opened, insufflation will be lost. Putting two fingers into the stoma site and lifting will allow for visualization of the abdomen while the stoma is oriented.

Fig. 9.18 A loop ileostomy is created in a Brooke fashion, everting the proximal end of the stoma to facilitate pouching

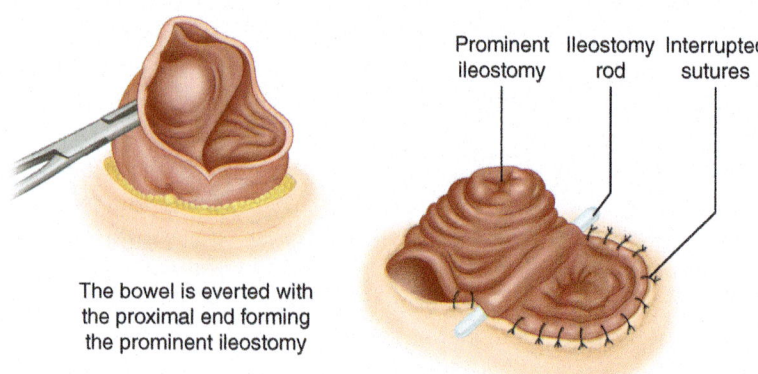

The bowel is everted with the proximal end forming the prominent ileostomy

Prominent ileostomy   Ileostomy rod   Interrupted sutures

It is critical that the proximal and distal sides of the stoma are identified and preserved. This can be checked laparoscopically prior to closure. By convention, the proximal aspect of the stoma is oriented superiorly when the stoma is externalized. This allows for easier pouching. Generally, a loop ileostomy is matured over a stoma rod, or stoma device, to ensure that the back wall is appropriately elevated. Elevation of the back wall will assist in preventing premature leakage of succus into the pouch. The stoma is matured in a Brooke fashion (Fig. 9.18).

Laparoscopic Lysis of Adhesions and Bowel Obstruction

Meagan M. Costedio and Anthony L. DeRoss

Introduction

Laparoscopic lysis of adhesions or treatment of bowel obstruction is performed for acute or chronic obstruction of the small bowel. The same techniques may also be used for cases of diagnostic laparoscopy.

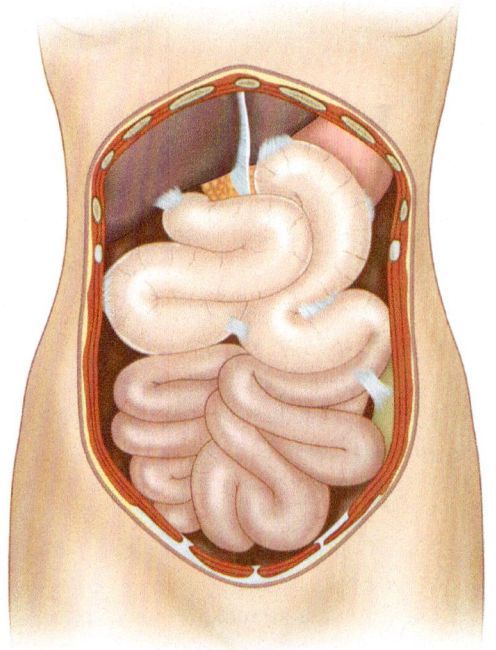

Indications
- Acute small bowel obstruction
- Chronic small bowel obstruction
- Chronic abdominal pain caused by adhesions
- Crohn's disease
- Meckel's diverticulum
- Postoperative peritonitis

M. M. Costedio (✉)
Division of Colorectal Surgery, University Hospitals, Cleveland, OH, USA
e-mail: meagan.costedio@uhhospitals.org

A. L. DeRoss
Pediatric Surgery, Cleveland Clinic, Cleveland, OH, USA

Patient Positioning for Laparoscopic Laparoscopic Lysis of Adhesions and Bowel Obstruction

The patient is positioned on the table using the split leg extenders with both arms tucked, followed by placement of a urinary catheter. The chest and the legs are secured to the table using tape or belt. The legs are draped separately to provide a sterile field between the legs where the surgeon can operate. Monitors are placed on the right and left sides of the patient at the mid-abdominal level. All operative cords, lines, and tubes should be run from the top of the operative field to the appropriate towers.

This arrangement allows the operating surgeon and assistant the freedom to move around the table during the operation based on the density and location of adhesions (Tip 10.1).

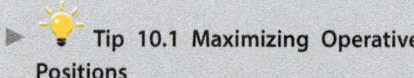

> 💡 **Tip 10.1 Maximizing Operative Positions**
> Tucking the arms and splitting the legs provides multiple positions for operating: left side, right side, and between the legs. Because adhesions may form at any location, the surgeon can change position to access the unpredictable anatomy of adhesions.

Operative Strategy

Step 1: Peritoneal Entry

A careful review of the chart and preoperative imaging is essential in planning safe operative entry to the abdomen for any reoperative surgery (Tip 10.2). For the reoperative abdomen, entry will be safest through a Hassan approach at the umbilicus. As this access point is frequently used during prior surgeries, preoperative imaging can identify bowel loops adherent to the midline incision.

> 💡 **Tip 10.2 Preoperative Planning**
> Invest the time to examine all prior operative notes and imaging prior to surgery. Understanding of anatomy will allow for better expectations of intraoperative findings and modifications to technique or practice that may be necessary.

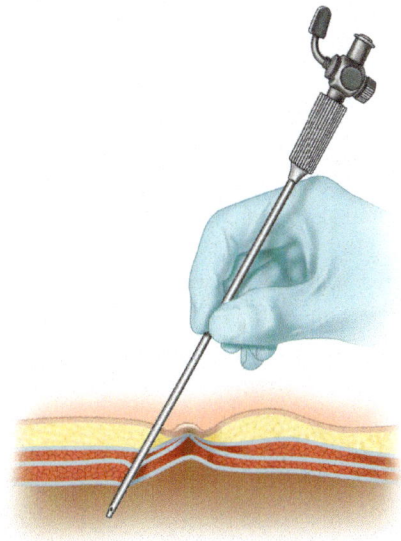

Fig. 10.1 Veress needle insertion. If inserted off the midline, a popping sensation will be encountered as the needle traverses each layer of the abdominal wall

In this case, the approach can be modified and a Veress needle inserted in the left upper quadrant. The left upper quadrant is used as fewer structures are at risk for injury during entry. If the left abdomen was the site of prior surgery, the right upper quadrant can be used.

If a Veress needle is used off midline (Fig. 10.1), a popping sensation will be encountered as the needle traverses each layer: the external oblique fascia, the internal oblique fascia, the transversus abdominis fascia, and finally the transversalis fascia and peritoneum together.

Once the Veress needle is inserted into the peritoneal cavity, sterile saline should be dripped into the needle and observed flowing freely into the peritoneum. The saline will not flow if the peritoneal cavity has not been entered or if the end of the Veress needle is not free.

A syringe is attached to the needle and aspirated, even if the saline does not flow through the needle. Aspiration of blood or succus is an indication of injury and may require conversion to open surgery for treatment. If the saline flows and there is no aspirate from the needle, the insufflation tubing is attached to the needle and insufflation started (Pitfall 10.1).

> ⚠️ **Pitfall 10.1 Veress Needle Aspiration**
> If blood or succus is encountered during aspiration, the site of injury is facilitated by leaving the needle in place. This facilitates localization of the injury after conversion to open surgery.

Initial intra-abdominal pressure should be between 4 and 5 mm Hg indicating correct intraperitoneal placement. Lifting of the abdominal wall with towel clamps anteriorly may help to create a free space for insufflation. Pressures greater than 10 mm Hg indicate that the tip of the Veress needle is in the abdominal wall or in an intra-abdominal organ. Insufflation should not be started until appropriate pressures confirm accurate placement.

Step 2: Initial Inspection and Port Placement

A 5 mm trocar can be placed at the umbilicus or site of the Veress needle. This trocar may be upsized later to a 5/12 mm port if necessary to accommodate a stapler. A 5 mm 30-degree camera is inserted, and the peritoneal cavity is inspected after pneumoperitoneum is established with pressures of 12–15 mmHg (Tip 10.3). Additional port placement is determined based upon existing abdominal wall adhesions.

> **Tip 10.3 Scope Choice**
> A 10 mm scope provides greater light, but a 5 mm 30-degree scope allows placement of the scope through any port. Changing the position of camera insertion may be especially helpful during lysis of adhesions.

A reasonable initial arrangement includes a 5 mm trocar in the left upper quadrant, a 5 mm trocar in the left lower quadrant, and a 5 mm trocar in the right abdomen based on the location and density of adhesions.

Right Side Adhesions

If the majority of adhesions are on the right side of the abdomen, the operating surgeon stands on the left side of the patient with an atraumatic bowel grasper in the nondominant hand and a scissor or energy device in the dominant hand using the left-sided ports. The assistant stands between the legs and controls the camera. The assistant uses a left lower quadrant port for an atraumatic bowel grasper.

Alternative Technique for Dense Adhesions

If adhesions are very dense, port placement may be altered. Additional ports should be placed under direct laparoscopic visualization through a clear segment of the abdominal wall.

If no free abdominal wall segment can be visualized for the second trocar placement secondary to dense adhesions, the scope itself can be used as an instrument (Pitfall 10.2). Careful, gentle sweeps with the scope along the abdominal wall can create enough additional domain to place a second trocar safely. Additional ports may be placed later to optimize working ports after the abdominal wall has been freed of adhesions.

> **Pitfall 10.2 Laparoscope**
> The light at the end of the scope can cause burns to tissue if contact is prolonged. When using the scope as an instrument, quick gentle sweeps should be used.

If no safe location can be found for additional port placement, if an injury occurs while entering the abdomen, or if adhesions appear too thick and impenetrable, it is appropriate to consider conversion to open surgery.

Step 3: Lysis of Adhesions

After the first two trocars are placed, adhesiolysis can begin. There are three techniques for adhesiolysis: blunt, sharp, and energy. A combination of these techniques is often used together (Tips 10.4 and 10.5):

> **Tip 10.4 Adhesions**
> Adhesions should be clear in color, not yellow or red. Yellow is the mesentery or fat, and red demonstrates vascularity. The correct narrow space is always clear and avascular.

1. Blunt adhesiolysis is best achieved using
   two atraumatic bowel graspers (Fig. 10.2).
   For tough omental adhesions to the abdominal wall, a bowel grasper and bullet grasper
   work well. The bowel grasper is placed in
   the nondominant hand and pushes anteriorly
   on the abdominal wall. The bullet grasper
   grips the adhesion near the omentum or
   bowel, and tension is used to divide the
   adhesion. Alternatively, the viscera may be
   grasped directly, but care should be taken to
   avoid injury to the bowel while trying to
   divide the adhesion. Having the assistant
   push externally on the abdominal wall at the
   location of adhesions may help in exposing
   the adhesions for dissection. Adhesions

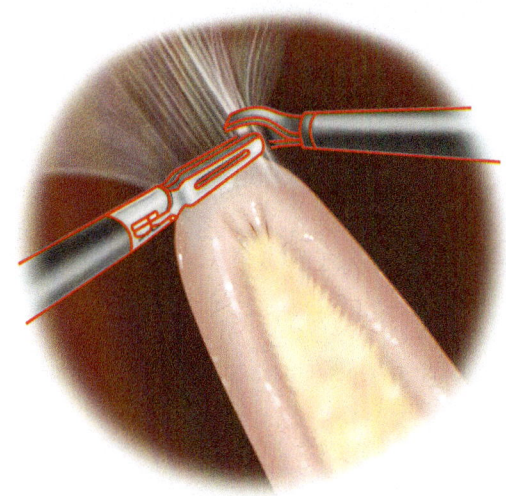

Fig. 10.3 Sharp dissection. Traction is created with the nondominant hand, and the scissors are used to cut adhesions at their origins

should separate with gentle tension. If the
adhesions do not separate easily at the inter-
face with the peritoneum, it is reasonable to
transition to sharp dissection.

2. Sharp dissection is important, particularly in
   close vicinity to fragile structures such as the
   bowel, gallbladder, spleen, or ureter. Traction
   is created with the nondominant hand, and the
   scissors are used to cut adhesions at their origins (Fig. 10.3). Dissection should take place
   in the avascular plane to minimize bleeding or
   injury to the mesentery. Most adhesions do
   not require cauterization if meticulously
   dissected.

3. Energy dissection. The plane between adhesions may be vascularized with small vessels. Lysis may require transection of the
   mesentery or omentum. These situations
   will necessitate use of electrocautery or
   other energy devices. Monopolar cautery
   should be set at a maximum of 30 watts of
   coagulation and may be used with the scissors for pure omental or abdominal wall
   adhesions to minimize bleeding (Pitfall
   10.3). Bipolar or ultrasonic energy devices
   can also be used for the same purpose and
   provide some protection of heat transfer, but
   they add expense, have a broader profile, and

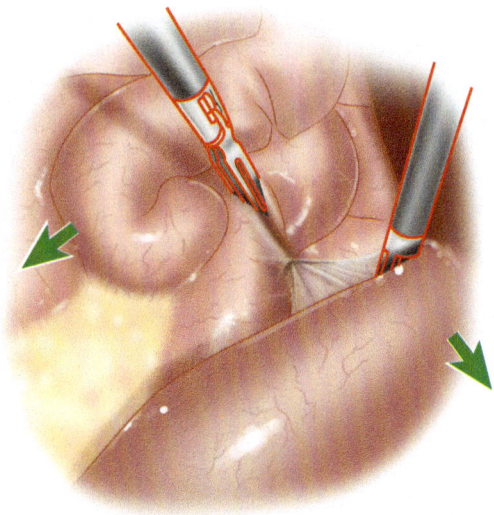

Fig. 10.2 Blunt adhesiolysis. A bowel grasper pushes anteriorly on the abdominal wall or bowel. Another grasper grips the adhesion near the omentum or bowel, and gentle traction is used to divide the adhesion

> ⚠️ **Pitfall 10.3 Monopolar Scissors**
> The monopolar scissors remain hot after use. Touching the bowel too soon after use can cause thermal injury even though no current is applied. This injury can present as a delayed bowel perforation.

can still cause thermal energy to delicate structures.

Visualization is key to successful adhesiolysis. When dissecting through thick adhesions, care must be taken to determine depth of tissue and whether structures are fused deep to the exposed tissue. A loop of the bowel may be fixed behind the omentum or mesentery. A 30-degree scope allows for changes in perspective to best visualize the adhesions and prevent inadvertent injury to the bowel (Fig. 10.4). Changing the camera location from one port to another provides a similar advantage.

Step 4: Running the Bowel

It is best to clear all omental adhesions from the anterior abdominal wall first to provide access and exposure of the bowel below. Relocation of the omentum superior to the stomach is the next step.

This step may require transection of the omentum from attachments in the lower abdomen and abdominal wall. The amount of devascularized omentum left behind should be minimized because of risk for necrosis and subsequent infection. Energy instruments are helpful for transection of the omentum. Care should be taken to ensure that all small bowel is safely freed from the omentum.

Once the omentum has been elevated and returned to the upper abdomen, the surgeon runs the small bowel to determine the source of obstruction. The bowel should be run from distal to proximal, starting at the terminal ileum identified by the antimesenteric fold of Treves. Distended small bowel is fragile and may be injured easily, even with gentle retraction (Pitfall 10.4). Care is taken to grasp the dilated bowel as little as possible, but grasps should be large enough so that the force is distributed to the majority of the bowel circumference. Grasping only a small portion of the bowel can lead to pinches, tears, and perforations.

Dilated bowel may obscure visualization. Adjusting the plane of the operating table left-side-down and/or into Trendelenburg position can

Fig. 10.4 Use of angled scope for better visualization. Rotating a 30- or 45-degree scope may provide additional perspectives and views of adhesions so that they can be divided safely and effectively

Range of different endoscopic viewing angles

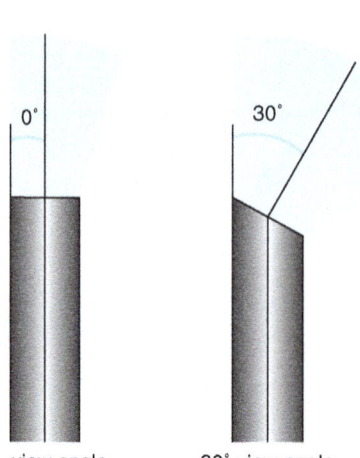

0° view angle   30° view angle   45° view angle

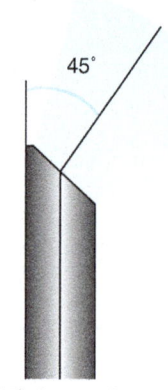

> ⚠ **Pitfall 10.4 Dilated Bowel**
> Dilated bowel is often edematous and fragile. The serosa can fracture easily even when handled carefully with atraumatic bowel graspers.

be helpful to augment retraction (Fig. 10.5). The surgeon starts running of the bowel while standing on the patient's left side. The cecum is identified, and the terminal ileum is grasped with the operating surgeon's left bowel grasper. In a hand-over-hand fashion, the decompressed terminal ileum is run proximally using two atraumatic bowel graspers (Fig. 10.6) until the ligament of Treitz or point of obstruction is identified.

Care should be taken to grasp the bowel itself, rather than the mesentery. The camera should be kept steady as possible, while the small bowel is displayed within the field of vision. This technique helps to prevent disorientation. If orienta-

tion is lost or bowel dropped during the process, the surgeon begins again at the terminal ileum.

As running the bowel progresses toward the upper abdomen, the surgeon may want to transition to standing between the patient's legs, using the right and left lower abdominal trocars for bowel graspers.

Adhesions are divided as they are encountered, taking care not to lose orientation of the bowel. The assistant's left hand retracts dilated small bowel that may be obscuring visualization as the surgeon provides tension and divides adhesions. The assistant controls the camera, angling it posteriorly.

Notes of pathology, such as areas of Crohn's disease, should be documented. The process is continued until all adhesions are lysed, the ligament of Treitz is reached, or the decision to convert to open procedure is made. All obstructing adhesions should be separated during the process. If a fistula is noted or a serosotomy is created, action must be taken. Repair can be performed laparoscopically or through a small midline extraction site after completion of the laparoscopic por-

Fig. 10.5 Changing the plane of the table. Adjusting the plane of the operating table left-side-down and/or into Trendelenburg position can be helpful to augment retraction

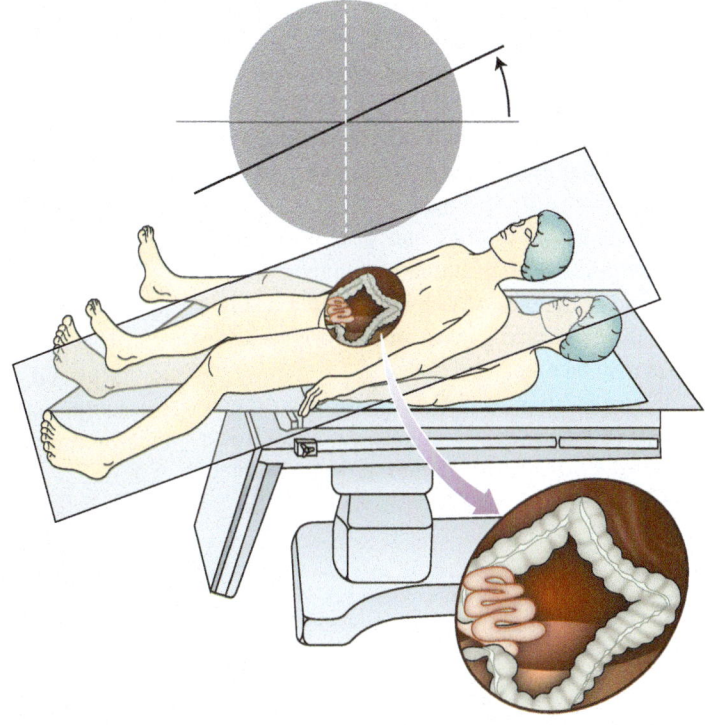

Fig. 10.6 Running the bowel laparoscopically. In a hand-over-hand fashion, the decompressed distal bowel is run proximally using two atraumatic bowel graspers

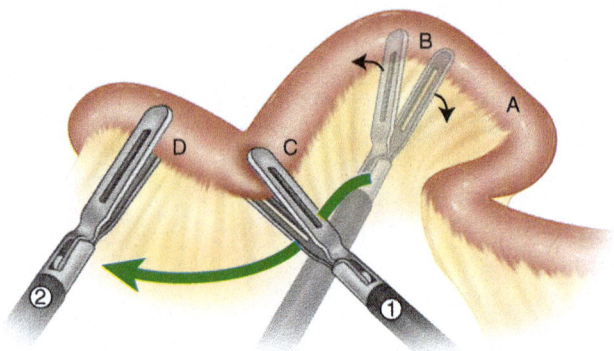

tion of the case. A suture is placed at the time of injury to mark the area of injury for repair.

Step 5: Repair of Serosotomy

Prior to closing, the surgeon should examine the entire small bowel for serosal tears or enterotomies. The bowel is inspected from the ligament of Treitz to the ileocecal valve making sure that all serosal surfaces are visualized. If a serosal tear is encountered, the surgeon can repair it using laparoscopic Lembert sutures. A 3–0 absorbable braided suture may be used, cut to 12–15 cm (Fig. 10.7). Seromuscular bites from either side of the serosal tear should be placed longitudinally, parallel to the lumen of the bowel, to prevent narrowing of the lumen.

Full-thickness injuries can also be repaired laparoscopically. Depending on surgeon experience and preference of technique, either a single layer of interrupted sutures or a two-layer technique may be used.

If visualization is difficult or a laparoscopic repair is not feasible, the 10 mm umbilical trocar site can be extended to 25 mm. A wound protec-

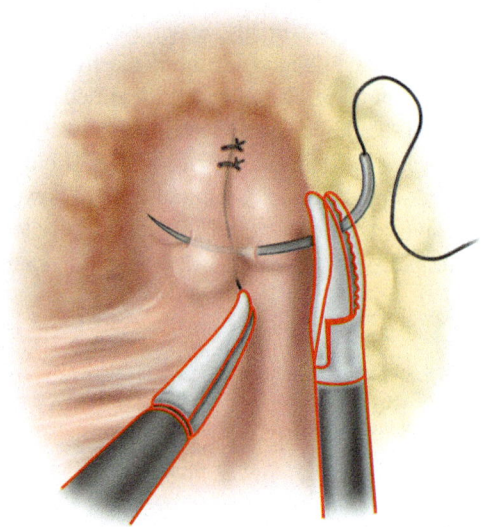

Fig. 10.7 Repair of serosotomies. Repair is done with laparoscopic Lembert sutures. Seromuscular bites from either side of the serosal tear should be placed longitudinally, parallel to the lumen of the bowel, to prevent narrowing of the lumen

tor is placed, and the small bowel can be run extracorporeally (Pitfall 10.5). Serosal tears or enterotomies can then be repaired in an open fashion.

> ⚠️ **Pitfall 10.5 Missed Enterotomy**
> An occult missed enterotomy can lead to a catastrophic complication. Risks can be minimized by using gentle traction during the procedure and inspecting the entire surface of the bowel either laparoscopically or extracorporeally at the end of the procedure.

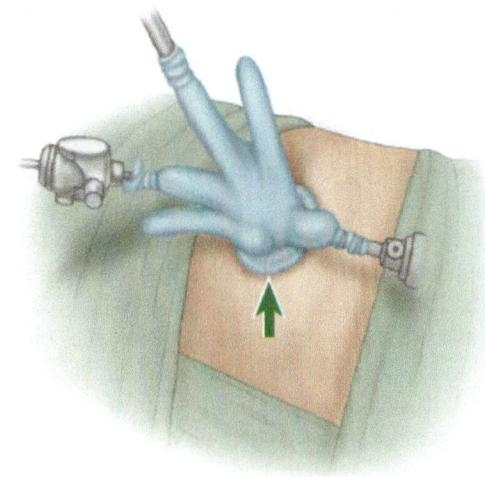

Fig. 10.8 Glove single-site platform. An inexpensive alternative to a commercially available single incision platform is a wound protector with a glove attached and trocars placed through the fingers for instruments

Step 6: Conversion to Open Surgery

When to convert? The simple answer is to convert whenever the thought of safety is entertained. Remember that the primary goal for every surgery is safe management of the patient. This aim should never be compromised in an attempt to limit the extent or number of incisions.

If the operation fails to progress laparoscopically, an intermediate step is to add an additional trocar. One extra instrument can make a significant difference in ability to accomplish the operative goals. If further steps in the procedure remain difficult, it is reasonable to set a time limit for progression. If the operation fails to progress, conversion should be considered.

A single incision port can be used initially if a larger incision will be needed for treatment of multiple inter-loop adhesions or bowel resection. An inexpensive alternative to a commercially available single incision platform is a wound protector with a glove attached and trocars placed through the fingers for instruments (Fig. 10.8). Once the omental and lateral adhesions are divided, the terminal ileum can be grasped through the glove and externalized. The bowel can be run, and the inter-loop adhesions can be lysed extracorporeally, saving time and aiding inspection for serosal tears and other pathology.

Conversion should be considered with any complication. Some complications may be managed safely laparoscopically, but the priority should be appropriate treatment and not stubborn maintenance of a laparoscopic approach.

Special Considerations

Single Band Adhesiolysis

Determining the source of obstruction is paramount to a successful surgery. Laparoscopic treatment of a single adhesive band is relatively straightforward. It can be transected, and the band remnants should be removed to prevent recreation of an adhesion.

The entire small bowel should then be run to ensure that there is not a secondary source of obstruction prior to closure.

Closed-Loop Obstruction

Closed-loop obstruction should be released and the bowel evaluated for viability. If there is question about bowel viability, the area should be evaluated extracorporeally for pulsatile blood flow or by using fluorescence to determine viability. If it is within the surgeons' skill set, an intracorporeal anastomosis may be performed should resection be needed. Viability of proximal and distal segments is vital to a favorable outcome.

Meckel's Diverticulum

A Meckel's diverticulum or omphalomesenteric duct remnant can be resected using a laparoscopic stapler. Generally located within several feet proximal to the ileocecal valve, this embryologic vestige can be a source of recurrent obstruction if there is a band extending from it to the abdominal wall. Once located, the area should be inspected and cleared of adhesions. An endo-

scopic linear stapler can be placed through a 12 mm port. The stapler should be aligned perpendicular to the normal bowel lumen to prevent narrowing of the intestinal lumen (Fig. 10.9).

Crohn's Disease

In the case of small bowel Crohn's disease, good preoperative imaging may decrease the need for surgery. Crohn's disease can produce dense adhesions that obliterate planes, leading to inadvertent injury of other organs. Decreasing inflammation preoperatively reduces the risk of operative complications and the need for conversion to open surgery.

A trial of nonoperative management including antibiotics, transcutaneous drainage of abscesses, bowel rest, and at least a 6-week waiting period gives inflammation a chance to subside. These measures maximize the chance for laparoscopic success.

There are times when waiting is not possible or when the inflammation is still severe despite an appropriate interval of time. In these cases, it is crucial to define normal anatomy prior to approaching the inflamed structures. The abdomen should be inspected briefly so that fistulas

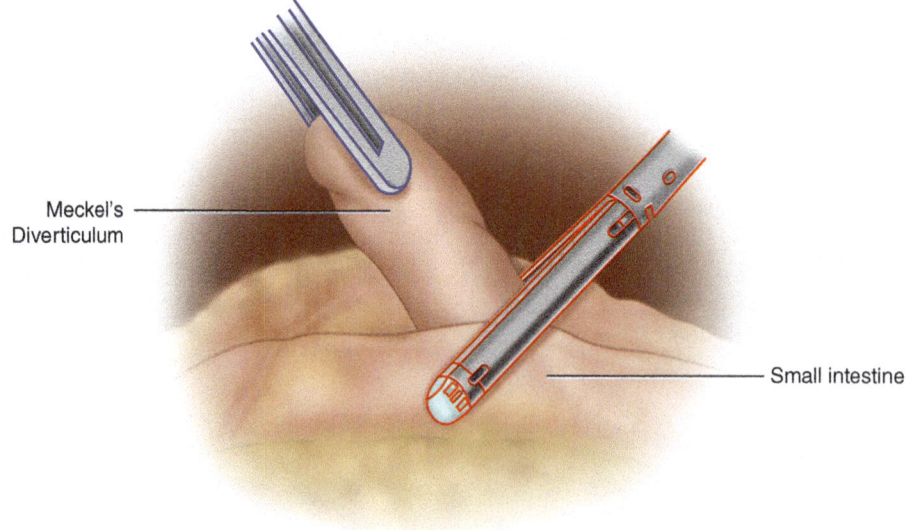

Meckel's Diverticulum

Small intestine

Fig. 10.9 Meckel's diverticulum. The stapler should be aligned perpendicular to the normal bowel to prevent narrowing of the intestinal lumen

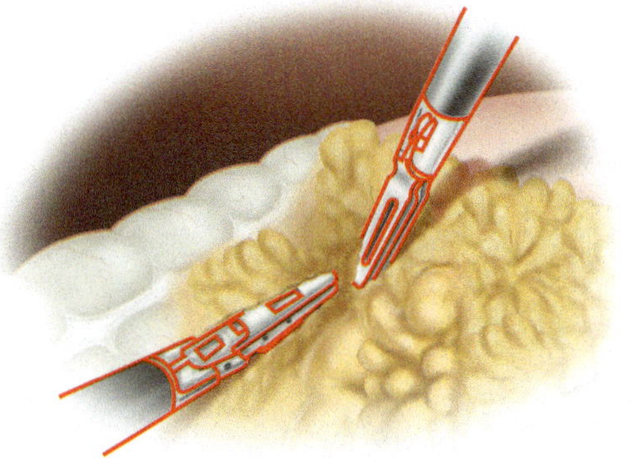

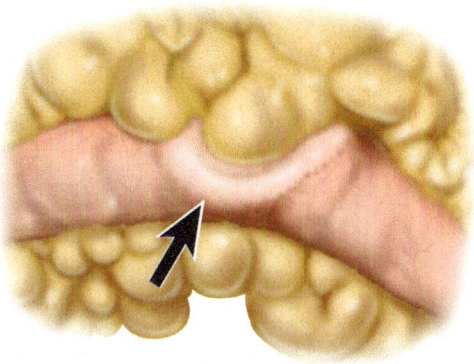

Fig. 10.10 Crohn's fistula. It is crucial to define normal anatomy prior to approaching inflamed structures

Fig. 10.11 Neoplasm. In the case of small bowel tumor, en bloc resection should be performed for oncologic completeness

can be located early (Fig. 10.10), proximity of disease to essential anatomy evaluated, and determination made as to whether conversion should be performed.

Upon completion of inspection and decision to proceed laparoscopically, a thorough lysis of adhesions can be performed.

Even if resection occurs using an open technique, advantages of laparoscopy include good visualization of the entire abdomen and small bowel as well as lysis of adhesions to minimize the size of laparotomy.

Areas of fistula formation may be ligated away from diseased bowel. Both proximal and distal ends of each fistula are inspected for primary disease and presence of a lumen. Any areas of primary disease and fistula will require segmental resection. Both ends of the fistula should be treated with either resection or appropriate closure.

Areas of affected bowel may require tactile evaluation to determine whether a pathologic stricture exists. The mesentery of the bowel may be too thick to allow for hemostatic ligation of vessels with sta-

plers or energy. Mini-laparotomy for assessment and resection is appropriate in these cases.

Neoplasm

In the case of small bowel tumor, en bloc resection should be performed for oncologic completeness. Any structures or loops of the bowel attached to the tumor should be removed without further dissection. All dense adhesions to the tumor should be considered malignant and should be removed with the specimen (Fig. 10.11). Adhesions near the mesentery should be incised away from the mesentery to avoid breaching of the mesenteric envelope surrounding potentially malignant lymph nodes.

Even if a clear source of obstruction is found, it is important to run the whole bowel and identify any additional sources of obstruction. Downstream areas of narrowing, adhesion, or stricture may not be apparent until after upstream problems are resolved.

Complications

11

Justin A. Maykel and Andrew T. Schlussel

Introduction

Intraoperative complications occur, even to the most careful of surgeons. Potential complications can be prevented by having a thorough understanding of anatomy and technical variations that help avoid these adverse events. In addition, maintaining a high level of vigilance allows for early identification of complications in efforts to prevent further sequela. This chapter will provide tips on how to reduce the incidence and manage some of the more common intraoperative complications related to laparoscopic colorectal surgery.

Common Complications

- Entry complications.
  - Bowel injury during entry into the abdomen
  - Bleeding from abdominal vessels
  - Bleeding from abdominal wall vessels

J. A. Maykel (✉)
Department of Colon and Rectal Surgery, University of Massachusetts Medical School,
Worcester, MA, USA
e-mail: Justin.Maykel@umassmemorial.org

A. T. Schlussel
Division of Surgery, Madigan Army Medical Center,
Tacoma, WA, USA

© Springer Nature Switzerland AG 2020
S. L. Stein, R. R. Lawson (eds.), *Laparoscopic Colectomy*,
https://doi.org/10.1007/978-3-030-39559-9_11

- Complications during dissection.
  - Bleeding
  - Injury to the bowel
  - Injury to the ureter
  - Splenic injury during flexure mobilization.

Entry Complications

The Complication: Bowel Injury During Entry into the Abdomen

Injuries to the bowel may occur with use of an open or a Hassan technique. These injuries are most common if there are abdominal adhesions preventing the bowel from dropping away during entry. This is noted primarily in reoperative surgery, but inflammation, infection, and even neoplasia can also cause adhesions.

Prevention of the Complication

- Blind entry into the abdomen should be avoided as this can increase the risk of inadvertent injury during entry. If the patient has had prior surgery, an open cutdown technique is typically used.
- New trocars with in-line visualization systems are commercially available and allow trocar advancement with direct camera view of each of the layers of the abdominal wall. These access methods require training and experience and have not been adequately

studied as a safer alternative to traditional entry methods.

- Avoid prior incisions sites. Alternate points of entry away from the existing incisions should be considered. The intra-abdominal location of prior surgery should also be considered. For example, if the patient had a prior cholecystectomy, consideration of placing a left upper quadrant port may decrease the chances of injuring a fixed loop of the bowel adhered to the abdominal wall from the prior operation.
- An open cutdown can be performed in any quadrant of the abdomen, although entry is typically performed in the midline, where the

rectus sheath is fused. Use of small vein retractors can help visualize the layers of the abdominal wall during entry to prevent injury.

Recognition of the Complication

After insertion, the abdominal cavity should always be thoroughly examined using the laparoscope to evaluate below and lateral to the entry site prior to continuing the operation or rotating the table. This prevents displacement of a loop of the bowel that may have been injured during entry.

If succus, bile, stool, or significant bleeding is seen after entry, an injury must be suspected and identified (Fig. 11.1). Immediately evaluate

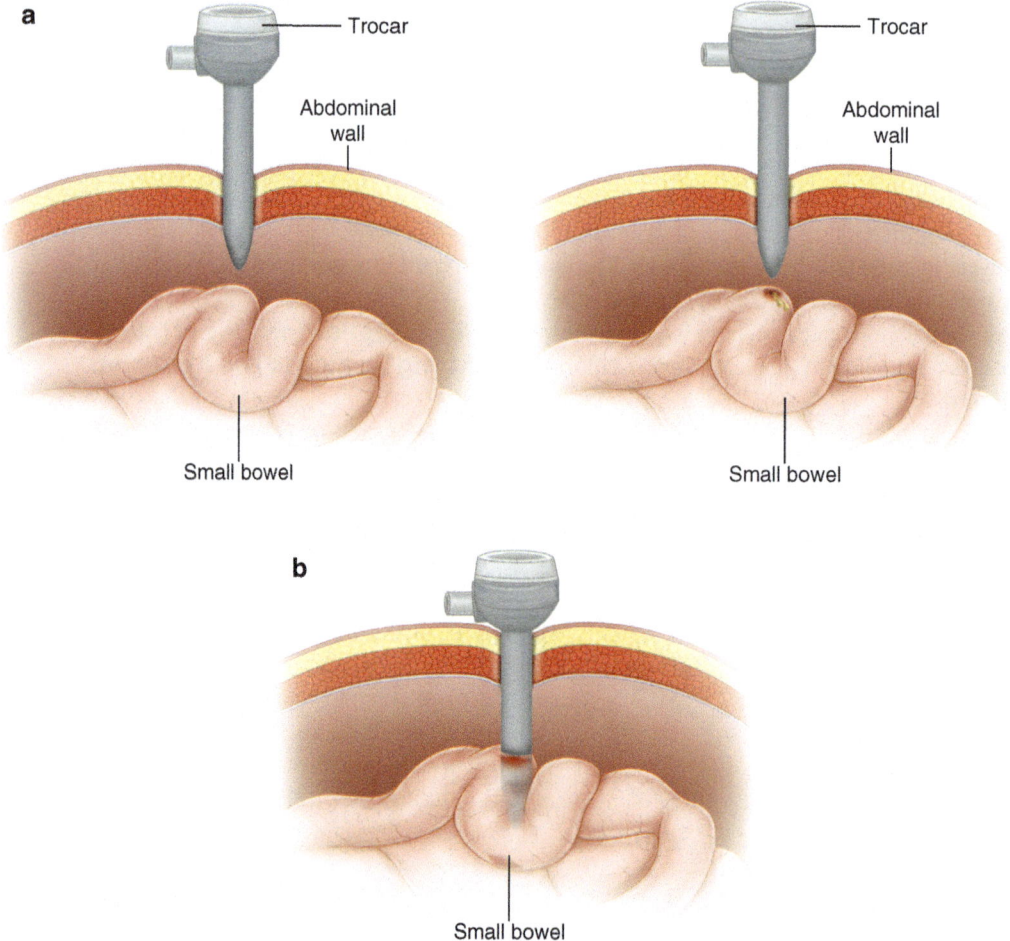

Fig. 11.1 (a) Trocar injury to the anterior surface of the small intestine. This may be recognized if bile, succus, or bleeding is seen after entry into the abdominal cavity. (b) Example of a penetrating intestinal injury to both the ante-rior and posteriors walls. An injury to the posterior surface should still be suspected even if the full thickness of the wall is not violated

the location of injury prior to rotation or tilting the operative table.

Treatment of the Complication

Typically, the injury occurs at the time of initial port placement, and only the laparoscopic port has been placed into the abdomen. The decision must be made at this time to continue laparoscopically or to vary the approach to open surgery to treat the injury. This decision will be based on the size of the injury, the surgeon's comfort in assessing the extent of the injury, managing contamination, and skill in repairing the injury laparoscopically.

If the decision is made to proceed laparoscopically, place additional ports to isolate the injury. Avoid grasping the bowel wall and instead grasp the mesentery or epiploic appendages adjacent to the injury. If the bowel must be handled, maintain a broad grasp on the bowel, as this will disperse the surface area and prevent additional injury. The grasper may be used to occlude the enterotomy, or a stitch can be placed to prevent ongoing leakage of succus or stool (Fig. 11.2). Leave the marking stitch long to facilitate identification of the injured segment of the intestine.

Three aspects of the injury must be identified: the location of the injury, the etiology of injury, and the severity of the injury:

1. *Location of the injury.* Gastric injury and small bowel injuries generally heal more readily than a colon injury, decreasing the chances of

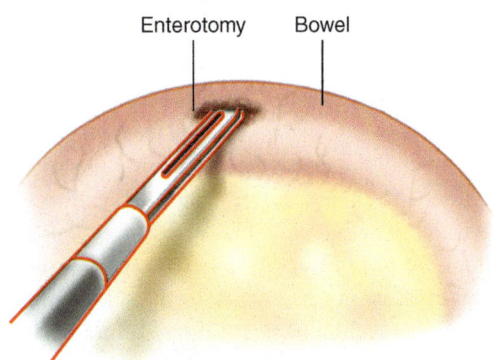

Enterotomy   Bowel

Fig. 11.2 Occlusion of intestinal lumen by laparoscopic bowel grasper to prevent leakage of intestinal contents

subsequent leak from the injury. Mobilization of the specific area of the bowel is also important. A serosal injury at the ligament of Treitz may be challenging to address based on the lack of mobility of the small bowel at this location. Alternatively, a mid small bowel injury can easily be externalized and inspected extracorporeally. In addition to the primary injury, the surgeon should inspect the adjacent bowel as well as any evidence of a mesenteric hematoma, as these may be additional injury sites. Finally, penetrating injuries are notorious for creating a second injury on the opposite side of the bowel lumen; therefore, the back side of the bowel needs to be inspected to rule out a simultaneous contralateral injury.

2. *Etiology of the injury.* Injuries that occurred sharply, with a knife or scissors, are generally straightforward and may be repaired primarily. If the injury occurs with electrocautery, an extra level of caution should occur as the extent of visualible injury may not reflect the full extent of damage. If a blood vessel is penetrated and insufflated during Veress needle entry, an air embolism can occur, leading to a life-threatening complication.

3. *Extent of the injury.* For an injury that is isolated to the serosa, interrupted Lembert sutures can be placed for repair. A 3–0 absorbable braided suture such as Vicryl is generally used to place seromuscular bites completely covering the injured serosa. Care should be taken to ensure that the bowel lumen is not narrowed; this is typically accomplished by placing sutures so the bowel is reinforced or closed transversely (Fig. 11.3).

A full-thickness injury involving less than 50% of the circumference of the bowel wall can generally be repaired as long as the mesentery is not involved. For a single-layer closure (preferred), 3–0 Vicryl Lembert sutures are placed to close the lumen transversely. When a double-layered repair is chosen, the first layer is placed in a running or interrupted fashion across the injury including all layers of the bowel wall. A second layer of Lembert suture is then placed to imbricate the defect.

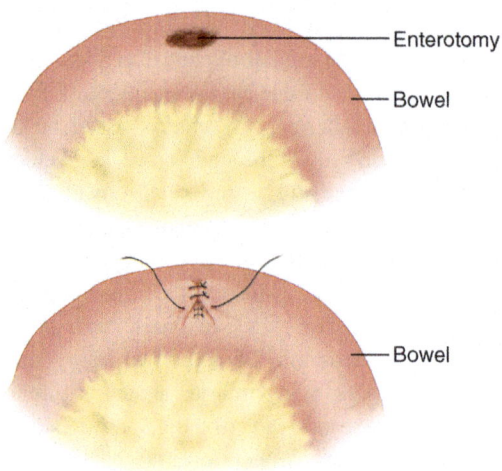

Fig. 11.3 A full-thickness injury may be repaired with a single-layer closure using monofilament absorbable suture, or a two-layer repair can be performed. Sutures are placed in a transverse fashion. Lembert suturing utilizes seromuscular purchases of intestinal wall to imbricate the initial full thickness closure of the enterotomy. Care must be taken not to narrow the lumen

If greater than 50% of the bowel lumen is injured or the mesentery has been disrupted with vascular compromise, a formal bowel resection should be considered. Intracorporeal resections may be done using endolumenal staplers as noted in Chap. 2 (right colectomy, intracorporeal anastomosis). It is also relatively easy to externalize the small bowel through the extraction incision and perform a small bowel resection. If the colon is affected and requires resection, keys for mobilization can be found in the chapter covering that portion of the colon.

The Complication: Bleeding from Abdominal Vessels During Entry

During initial entry into the abdomen, injury can occur to the aorta, inferior vena cava, and iliac or mesenteric vessels. This is most common when Veress needle entry, Optivue ®, or Sight-right ® access are employed.

Prevention of the Complication

Strategic location of the initial blind port may also decrease the risk of vessel injury. Placing the Veress needle in the left upper quadrant, at Palmer's point, may help to decrease this risk of injury in most patients. Based on simple anatomy, this location decreases inadvertent injury to the aorta, inferior vena cava, and iliac vessels. The Veress needle should always be inserted at right angles to the abdominal wall, to prevent angling toward the iliac vessels.

During entry, the Veress needle should be passed in a controlled fashion through each layer of the abdominal wall, feeling each click of the device during advancement. Repeated pushing or manipulation can increase the risk of injury during placement. Verification of successful placement is paramount prior to insufflation to prevent air embolism. An empty syringe is aspirated and should return air rather than blood or succus (see Chap. 1).

Another potential source of injury is placement of the Optivue ® or Sight-right ® trocars too deeply into the abdomen. To prevent this, once pneumoperitoneum is established, a trocar can be placed over the laparoscope. The Optivue ® or Sight-right ® trocar can then be advanced through each layer of the abdominal wall. Each layer should be clearly visualized. As soon as the peritoneal cavity is entered, the obturator of the trocar is removed. Advancing the trocar too deeply into the abdominal cavity is a typical cause of a major vascular injury, particularly when the abdominal wall is relaxed and excessively mobile.

Lifting the abdominal wall away from the viscera may also decrease rate of injury. A penetrating towel clamp can be attached to the skin and fascia adjacent to the entry port and create upward pressure during entry to reduce rate of injury.

Recognition of the Complication

Return of blood during Veress placement is a sign that a vessel has been injured during placement. Reinsertion of the Veress needle should not be considered at this time. The Veress needle or port should be left in situ to identify location of injury after opening. An alternative location for entry by a different technique is considered. Immediately following placement of the laparoscope, the abdomen should be inspected. The source of any bleeding should be identified.

Treatment of the Complication

If the surgeon feels that control may be obtained laparoscopically, additional laparoscopic ports can be placed rapidly to grasp the vessel and occlude the vessel while the abdomen is opened. A Ray-tec® sponge can be placed in the abdomen to control bleeding and create pressure until more precise control is obtained.

The surgeon should consider immediate conversion to laparotomy for any major vascular injury. After identification of the injury, communicate concerns immediately, and clearly, to the anesthesia and operative team. Conversion to open may take several minutes, especially if the team was not well prepared for open surgery. Rapid conversion to open surgery and preservation of patient stability will take a team approach. Call for any additional assistance including an experienced surgeon and additional runners for supplies or anesthesia help. Ensure that blood products are immediately available.

During conversion, if the patient is stable and bleeding is controlled, pneumoperitoneum should be maintained while the operating room team is preparing. The pressure gradient of the pneumoperitoneum will provide a tamponade effect and limit bleeding. Constant control of a major venous injury must be maintained at this time in order to prevent an air embolism.

Once the abdomen has been opened, proximal and distal control of the vessel should be obtained. Evaluation of the extent of injury and options for repair including consultation of a vascular surgeon should be considered. Primary repair, if feasible, can then be performed with a nonabsorbable polypropylene suture.

The Complication: Bleeding from Abdominal Wall Vessels During Port Placement

Most commonly, the inferior epigastric artery can be injured during placement of secondary ports for laparoscopy. Unlike injury to a major vessel, this complication can generally be treated using laparoscopic techniques.

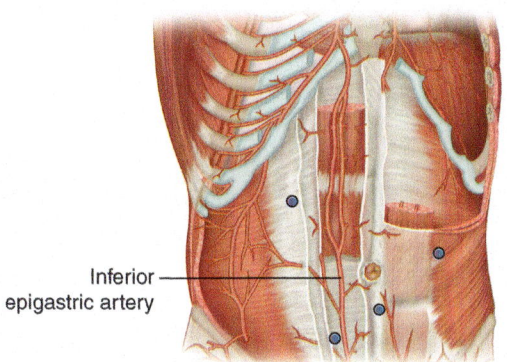

Fig. 11.4 Vascular anatomy of the abdominal wall and epigastric arteries. Below the umbilicus, there is generally a single epigastric artery running through the rectus sheath. Above the umbilicus, this splits into multiple branches

Prevention of the Complication

The epigastric vessels traverse the medial aspect of the rectus sheath (Fig. 11.4). Generally, the rectus sheath runs within 10 cm of the midline on either side. Placing ports lateral to this landmark reduces the risk of injury to the inferior epigastric artery.

In a patient with a thin abdominal wall, both superficial and deep vessels may be visualized using trans-illumination of the laparoscope. Prior to port placement, shine the light toward the abdominal wall in the location of planned trocar insertion. Check both internally, via the laparoscope, and externally, for vessels in the trajectory of trocar insertion. In obese patients, the course of the inferior epigastric artery may still be noted on the anterior abdominal wall, though visualization may not be as good (Fig. 11.5).

Recognition of the Complication

If the inferior epigastric artery has been injured, bleeding will generally be seen from either the external incision or running internally from the trocar. Occasionally, the vessel itself will be visualized prior to transection when caught on the end of the trocar during insertion. As opposed to a small superficial vessel injury, this bleeding is generally continuous and may be relatively significant.

Treatment of the Complication

Ligation of the inferior epigastric artery does not have significant morbidity unless the patient has

Fig. 11.5
Representation of the
course of the inferior
epigastric artery along
the posterior aspect of
the abdominal wall

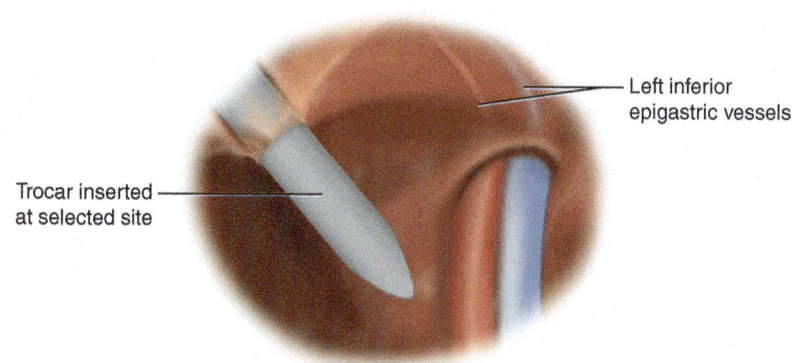

Left inferior
epigastric vessels

Trocar inserted
at selected site

Fig. 11.6 A Maryland
dissector with
electrocautery or bipolar
device may be used to
cauterize both proximal
and distal to the injured
vessel

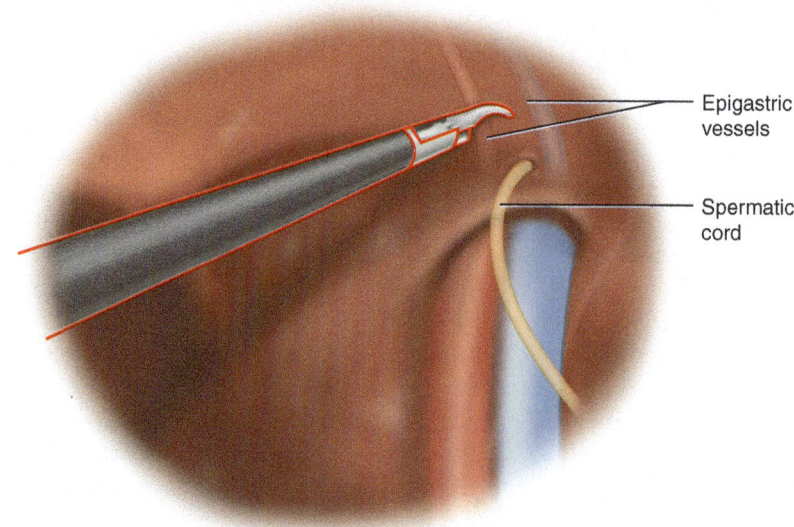

Epigastric
vessels

Spermatic
cord

a rectus abdominal flap. Superficial bleeding from a port site can be treated with cauterization. If the bleeding is deeper, extend the port site to improve visualization and allow for appropriate retraction. Small retractors such as vein retractors, ladyfingers, or even retraction with the tip of a suction device can help optimize visualization of the bleeding. A figure of eight suture can be used for vessels that are seen externally.

When the site of bleeding is not well visualized through the incision, a transabdominal suture ligation can be placed across the epigastric vessel. This can be done using a Carter-Thomason® or Gore® suture passer. The suture is inserted as a figure of eight around the injured

vessel (see Chap. 1). Laparoscopic guidance can help ensure that the vessel is securely ligated and does not cause further bleeding or an abdominal wall hematoma.

If the disrupted vessel is visualized laparoscopically on the end of the trocar, either electrocautery or a bipolar device can be used to ligate the vessel. Once the energy instrument of choice is positioned, retract the trocar slightly, creating a bit of laxity on the vessel. This may transiently increase bleeding that the trocar previously controlled. The Maryland dissector connected to electrocautery is placed around the vessel, and the vessel is cauterized both proximal and distal to the injury (Fig. 11.6).

Fig. 11.7 The figure represents the division of the proximal ileocolic pedicle close to the duodenum. Avoid dissecting and dividing the mesenteric vessels at an excessively proximal location. The vessel should be ligated with enough room to allow for proximal occlusion in case of incomplete hemostasis

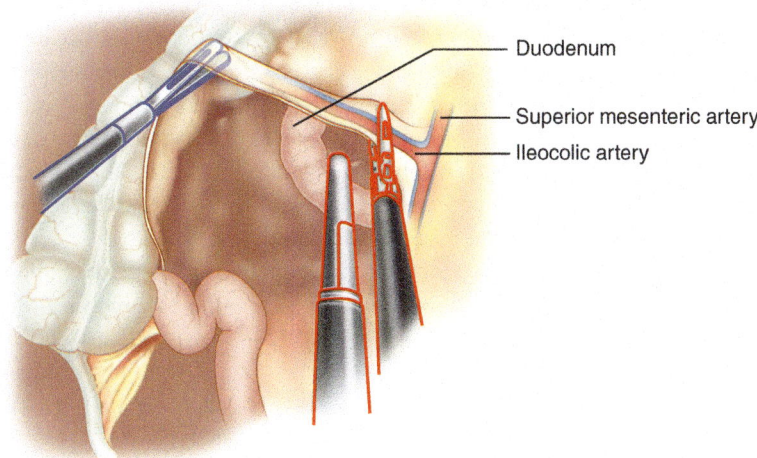

Duodenum

Superior mesenteric artery

Ileocolic artery

Complications During Dissection

Bleeding

Intraoperative hemorrhage can occur during any portion of a laparoscopic colon or rectal resection. This section will discuss the following situations:

- Bleeding to mesenteric vessel during ligation.
- Bleeding secondary to excessive traction.
- Presacral bleeding.
- Intra-abdominal bleeding noted during extraction.

The Complication: Injury to a Mesenteric Vessel During Ligation and Division

Injuries can occur because of improper ligation technique, failure of technology, or calcifications in the vessels.

Prevention of the Complication

Maintaining control of regional arteries or veins is crucial during ligation. Proximal control of the vessel should be maintained until hemostasis is obtained. Always check the proximal end of a vessel during ligation to ensure adequate hemostasis.

Avoid dissecting and dividing the mesenteric vessels at an excessively proximal location. The vessel should be ligated with enough room to allow for proximal occlusion in case of incomplete hemostasis (Fig. 11.7). This provides an opportunity for proximal vascular control and should not significantly sacrifice oncologic margins or lymph node yield. It is remarkable how the divided vessel may retract once divided and is no longer under the tension provided by retracting it up and away from the retroperitoneum.

The peritoneum and underlying mesentery should be scored and opened parallel to the vessel prior to transection. Exposure is critical. This allows for isolation of the vascular pedicle away from neighboring structures and control of the vessel. The vessel can then be controlled with clips, a stapler, or an advanced energy device. An Endoloop® should always be accessible in case the primary device fails.

The surgeon should understand the limits of instrumentation and techniques. Understanding how to work the bipolar, clips, stapler, or Endoloop® is imperative. Injuries occur more frequently if the surgeon does not understand the technology. Explanations should be provided to trainees or assistants who are unfamiliar with the instrumentation prior to allowing them to use the device, and practice with the instrument should occur prior to intra-abdominal use. Each instrument, especially an energy device, has a recommended maximal size of vessel ligation. These guidelines are provided in Chap. 1.

During dissection, the surgeon should note if there is excessive calcification in the vessel. If the vessel feels firm during palpation, the surgeon must choose the right instrumentation for transection. Energy instruments are generally not recommended for calcified vessels; the calcium deposits prevent complete occlusion of the vessel during the cauterization phase of the instrument. Staplers with vascular loads may be used but may still have some back bleeding. Endoloop® is generally a good method of vessel ligation for calcified arteries.

Recognition of the Complication

After ligation of a vessel, watch the portion of the vessel that will be remaining in the patient, to evaluate for bleeding. Do not move on too quickly to the next phase of the operation. Bleeding should be dealt with immediately.

Treatment of the Complication

If bleeding occurs following transection, the first objectives are to gain control of the bleeding vessel, determine what is bleeding, and have the entire team on standby for urgent needs. Communicate with the team as appropriate. Ensure the circulator is available to obtain additional equipment or assistance. Inform the anesthesia provider to advise them of the situation. Ensure all members of the team are properly prepared, and blood is available, if needed.

Blood loss obscures laparoscopic visualization. Blood absorbs light, decreasing differentiation within the abdomen. If blood splatters on the laparoscope, visualization becomes impossible. Swift removal and replacement of the laparoscope becomes necessary. A laparoscopic suction-irrigation system helps to improve visualization and exposure. Using irrigation helps to remove excess clots and to identify the location of bleeding. The exact site of bleeding should be identified by maintaining adequate exposure and with targeted suctioning.

Ideally the source of bleeding is quickly identified, and proximal control of the bleeding is obtained with a bowel grasper. Prior to treatment it is important to determine what is bleeding and identify any surrounding structures which may

be injured during manipulation. For example, the location of the duodenum should be identified prior to treatment of bleeding from the ileocolic artery or middle colic arteries, and the location of the ureter should be established during cases of bleeding at the inferior mesenteric artery.

A Maryland dissector with its angulated tip can be used to precisely grasp the bleeding end of the vessel and cauterize to coagulate the vessel. If the bleeding is from a small vessel, electrocautery may be sufficient. If the bleeding is thought to be from a larger vessel, this may actually increase injury to the vessel, and consideration of a bipolar, stapler, Endoloop®, or laparoscopic clips may be used to occlude the vessel.

If bleeding cannot be controlled (the vessels are avulsed or extensively damaged), laparoscopic control should be obtained followed by immediate conversion to an open technique.

The Complication: Bleeding Secondary to Excessive Retraction or Force

The hepatic and splenic flexures are potential sources of intra-abdominal bleeding, typically related to traction injury. Excessive force resulting in a tear of the mesenteric vessels can occur during exteriorization of the diseased segment.

Prevention of the Complication

At the splenic and hepatic flexures, the attachments to the colon tend to be short and may contain some small unnamed vessels which are particularly vulnerable to bleeding (Fig. 11.8). These vessels, if inadvertently divided, can retract and result in bleeding that may be challenging to control due to poor visualization. Therefore, it is imperative to ensure these vessels are adequately ligated during initial transection.

To decrease tension on these vessels, the surgeon may place the patient in reverse Trendelenburg during dissection. This can optimize exposure and therefore minimize excessive retraction tension while exposing the flexures. If reach to the flexure is difficult, consider using long bowel graspers or bariatric instrumentation

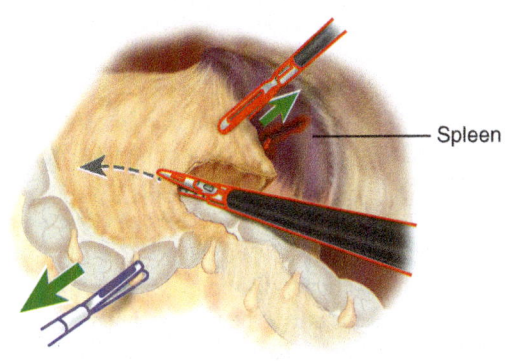

Spleen

Fig. 11.8 Short attachments to the colon at the splenic flexure may contain small vessels which are vulnerable to bleeding

for additional length which may reduce tension on the splenic or liver capsule.

When the colon mesentery is thickened or foreshortened, the colon should be fully mobilized intracorporeally prior to extraction to prevent tearing or shearing. Complete mobilization is assured when the colon can be retracted past the midline, and proximal and distal resection margins can reach the predetermined extraction site without tension.

If tension on the colonic mesentery prevents exteriorization, start transection at the free edge of the mesentery, where the vessels have been ligated, and use the energy instrument to divide the mesentery parallel to key vessels all the way to the colon wall. If the bowel still does not reach easily, the bowel itself can be transected intracorporeally, using a laparoscopic stapler. The transected end of the colon is generally easier to bring to the incision than a loop of the bowel, particularly when there is a thickened segment as a result of inflammation or malignancy.

The extraction site should be large enough for the bowel and mesentery to be extracted without tearing of the mesentery. A wound protector is used to optimize the size of the wound as well as prevent contamination. Using a wound protector that is slightly larger than the incision size will optimize retraction of the skin and soft tissue.

Recognition of the Complication

If the mesentery has been torn during retraction, bleeding will be seen. It is important to look around the abdomen to identify bleeding prior to moving on to the next phase of the operation. Laparoscopy can create tunnel vision – only a small portion of the abdomen is seen at any time. The operative field should be kept clean and without bleeding, which helps to highlight even the smallest quantities of blood.

If the bleeding occurs during extraction, the surgeon will generally see bleeding around the extracted portion of the bowel in the wound protector. Additionally, if bleeding is suspected, the mesentery should be inspected laparoscopically after returning the bowel to the abdomen prior to closure.

Treatment of the Complication

If the bleeding is relatively minor, it may stop spontaneously. Further manipulation may simply exacerbate the bleeding. If watchful waiting is thought to be best, the area of bleeding should be checked after several minutes and also after insufflation is released to ensure it has stopped prior to closure. Insufflation may tamponade bleeding, and bleeding can recur after abdominal pressures remain to normal levels.

Areas of continued mesenteric bleeding can often be stopped with simple pressure, using a Ray-tec® or sponge to compress the area, in some cases. If the precise area of bleeding is grasped with a laparoscopic instrument and held 3 minutes, the bleeding will often stop spontaneously.

If the bleeding is significant but controlled with pressure, continue to grasp the vessel while considering options to improve visualization. This includes adding additional ports for further dissection/mobilization to better control the bleeding. The surgeon should consider conversion to open surgery to control the bleeding. Electrocautery, bipolar energy, and suture material are also appropriate tools.

If the bleeding has come from mesenteric vessels, the viability of the neighboring colon or small bowel should be evaluated. Proximal ligation of a mesenteric vessel may result in further colonic devascularization and compromise of the potential conduit. Verifying blood supply prior to closure can be done by external evaluation of marginal artery, evaluation of mucosa, or fluoroscopic techniques.

The Complication: Presacral Bleeding During Proctectomy

The presacral fascia covers the presacral venous plexus, which is in continuity with the basivertebral veins. This plexus of veins extends the entire length of the spine and contains no valves. This allows for bidirectional flow resulting in massive bleeding if these vessels are torn.

Prevention of the Complication

Remaining in the proper mesorectal plane between the mesorectal fascia and the presacral fascia can prevent bleeding. Tips for maintaining this plane are provided in chapters on proctectomy (Chaps. 6 and 7).

The most likely area of injury to the presacral veins is the lower pelvis where Waldeyer's fascia can attach directly to the presacral fascia. This area should be dissected sharply, as blunt dissection can result in tearing of these vessels, particularly as the sacrum takes an anterior turn toward the coccyx.

If radiation was given preoperatively, these planes may become more fused and difficult to dissect. Greater care should be taken in these cases.

Recognition of the Complication

Presacral bleeding is generally conspicuous and seen at the time of injury. Any small amount of bleeding during the time of dissection should be promptly treated before tension is released and vessels retract.

Treatment of the Complication

Options for treatment include pressure, electrocautery, packing of the pelvis, hemostatic agents, or clamping with suture ligation.

Bleeding can be controlled initially with instrument pressure, providing an opportunity to optimize exposure and initiate resuscitation. The suction irrigator is often used to put pressure and tamponade the area of bleeding. A laparoscopic peanut can also be used. After several minutes of holding pressure, the pressure can be released to determine if bleeding is ongoing. If pressure is inadequate to control bleeding or bleeding continues after attempts at control, conversion to open surgery should be considered.

While pressure is held, the electrocautery coagulation setting is placed on 80 watts. This will provide a greater degree of char and obliteration of bleeding area. The electrocautery is generally placed on a flat instrument, such as the paddle. The instrument is then used hovering over the area of bleeding, rather than pressing directly on the area. This allows the current to arc over the area and seal the vessel. If the area of bleeding is touched directly with the instrument, the eschar which has developed will be removed when the instrument is withdrawn. This will cause the bleeding to recur. Prior to resuming the case, the electrocautery settings should be returned to the surgeon's regular levels.

If the presacral veins retract into the bone and electrocautery is unsuccessful, alternative techniques should be attempted. This typically requires converting to an open approach in order to obtain optimal exposure. Consider calling a colleague for an extra pair of experienced hands to assist. Some of the most common and successful alternative techniques are:

- Multiple cellulose or thrombin-based hemostatic agents can be applied and packed in the pelvis. A Ray-tec® or lap pad should be placed over them to apply pressure for 5 to 10 minutes.
- Titanium thumbtacks and table fixation staples have been developed to aide in the control of massive presacral hemorrhage but can be difficult to maneuver and position in a narrow pelvis (Fig. 11.9).
- A pledget of Surgicel® can be positioned and secured with lateral sutures to compress the bleeding vessels.
- A long Kelly clamp and a cotton peanut sponge may be positioned on the bleeding vessel. This will facilitate exposure, improving opportunities to suture ligate bleeding the lateral tissue.

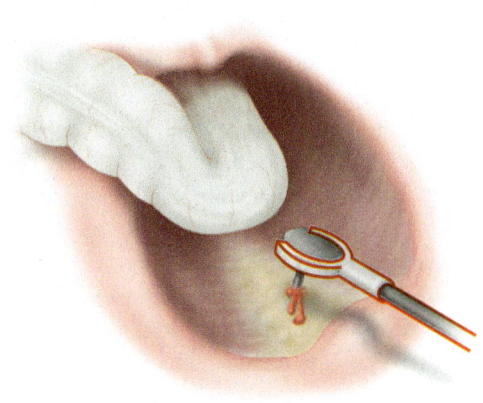

Fig. 11.9 Tamponade of presacral vessels

- A small piece of the rectus abdominis muscle can be sutured or coagulated on top of the presacral fascia to successfully control hemorrhage. As this maneuver takes time, manual compression should be used while the rectus muscle is harvested.
- If all of these maneuvers fail, the pelvis should be packed, the patient stabilized in the ICU, and a return to the OR is planned for the following day at which time the bleeding has generally stopped.

Complication: Injury to the Bowel

While the rate of an iatrogenic puncture or laceration to an abdominal organ is low, injury to the small or large intestine is a potential risk at any portion of the operation. Failure to recognize this complication can have devastating consequences such as enteric leak, fistulization, or abscess, potentially requiring a prolonged hospital stay, reoperation, or need for an intestinal stoma.

Prevention of the Complication
When moving instruments into or out of the operative field, the surgeon and assistant must constantly be aware of the surrounding tissues. Novice surgeons and assistants should watch the instruments pass from the trocar to the operative field, to ensure the pathway is clear. As surgeons become more comfortable laparoscopically, blind

insertion may occur. During insertion, instruments should be aimed anteriorly, away from the bowel and abdominal structures. This is particularly important when placing an instrument through a dependent port, such as a suprapubic port when a patient is in the reverse Trendelenburg position. Any tension during instrument insertion should be immediately inspected to ensure that no injury occurred. The camera should immediately be pulled back to view any instruments that have not easily reached the field of view.

Blunt grasping or retraction can also cause injury to the bowel. As a general principle, it is safer to grasp the mesentery or epiploic appendages to retract the bowel as opposed to grasping the bowel itself. The bowel or mesentery should never be pulled or grasped with excessive force. Graspers can be used without utilizing the lock function – better to lose retraction than to pull too hard and tear tissue. Wider and longer bites on the bowel tend to be less prone to inadvertent injury. Each surgeon develops a preference for specific graspers. Familiarity with the mechanics of a grasper helps to prevent inadvertent injury.

Electrocautery is another potential source of injury. Insulation failure can result from a break or defect in the instrument coating, and this is a potential site for thermal conduction and tissue injury. Instruments should be routinely inspected at the start of each case to ensure that insulation is intact.

During application of electrocautery, the entire metal portion of the device should be maintained under direct laparoscopic visualization. The angle of instruments should be evaluated. If the angles are too obtuse, the instrument may rest on a piece of the bowel or mesentery, causing injury away from the intended field of dissection (Fig. 11.10). Although instruments generally cool down rapidly after use, electrocautery and ultrasonic instruments are hot immediately after activation. Avoid immediate use on the bowel or tissues.

Recognition of the Complication
As with all injuries, a high level of suspicion should be maintained at all time. By keeping the

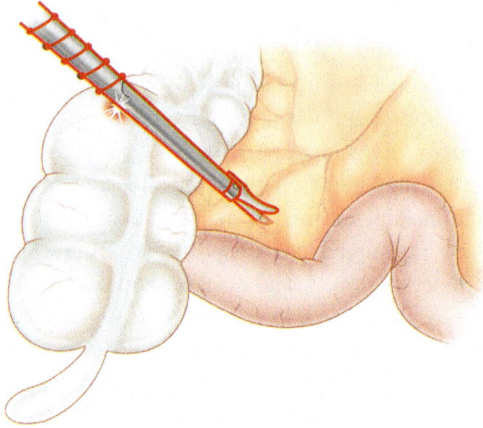

Fig. 11.10 Electrocautery injury to the bowel

laparoscopic instruments in view, the surgeon and assistant should be able to recognize the injury and provide immediate treatment.

Any visualization of succus should be investigated immediately and the source determined. If a mesenteric hematoma is identified, it should be evaluated as well – mesenteric hematoma is often a sign of occult injury to the bowel wall.

Treatment of the Complication

If there is suspicion of an intestinal injury, the bowel should be inspected. The bowel is visualized either laparoscopically or through a small incision and inspected carefully. Injured bowel should be handled with care to ensure the defect is not enlarged. An atraumatic grasper is used to gently occlude any enterotomy and prevent any further contamination. Any spillage of intestinal contents should be evacuated from the abdomen using a suction-irritation device.

Once an area of injury has been identified, it should be determined if the injury is full thickness or partial thickness. If partial thickness, serial Lembert sutures can be placed to close the injury. A braided absorbable or silk suture is generally used. Sutures are placed in a longitudinal manner to prevent narrowing of the bowel lumen. If the injury is full thickness, a single-layer closure using monofilament absorbable suture or a two-layer repair can be performed. If there is a significant injury involving greater than 50% of

the lumen, consideration of resection and anastomosis should be made.

Special evaluation is made at the source of any cautery injury. Burns continue to progress after the initial injury and may not have adequate integrity to tolerate repair. If the injury was caused by monopolar, bipolar, or ultrasonic instrumentation, it should be assumed that the actual damage to the bowel is greater than the visualized injury. It is always safer to assume a greater field of injury and err on the side of caution. Repairs can be made using single-layer Lembert, two-layer closure, or resection as appropriate.

Repair can be performed using a laparoscopic or open approach. The method of repair and technique used should be based on surgeon experience and comfort level. If there is any question, the extraction site for the intended operation can be used to inspect the bowel and perform resection and primary anastomosis.

Injury to the Ureter

While ureteral injury is a rare complication of colon surgery, there are situations in which the risk is increased. The rate of injury is greater in pelvic operations, including patients with rectal cancer and diverticular disease, secondary to the anatomic location of the ureter close to the field of dissection. The most common locations of injury are at the pelvic brim, during dissection of the inferior mesenteric artery, and low in the pelvis, during rectal dissection. In addition, any case of inflammatory disease, on the right or left side of the abdomen, may distort the normal anatomy, displacing the normal course of the ureter and increasing the risk of inadvertent injury. Injuries can occur in patients with no risk factors. Meticulous surgical technique must always be utilized to prevent this injury.

Prevention of the Complication

The preoperative planning phase provides the best opportunity to prevent ureteral injury. It is important to first review images to identify cases where the ureter may be involved due to inflam-

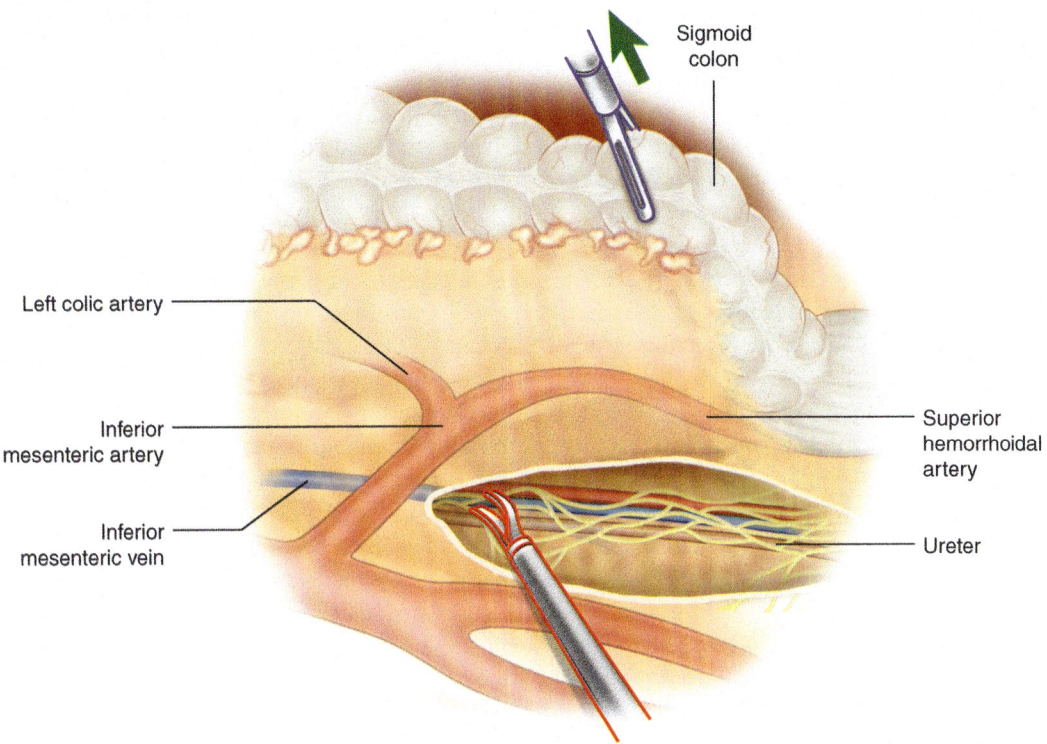

Fig. 11.11 Careful mobilization of the sigmoid colon and its mesentery allows for identification and preservation of the left ureter

mation or malignancy. Careful inspection of images can identify areas of concern for ureteric involvement prior to surgery, and often these are cases that should not be attempted laparoscopically by the novice surgeon.

Iatrogenic injury to the left ureter is most commonly seen during mobilization or devascularization of the left colon (Fig. 11.11). The injury typically occurs by crushing, lacerating, or ligating the ureter. To reduce this risk, the ureter should always be identified prior to division of the inferior mesenteric artery or superior hemorrhoidal artery. Performing a circumferential dissection of the mesentery surrounding the colon prior to application of a linear stapler will help to ensure the ureter is not clamped, crushed, or stapled with the device.

The right ureter is also at risk during cases of inflammatory or malignant diseases, as well as following radiation or in reoperative surgery. Just as in cases of left-sided disease, proximal identification of the ureter, placement of a stent, and consideration of conversion to open technique may be appropriate.

In cases of benign disease, the ureter may be identified proximal to the inflammation and freed from the resection plane through its course. Again this may require advanced laparoscopic experience and consideration of open technique may be appropriate.

In malignant disease, the ureter may need to be resected with the tumor and may be more appropriately handled with an open technique.

The use of prophylactic ureteral stents is often debated. While stents will assist in the recognition of a ureteral injury, their use is not routinely supported as a tool for prevention. In addition, they present additional risks that must be considered. These include iatrogenic ureteral perforation, transient hematuria, urinary tract infections, and hydronephrosis due to edema from stent placement. The placement of ureteral stents incurs an additional cost and adds to the patient's time under general anesthesia. Stents should be placed on a case-by-case basis and should be considered in reoperative surgery or when there is a high inflammatory burden.

If the surgeon is unable to visualize the ureter, a stent can be placed intraoperatively. This can help the surgeon clearly identify the course of the ureter as the urologist advances the stent under laparoscopic visualization.

Recognition of the Complication

Rapid and early identification of an iatrogenic ureteral injury is critical to ensure the most successful repair. If there is any concern, the surgeon should follow the course of the ureter and evaluate its integrity. Blood in the Foley catheter or decreased urine output are nonspecific signs of potential injury.

If an injury or potential injury is suspected, several options are available to better characterize the injury:

- A cystoscopy and stent placement can be performed intraoperatively to evaluate the location of the ureter and visualize an injury. Visualization of the stent is a clear indication of injury.
- Injection of methylene blue by injection through the IV may be helpful in further elucidating the injury. Visualization of blue liquid is conclusive for an injury.
- Alternatively, IV contrast can also be injected intraoperatively, followed by an X-ray of the abdomen while in the operating room.
- A retrograde pyelogram can be performed through the urethral catheter using methylene blue. The bladder should be filled sterilely using diluted methylene blue to evaluate for any leak. The bladder is filled until distended and the bladder and ureter can be inspected for any leakage of blue dye.

Ideally, a ureter injury is identified intraoperatively and treated immediately. When missed intraoperatively, signs of urinary tract injury include a fluid collection, decreased urine output, and ileus. If a drain was left postoperatively, clear copious drainage may be a sign of urinary injury. Testing the fluid collections for creatinine levels may confirm the diagnosis.

Treatment of the Complication

If an injury to the ureter is discovered intraoperatively, consultation with a urologist is recommended. Only the most experienced surgeons should attempt a laparoscopic repair.

Options for treatment of a ureter repair include primary anastomosis over a stent, psoas hitch, and Boari flap. These are beyond the scope of this chapter.

If there is concern for devascularization or narrowing of the ureter, without a full-thickness injury, a stent can then be passed across the injury. A closed suction drain should be placed in the area of repair to monitor for signs of a urine leak postoperatively.

Postoperatively, a Foley catheter should be left in place beyond the typical 48 hours recommended for most surgeries. Duration of the catheter is dependent on the type of injury and surgeon choice and should be discussed with urology. Stent removal is recommended in 4 to 6 weeks following the repair.

Splenic Injury

Splenic injuries are rare complications that can occur during mobilization of the left colon, particularly the splenic flexure. Laparoscopy may provide better visualization and allow for fine dissection, which contributes to a lower rate of complications. Despite the risk of this potentially catastrophic complication with mobilization of the splenic flexure, it may be a necessary part of the operation, and therefore it is important to understand how to address this injury if it occurs.

Prevention of the Complication

The most common cause of iatrogenic splenic injury is excessive traction on the splenocolic ligaments. Pulling too firmly on the omentum or ligaments may tear the capsule of the spleen.

Excessive tension and traction on the spleen can be minimized during a laparoscopic approach. Positioning the patient in reverse Trendelenburg and right side down will allow gravity to pull the colon away from the left upper quadrant and provide better exposure of the spleen. Using longer bowel graspers, such as bariatric bowel graspers, may prevent excessive tension in patients with tall torsos or wide abdomens.

Understanding multiple approaches, as described in Splenic Flexure Mobilization Chap. 4, may help decrease the chance of injury. By varying approach from medial to lateral or top down, the surgeon has multiple options for dissection. This can help prevent injury to the spleen if one technique is difficult, or the operation is failing to progress, or move forward in an appropriate and timely manner.

Identification of the Complication

Generally, the surgeon will see bleeding in the left upper quadrant. The surgeon must remain vigilant in looking for bleeding in this area. Small vessels may retract under the spleen, and splenic capsule injuries can be obscured by the adipose tissue, omentum, and mesentery. Laparoscopic visualization is limited to one quadrant at a time, making it easy to miss bleeding away from the surgeon's field of view. Prior to leaving the left upper quadrant and again prior to closure, the surgeon should make a point of evaluating all quadrants for bleeding. If bleeding is noted, the surgeon should reposition the patient to inspect for the source of bleeding.

Treatment of the Complication

Identification of the extent of injury will be helpful in determining the best method for salvage.

A small bleed, with minimal but continuous bleeding, can often be treated laparoscopically. A suction irrigator is used to identify the source of bleeding and evaluate quantity of bleeding. If the bleeding is secondary to small vessels from the splenocolic ligaments or omentum, these can be treated with the bipolar instrument. The area

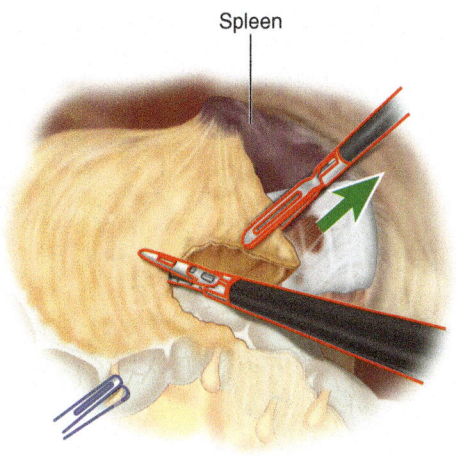

Fig. 11.12 Treatment of splenic injury with electrocautery and manual tamponade

should be irrigated, all blood and clot evacuated and inspected to ensure it is hemostatic.

If the bleeding is coming from a small capsular tear, the surgeon can place a Ray-tec® sponge through the 10/12 mm trocar in order to apply pressure on the spleen using either a grasper or laparoscopic peanut (Figs. 11.11 and 11.12). The cautery can be increased to 80 watts and applied to the area of bleeding. Ideally, rather than touching or pushing on the spleen or capsule, the cautery is held slightly above the bleeding, arcing to the area of injury. This prevents sticking of the cautery tip to the spleen and subsequent removal of eschar when the instrument is withdrawn.

Hemostatic agents such as fibrin, Gelfoam® or Surgicel®, or thrombin can be applied to the area to cause coagulation. Some of these are available in powder or spray form that may be more easily applied laparoscopically. The area should be reinspected after several minutes to ensure it is hemostatic.

For larger injuries, including fracture of the spleen, or ongoing significant bleeding, the surgeon should consider open splenorrhaphy with pledgeted sutures or splenectomy. These are beyond the scope of this chapter.

Index

© Springer Nature Switzerland AG 2020
S. L. Stein, R. R. Lawson (eds.), *Laparoscopic Colectomy*,
https://doi.org/10.1007/978-3-030-39559-9

The manufacturer's authorised representative in the EU is Springer
Nature Customer Service Centre GmbH, Europaplatz 3, 69115 Heidelberg,
Germany. If you have any concerns regarding our products, please
contact ProductSafety@springernature.com

Printed and bound by CPI Group (UK) Ltd, Croydon, CR0 4YY
29/04/2026
02099466-0013